T0332108

THE ART OF

COOKING

with

CANNABIS

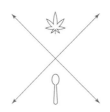

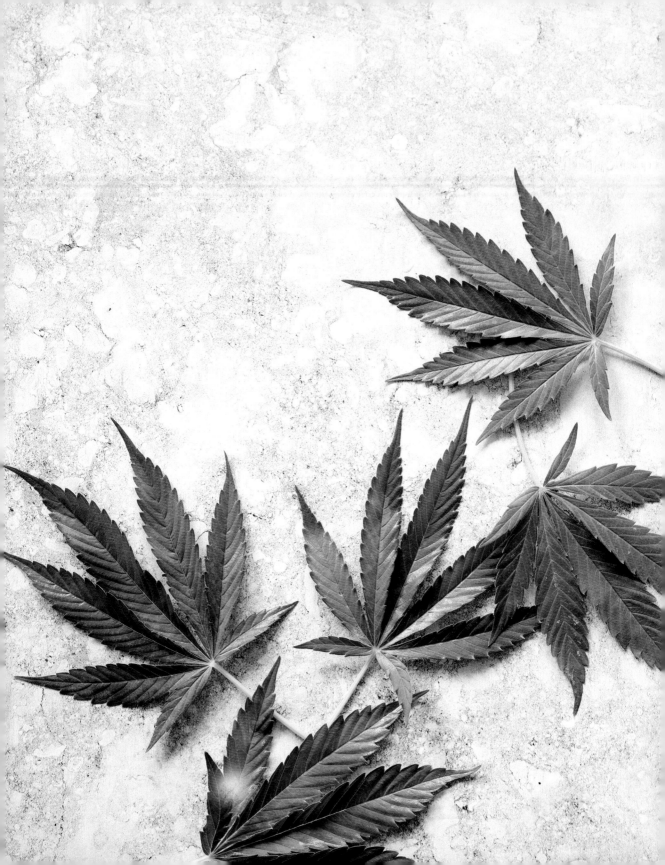

THE ART OF
COOKING
with
CANNABIS

CBD and THC-Infused Recipes from Across America

TRACEY MEDEIROS

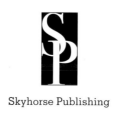

Skyhorse Publishing

Visit our website at www.skyhorsepublishing.com.

10 9 8 7 6 5 4 3 2

Library of Congress Cataloging-in-Publication Data is available on file.

Cover design by Daniel Brount
Cover image by Clare Barboza

Print ISBN: 978-1-5107-5605-2
Ebook ISBN: 978-1-5107-6411-8

Printed in China

Note: The cannabis recipes in this book are only intended for those who have obtained cannabis legally under applicable federal and state law.

Photo Credits:
All photographs are by Clare Barboza with the following exceptions:
Page 26, Jamaican Me Shake and page 43, Vermont Milk Punch: Photo courtesy of Brent Harrewyn
Pages 90–93, Blue Sparrow Coffee: Photos courtesy of Blue Sparrow Coffee
Page 158, deadhorse hill: Photo courtesy of Brian Samuels
Page 170, Vegetarian Stuffed Sweet Potatoes, and page 172, Spicy Maple Cauliflower "Wings": Photos courtesy of Eaton Hemp
Page 208, OrcaSong Farm: Photo courtesy of OrcaSong Farm
Page 214, Rainshadow Organics: Photo courtesy of @juliadukephoto
Page 320, Parsley Root Salad: Photo courtesy of Opulent Chef
Page 334, Chef Daniel Asher: Photo courtesy of River and Woods
Page 375, Chef Jazmine Moore: Photo courtesy of Jazmine Moore/Green Panther Chef

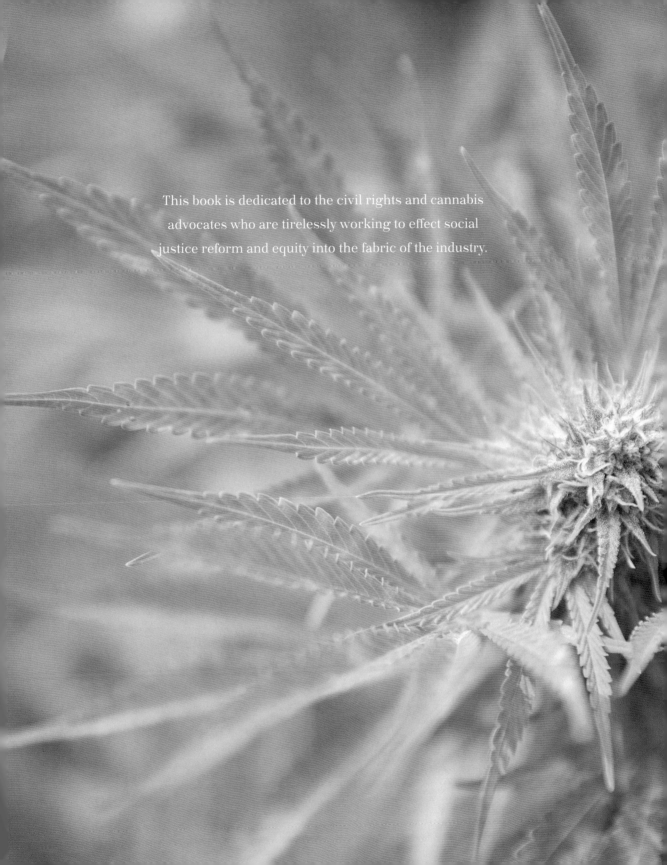

This book is dedicated to the civil rights and cannabis advocates who are tirelessly working to effect social justice reform and equity into the fabric of the industry.

CONTENTS

ACKNOWLEDGMENTS

Where to begin? So many people have helped to make this book a reality! Thank you to the folks at Skyhorse Publishing who encouraged me to, "Go For It." My editor, Abigail Gehring, always there to lend a helping hand, along with cover designer Daniel Brount and interior designer Laura Klynstra who have helped to make this cookbook a work of art. My photographer, Clare Barboza, whose beautiful photographs brings new meaning to the phrase, "A picture is worth a thousand words." Food stylist, Gretchen Rude, who has captured the essence of each dish.

A special thanks to my very able recipe tester, Sarah Strauss, who patiently tested, and many times retested, each recipe so that the reader would have smooth sailing. To all the book's contributors who very generously agreed to be part of this project, taking time out of their busy schedules to share recipes and snapshots of their lives. This was done during the COVID-19 pandemic that threatened all that they hold dear. You are the heart and soul of this project. I am in awe of your generosity and so very grateful!

Heartfelt gratitude to my family, including my husband, son, and mother, who stood by me every step of the way. Thank you for being you! I could not have done this book without your support and never-ending patience. I love you all so very much!

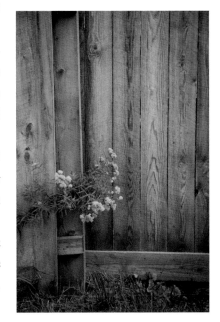

During this unprecedented time in all of our lives, I would like to extend a world of thanks to each and every one of you. It has been an absolute pleasure working with you!

A portion of the proceeds from the sale of this book will be donated to **Open for Good**. Open for Good is a campaign to help independent restaurants to survive, rebuild, and thrive for the long term.

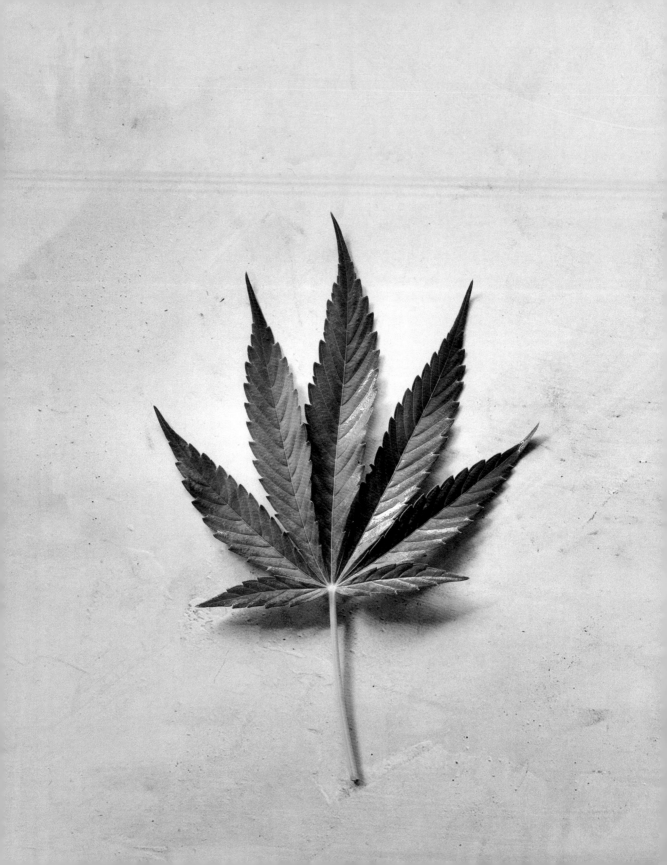

INTRODUCTION

I consider myself extremely fortunate to be able to live in the state of Vermont with its many farms and enduring sense of community. Over the past sixteen years of my life, this place has been a muse of sorts for me, fostering inspiration for my writing and book projects. In fact, three of my cookbooks have been dedicated to these magical surroundings that I call home.

The Green Mountain State was the first in our nation to legalize marijuana legislatively. It was during this period that I found myself reading time and time again about the cannabis plant's potential for medicinal benefits. The thought that this plant could serve as an effective treatment for epileptic seizures, anxiety, and inflammation, among other medicinal benefits, really made me sit up and take notice. These occurrences gave me cause to embark on a cannabis journey, reaching out to folks across the United States who use this plant to create delicious meals that aid with certain aspects of health and wellness. I wanted to hear their heartfelt stories and learn about their experiences firsthand. It was my goal to have these creative individuals share their culinary techniques, innovative methods of preparation, and progressive philosophies on unique ways to use this plant thoughtfully and responsibly. And share they did!

Throughout the course of my many conversations with these dedicated contributors, I was truly amazed to find how this single ingredient, this one plant, was being used as a creative art form that was transforming and elevating the culinary landscape right before my eyes. I became passionately curious about the artistry of cannabis and its wellness properties. It was for this very reason that I decided to write *The Art of Cooking with Cannabis*.

All across the United States, the general opinion of cannabis is moving in a positive direction. Hemp and marijuana are derived from this tall plant with its distinctive coarse leaves. This cookbook, with its collection of 125 authentic recipes and forty-five skillful contributors, is a testament to the fact that the world of cannabis is no longer shrouded in mystery, a sensitive subject that folks chose at one time to discuss behind closed doors.

One of the pivotal factors behind this change is attributed to the Hemp Farming Act of 2018, which has reclassified hemp with less than 0.3 percent THC, from a Schedule 1 controlled substance to that of an ordinary agricultural product. Under this 2018 act, hemp can now be commercially grown and transported across state lines to be manufactured into CBD products, which can be sold to the public. States are required to have a system that maintains information on all land where cultivation takes place, as well as the procedures for testing. If consumers are compliant with their state's rules, they can legally grow and use hemp products, including CBD. It is left to each state to set their own policies.

It should be noted that even though marijuana and hemp are different varieties of the *Cannabis sativa* species, hemp is not marijuana. Both contain CBD, with a much higher percentage found in hemp, which also contains lower levels of THC (less than 0.3%) when compared to marijuana. THC is the psychoactive element of the cannabis plant that produces a high or euphoric feeling. CBD is associated with the therapeutic effects of the plant without the high.

CBD and THC are not different types of cannabis; they are different components. The cannabis plant contains more than eighty-five known chemical compounds, which are called cannabinoids. The best known are tetrahydrocannabinol (THC) and cannabidiol (CBD). A cannabinoid is a compound that interacts directly with our body's endocannabinoid system, which helps support vital functions throughout our body such as mood, pain sensations, stress, appetite, and sleep.

Cannabis is categorized into three basic plant types or species: indica, sativa, and hybrid. Indica is associated with producing a physical effect felt throughout the body, sativa impacts mood and emotion, while hybrid contains similar levels of both, offering a balance of benefits. The distinguishing factors between these species are their respective levels of terpenes and cannabinoids and combination of CBD and THC.

Terpenes determine the smell of many plants and herbs, such as rosemary and lavender. The cannabis plant contains a high concentration of terpenes. These organic hydrocarbons are found in the essential oils of plants and can intensify or downplay the effects of cannabinoids. When the terpenes and cannabinoids found in cannabis are used together, they produce a synergistic result called the entourage effect, which magnifies therapeutic benefits. Terpenes are the aromatic oils that give cannabis its distinctive scent and flavors such as citrus, berry, mint, and pine. (See Common Cannabis Terpenes: Aromas, Flavors, and Therapeutic Effects, page 116.)

CBD oil is extracted from hemp leaves and flowers and can be found as full spectrum, broad spectrum, and isolates. Many find full-spectrum oils to be more effective because they contain a wide range of beneficial plant parts. Full spectrum preserves all the cannabinoids in the final product, making this the ideal option for CBD's best therapeutic effect, while with broad-spectrum products, only the THC cannabinoid that is removed. CBD isolates contain only CBD and have no THC, terpenes, or other cannabinoids. Isolates begin as a full-spectrum oil before all of the plant's natural compounds, except for CBD, are removed, leaving a pure crystalline powder. Because isolates are colorless, odorless, and tasteless, this broadens their versatility and ease of use, making them extremely popular. The powder can be stirred into food and drink, infused into oils to make edibles, added to CBD products to increase potency, and vaped.

Cannabis oil is extracted from the marijuana variety of the cannabis plant. These oils can vary in composition, usually having a percentage of THC, CBD, and other healthful plant compounds. Technically, CBD oil can be made from marijuana as it is also rich in CBD, but most CBD oil obtained from marijuana is called cannabis oil or marijuana oil. Unless you go to a marijuana dispensary to purchase your CBD oil, the products you will find at other stores come exclusively from the hemp plant and are referred to as hemp oil, CBD oil, or CBD hemp oil. The main difference between CBD oil from hemp and oil from marijuana lies in the ratio between their THC and CBD. Hemp-derived CBD oil has a high concentration of CBD with THC that does not exceed 0.3 percent. Marijuana-derived oil is high in CBD, with a wide range of THC levels. Because of this fact, it is always important to ask for as much information as possible on the product that you are buying.

CBD tinctures are extracts of hemp in liquid form combined with alcohol, glycerin, and cinnamon or peppermint oil. Unlike CBD oil, tinctures contain a low potency of CBD. The ratio of CBD in tinctures is less than that found in the oil because other substances have been added to enhance its flavor. You can cook with tinctures by using water-soluble CBD. They can also be used sublingually by placing a few drops under the tongue and holding them there for at least a minute before swallowing. The alcohol in tinctures enhances the life of the CBD.

CBD oil, also called CBD isolate, is pulled from *Cannabis sativa* using a CO2 extraction method and then diffused into an oil for easier consumption. Tinctures are extracted by using alcohol-based products which may make the CO2 method better for folks who have a sensitivity to alcohol. The price of CBD products depends on strength, potency, and extraction method. Usually, CBD oil is more expensive than tincture. To extend the life of any CBD product, it is always best to keep the container away from direct sunlight. Tinctures and oils have similar packaging and uses, both stored in tinted glass bottles that help to keep out sunlight.

CBD edibles are a popular way for first-time users to gradually get used to the new substance. CBD that is found in food usually comes in two forms, oils and tinctures. Oils have varying intensities of cannabis flavor. It is common to purchase edibles from local dispensaries, where a wide range of products and dosages are available. Selections of edibles include gummies, cookies, brownies, hard candy, chocolates, sauces, dressings, coffees, and teas, as well as a host of other products. CBD edibles are generally infused with CBD hemp oil and are nonintoxicating. It is always best to choose edibles that use natural ingredients. CBD hemp oil can be mixed into almost any prepared food. This oil evaporates at high temperatures, so sautéing CBD-containing food in an open pan is out of the question.

Phytocannabinoids are cannabinoids that occur naturally in the cannabis plant. They each have a specific boiling point. If you go beyond this boiling point, they will lose their effectiveness. For CBD, the boiling point is 320–356°F or (160°C–180°C). THC's boiling point is 315°F (157°C). (See Phytocannabinoid Boiling Points and Why They Matter, page 19.)

Marijuana edibles differ from those of cannabidiol (CBD) in that they contain a high concentration of THC and are used for their euphoric effect. These edibles have the benefit of offering precise dosages, a control of ingredients, and longer-lasting effects. An intoxicating end result may take hours to set in. Because of this delay, users must employ trial and error to see what regimen works best for them. When you consume the edible on an empty stomach, the results will be felt much more quickly than if you have recently eaten a big meal. For beginners, the general rule is to start with the lowest dose of THC and then wait 2–4 hours to observe the effects before taking more. A person's body mass, metabolism, and genetics are all part of the equation. The general rule is to start low and go slow.

Always review a product's packaging information to be educated on milligram dosages, remembering that this is not "one dose fits all." Do your homework; not all companies are honest on their labels. Find out where the manufacturer sources their CBD and make sure that your selection has come from organic farmland that is free from toxins. Purchase from brands that offer a certificate of analysis (COA), which ensures that the product you buy is safe and has been tested. Reliable companies send their products for third party testing before putting them on the market. The label on your CBD product, food, or drink should indicate these details.

CBD and THC are never a substitute for professional health care. Be sure to consult with your health-care provider before trying CBD oil or any other cannabis products. Some herbal medications, including CBD oil and cannabis, can have interactions with other medicines. It is always safer to seek your doctor's advice before introducing any new substance into your body.

The Art of Cooking with Cannabis introduces the reader to the ever-evolving world of cannabis. Its generous contributors, who have helped to make this book possible, stretch across the United States from coast to coast. Each award-winning chef, organic farmer, artisan, and food producer is introduced to the reader through a descriptive profile that offers a brief synopsis of the personal journey that has led these folks to explore the world of cannabis. These individuals come from rural and suburban communities, as well as the bustling cities that stretch over the length and breadth of the United States. Taking time from their busy lives, they have kindly agreed to share their inspiring stories and nourishing recipes, enabling others to gain insight into the world of cannabis and the role that it plays in our society.

I have organized the recipes into three sections: CBD, Hemp, and THC. Within each chapter, I have categorized the contributors by four main regions in the United States: Northeast, Midwest, South, and West. Insightful sidebars seek to demystify the world of cannabis by offering tips and how-tos that will help both beginners and seasoned participants to cook with ease and confidence. By destigmatizing the use of the plant, I am encouraging readers to learn more about responsible cannabis consumption, with its many health and wellness benefits. It is important for readers to understand that the cannabis dosage listed in the ingredient section of any recipe in this cookbook is only a suggestion that is to be used as an approximation.

I have filled each chapter with carefully curated dishes, the ones I would make again and again, such as Smoked Mussels with Roasted Corn Purée and Peppers (page 7), created by Chef David Ferragamo of Euphoric Food in Haverhill, Massachusetts. I offer choices to suit everyone's lifestyle; a vegan Raw Hemp Leaf Pesto (page 185) by Hudson Hemp, located in New York's Hudson Valley, will have folks asking for seconds. Chef Unika Noiel of LUVN Kitchn in Seattle, Washington, shares her decadent Blackberry Cobbler dessert (page 307), while Sama Sama Kitchen offers Soto Ayam, an Indonesian Chicken Soup with Noodles and Cannabis (page 343) from their Santa Barbara, California, location. The cookbook's selection of culturally diverse recipes is sure to pique the reader's interest and appetite and are intended for use by those who have obtained cannabis legally under applicable federal and state law. The reader should be aware that statements made in this cookbook have not been evaluated by the Food & Drug Administration.

This collaborative act captures the profound shift in attitude that has occurred within the cannabis scene. Both older and younger people have developed more liberal views, overcoming their trepidation about its legalization and use. With help from advocates around the world—scientists, doctors, farmers, and citizens—our access to cannabis-based products and knowledge is increasing. These infused products can be found in dispensaries, pharmacies, health food stores, and, depending upon state legislation, a wide range of other businesses.

By offering a simplified explanation of the plant and its use, my desire is to inspire folks to rethink cannabis as a culinary ingredient. With pleasure, I applaud the book's forward-thinking contributors who are using their voices and recipes for positive change, making a significant impact within the food and cannabis industry. It is my hope that *The Art of Cooking with Cannabis* will take its readers on an unforgettable culinary journey of discovery.

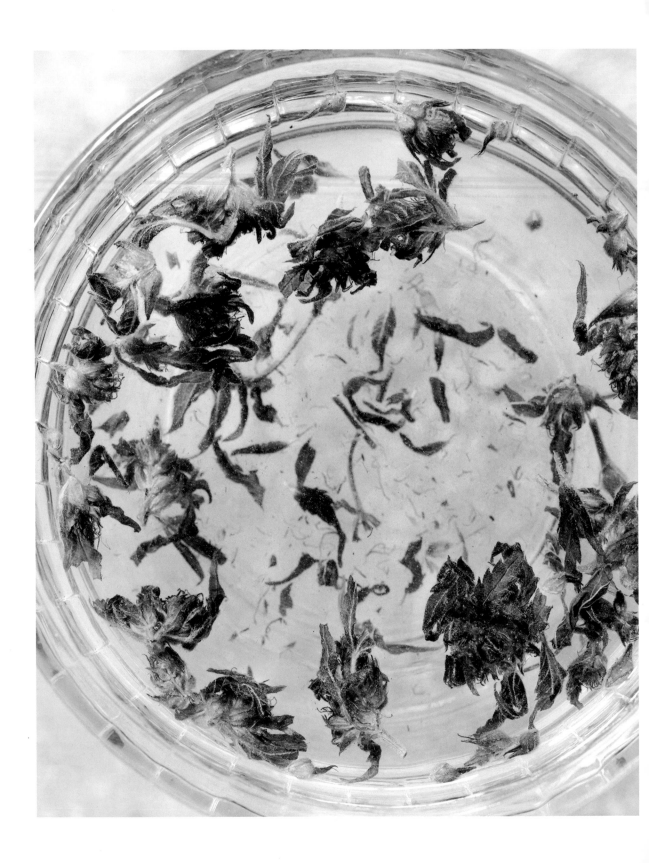

CHAPTER 1

CBD—CANNABIDIOL

CBD is the abbreviation for cannabidiol, one of the cannabinoids or chemical compounds found in the cannabis plant. CBD is not psychoactive, meaning that it will not cause you to feel high or intoxicated. It is a safe, nonaddictive substance, one of more than a hundred phytocannabinoids that are unique to cannabis and endow the plant with its powerful therapeutic profile. CBD oil is extracted from the flowers and leaves of *Cannabis sativa* (hemp plant).

Because CBD does not have the side effect of causing someone to feel high, it is a popular option as a natural alternative for helping certain conditions like chronic pain, multiple sclerosis, PTSD, epilepsy, and mental disorders. Sought after because of its versatility and ease of use, it can be employed in different ways: edibles (gummies are the most popular), tinctures, topicals, capsules, and vaping. CBD inherits many of the medicinal, anti-inflammatory, and anxiolytic properties of cannabis, also providing relief from natural stress, anxiety, and pain. What allows CBD to treat so many conditions and maintain health and wellness in the body is the unique way it interacts with the receptors throughout our system. CBD can deliver many of the same benefits as THC without the psychoactive effects.

CBD that is used in food and drink is oil- or alcohol-based. CBD tinctures that are alcohol-based dissolve more easily than oil-based tinctures, which are not water-soluble. Both CBD oil and tinctures can be used in an assortment of cocktails, beer, wine, smoothies, and milkshakes. The two are also a popular addition to kombucha (a tea-based beverage), cold brew coffee, salad dressings, certain sweets and desserts, edibles, and a variety of infused dishes. Foods that are infused with CBD are becoming more readily available.

The benefits that come from infused foods and beverages depend upon the quality of the CBD that is used. Buying organically grown CBD that is full spectrum (contains all the cannabinoids in the plant without the THC) is the best policy. It is always wise to make sure that you are buying from a reputable company that provides lab-documented results that validate the contents listed on the label. When working with CBD, the focus is on dosage, making it important to use a product that has a verified CBD concentration to avoid the risk of using too much or too little.

NORTHEAST

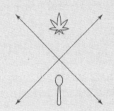

CHEF DAVID FERRAGAMO

Chef/Owner, Euphoric Food

Chef David Ferragamo was born and raised in Haverhill, Massachusetts. Even as a teenager, Ferragamo was drawn to cannabis-infused cooking. At the age of sixteen, eager to learn about the science of cannabis, he was enthusiastically exploring his passion for the culinary world by creating infused butters and Everclear tinctures.

Ferragamo started a private chef company at the age of eighteen while still attending culinary school at Le Cordon Bleu College of Culinary Arts in Boston. He partnered with a Harvard alumnus to start Euphoric Food, a private catering company based in his hometown of Haverhill, Massachusetts. The hardworking student graduated from culinary school in 2017. Always intrigued by the word "euphoria," Chef Ferragamo decided to use the name Euphoric Food when he entered the realm of cannabis-infused food. For the young entrepreneur, the word "euphoric" represents the type of experience that he strives to provide. At Euphoric Food, gourmet memories are created through the combination of cannabis and food. The company's team uses communal kitchen space to do their prep work when holding events at public venues or in the comfort of a patron's home. The staff have been trained to create memorable dining experiences that fascinate guests with well planned, multicourse meals highlighted by the addition of cannabis.

Every private dinner is different. The staff works with the host to create a menu that is customized for that specific event. That menu will never be reused for future occasions. Beforehand, the team gets to personally know each dinner guest, making it a priority to educate them on the proper consumption of cannabis. During each course, there is a strict procedure for dosing that has been discussed with the guests prior to the event.

Chef Ferragamo's cooking style is constantly changing; he never sticks with the same cuisine. His inspiration comes from memories and seasonality. When creating a new dish, he first develops a profile of flavors. The goal is to keep each course simple and ingredient driven. The focus is on creating multiple textures of usually one ingredient. As the chef is passionate about combining fresh local produce with cannabis, seasonal availability is always at the forefront when planning a menu.

The dedicated chef considers farmers to be his primary source of inspiration. He believes himself fortunate to have the opportunity to live in Massachusetts, surrounded by a landscape of fertile farmland. Ferragamo has no doubt that all of us need to do our part to create a sustainable future for ourselves and future generations. By buying local produce, we are helping to support the caretakers of the land and their farms. The chef visits numerous farmers' markets and farm stands each week to build and strengthen relationships with these folks. Every menu that Euphoric Food creates credits its specific ingredient to the farm from which it came. Chef David Ferragamo's mission is to sustain local farms, create beautiful memories, and heal through the power of food and herbs.

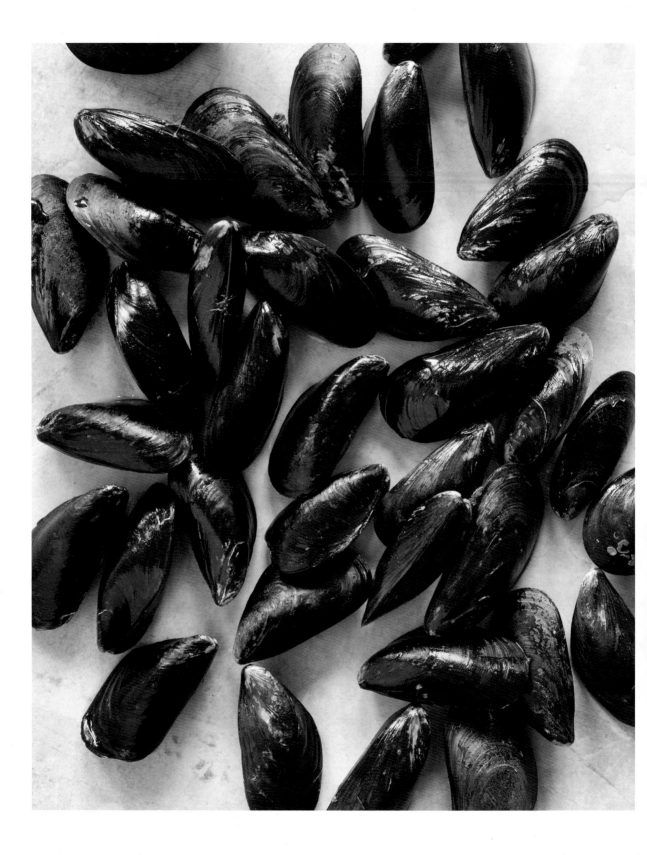

SMOKED MUSSELS
with Roasted Corn Purée and Peppers

by CHEF DAVID FERRAGAMO, EUPHORIC FOOD **MAKES** 4 servings, 15 milligrams per serving

CHEF DAVID FERRAGAMO: During the winter months, we harvest and cure the wood that is used for smoking. Because we live just minutes from the beach, when summer arrives there is access to an incredible bounty of fresh seafood. I spent this past summer working on a farm where everything just came together so naturally, transforming some of the season's best into this mouthwatering dish.

SMOKED MUSSELS

Note: You will need to soak the mussels at least 2 hours before you intend to serve them.

2 cups water

¼ cup salt

2 pounds fresh mussels

½ cup unsoaked wood chips, such as oak or pecan wood

ROASTED CORN PURÉE

Makes ⅔ cup

2 (medium-large) cobs of corn, with husks on

2 tablespoons unsalted butter, softened

¼ teaspoon salt

⅛ teaspoon freshly ground black pepper

ROASTED PEPPERS

2 medium red bell peppers

1. To prepare the mussels: Fill a large bowl with 2 cups of water, just warmer than room temperature. Whisk in ¼ cup of salt until it has fully dissolved. Add the mussels, then add just enough cold water to cover them. The mussels will start to release their sand into the water. Allow the bowl of mussels to sit on the counter, at room temperature, for 20 minutes, then transfer to the refrigerator and chill for 2 hours.

2. Preheat the oven to 400°F. Line a rimmed baking sheet with parchment paper or a silicone baking mat. Set aside.

3. To roast the corn and peppers: Roast the corn and red bell peppers at the same time in the oven. Place the corn with its husks and silks attached directly on the middle oven rack, lengthwise, parallel to the bars on the oven rack. Place the whole peppers on the prepared baking sheet and roast on another oven rack, turning occasionally. Roast until the pepper skins are wrinkled and slightly charred, and the corn husks are browned, about 30 minutes. Note: Corn should be bright yellow and the kernels swollen and tender. Remove the corn and peppers from the oven and allow to cool for 15 minutes.

4. While the corn and peppers are roasting, remove the mussels from the refrigerator. Using a slotted spoon, gently remove the mussels, discarding any that may be broken or do not close when tapped. Scrub the mussels

Ingredients list continues on next page

Recipe continues on next page

TOASTED MARCONA ALMONDS

½ cup raw Marcona almonds, coarsely chopped

GARLIC-INFUSED SUNFLOWER OIL

5 medium cloves garlic

6 tablespoons sunflower oil, divided

HERB MIXTURE

⅓ cup fresh chives, loosely packed

⅓ cup fresh Italian parsley leaves, loosely packed

⅓ cup fresh dill, loosely packed

⅓ cup fresh bronze fennel fronds, loosely packed

⅓ cup fresh tarragon leaves, loosely packed

60 milligrams broad-spectrum CBD oil, preferably The Healing Rose

3 tablespoons fresh lemon juice, or to taste

½ teaspoon salt

¼ teaspoon freshly ground black pepper

Rock salt, such as Pink Himalayan, for garnish

Grilled sourdough bread, optional

with a brush under cold running water, and remove the beards by pinching them with your fingertips and pulling firmly toward the hinge of the shell until they come off, or remove the beards with sharp kitchen shears. Rinse once more, and place in a colander to completely drain.

5. Reduce the oven temperature to 325°F. Turn on the overhead oven fan and leave on while smoking the mussels.

6. To smoke the mussels: Create an oven smoker. Sculpt a piece of foil into a shallow bowl and scatter the wood chips in the middle of the bowl. Set aside. Place the mussels in a baking dish that is big enough to hold all the mussels and the foil packet of wood chips. Place the foil packet with wood chips alongside and on top of the mussels, so that the smoke is not put out by the liquid released from the mussels as they cook. Using a kitchen torch, light the wood chips on fire, and let them burn until the edges of the chips are glowing and a good amount of smoke is produced. Cover and tightly seal the baking dish with aluminum foil, then create a tiny hole for ventilation so the chips have an oxygen supply. Transfer the baking dish to the oven and bake until all of the mussels have opened and the flesh is peeled away from the walls of the shells, about 30 minutes.

7. While the mussels are smoking, make the corn purée: Carefully remove and discard the husks and silks from the roasted corn. Using a small sharp knife, slice the corn from the cob, into a bowl, turning the ear as you go. Repeat with the remaining ear of corn. Place ½ of the roasted corn, 2 tablespoons of butter, salt and pepper into a blender or food processor and process until smooth and creamy. Set aside.

8. To prepare the roasted peppers: Remove the skin and seeds from the peppers. Coarsely chop and set aside.

9. While the mussels are smoking, toast the almonds. In a small dry nonstick skillet over medium heat, toast the almonds, shaking the pan often to prevent burning, until fragrant and light golden brown, about 4 minutes. Transfer the almonds to a paper towel–lined plate and allow to cool.

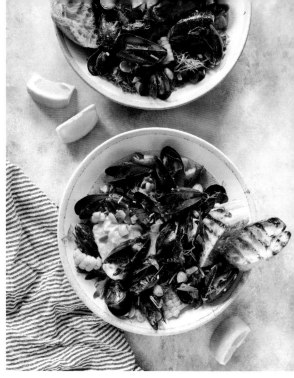

10. While the mussels are smoking, make the garlic-infused sunflower oil. Coarsely chop the garlic. Steep the garlic in hot water for 3 minutes. Using a small sieve, strain the garlic.

11. Heat 4 tablespoons of sunflower oil in a heavy-bottomed skillet over medium-high heat until hot, but not smoking. Add the garlic and fry until golden brown, about 1 minute. Using a small sieve, strain the garlic out then transfer to a paper-towel-lined plate and allow to cool. Remove the oil from the heat and reserve.

12. To make the herb mixture: Finely chop the chives, parsley, dill, fennel, and tarragon. Place the herbs in a small bowl and toss together until well combined. Set aside.

13. Carefully transfer the baking dish to a well-ventilated area (such as outside) before opening the foil, to avoid overwhelming your home with smoke. Using tongs, carefully remove the foil smoker packet and leave it outside before bringing the baking dish back in to work on the mussels. Discard any mussels that do not open. When cool enough to handle, carefully remove the meat from the mussels and place them in a bowl. Cover the mussels with foil to keep warm, and set aside. Strain the cooking liquid through a cheesecloth-lined fine-mesh strainer to remove any sand and detritus, and reserve.

14. To assemble: In a large bowl, combine the mussels, remaining ½ of the corn kernels, roasted peppers, almonds, fried garlic, garlic oil, herbs, CBD oil, lemon juice, the remaining 2 tablespoons of sunflower oil, salt and pepper. Gently toss until well combined.

15. To serve: Place some of the smoked mussel mixture in the center of individual bowls, lightly drizzle with some of the reserved cooking liquid, then top with a dollop of corn purée. Garnish with light sprinkles of rock salt. Serve with grilled sourdough bread on the side, if desired.

Recipe continues on next page

NOTES

If you can't find fresh bronze fennel fronds, you can substitute common fennel fronds.

An aluminum disposable pan, deep enough to hold all the mussels, works well for this dish. If using, when baking in the oven, place a baking sheet underneath the foil pan so it has more stability.

A smoking gun also works well for this dish.

When purchasing mussels, looks for shells that are tightly closed and that do not give off a bad, funky odor. They should smell like the sea, salty and clean.

ROASTED HONEYNUT SQUASH & RED PEAR SALAD

with CBD-Infused Pear Vinaigrette

by CHEF DAVID FERRAGAMO, EUPHORIC FOOD **MAKES** 4 servings as an appetizer or as a side salad

> **CHEF DAVID FERRAGAMO:** Pears have always been my favorite fruit. After hearing about Dan Barber's culinary journey with Honeynut squash, I couldn't stop roasting them—with both being abundant in my summer CSA shares, I was inspired to create this salad.

CHARRED SHALLOTS

3 medium banana shallot bulbs, halved lengthwise, peeled, roots intact

1 tablespoon sunflower oil

Kosher salt and freshly ground black pepper to taste

ROASTED HONEYNUT SQUASH

2 pounds, 6 ounces Honeynut squash, peeled, optional (see Note on page 13)

2 tablespoons sunflower oil

2 tablespoons pure maple syrup

1 teaspoon kosher salt

½ teaspoon freshly ground black pepper

¼ teaspoon freshly grated nutmeg

ROASTED RED PEARS

3 ripe red pears, such as Red d'Anjou or Red Bartlett

1 tablespoon sunflower oil

½ teaspoon kosher salt

3 tablespoons reserved pear juice

1. Preheat the oven to 400°F. Line a rimmed baking sheet with parchment paper or a silicone baking mat. Set aside.

2. To make the charred shallots: Heat a dry cast-iron skillet over medium-high heat until hot but not smoking. Reduce the heat to medium-low and add the shallots, cut-side down. Char, turning a few times until slightly blackened all over, about 15 minutes. When cool enough to handle, separate the shallot layers into individual leaves and place in a small bowl, then add the sunflower oil, salt, and pepper to taste, tossing until well combined. Cover the bowl tightly with plastic wrap, and set aside at room temperature for 1 hour.

3. To make the roasted Honeynut squash: Cut the squash in half lengthwise and scoop out the seeds and strings. Cut the squash into half-moon slices, about ½ inch thick.

4. With a sharp knife, score the squash on the diagonal in a crosshatch pattern so that the seasonings and oil can penetrate it. Pat the squash slices dry with paper towels.

5. In a medium bowl, toss together the squash, sunflower oil, maple syrup, salt, pepper, and nutmeg until well combined. Spread the squash slices out in a single layer on the prepared baking sheet and bake until fork-tender, about 25 minutes. Tent with foil and set aside.

6. Reduce the oven temperature to 375°F.

Ingredients list continues on next page

Recipe continues on next page

TOASTED WALNUTS

1 cup walnuts

SALAD

⅓ cup fresh celery leaves, loosely packed

¼ cup fresh flat-leaf parsley leaves, loosely packed

¼ cup fresh mint leaves, loosely packed

⅓ cup fresh watercress, tough stems trimmed, loosely packed

CBD-INFUSED PEAR VINAIGRETTE

Makes about 1 cup

½ of the roasted pear slices (12 slices)

3 tablespoons pear juice, reserved from roasted pear recipe

1 tablespoon white balsamic vinegar

½ tablespoon pure maple syrup

1 teaspoon chopped fresh flat-leaf parsley

½ teaspoon kosher salt

¼ teaspoon freshly ground black pepper

40 milligrams broad-spectrum CBD oil, preferably The Healing Rose

GARNISH

4 ounces hard aged sheep cheese, such as Queso Manchego, Pecorino Romano, or Pecorino Toscano

1 red pear, such as Red d'Anjou or Red Bartlett, cored, stems removed, unpeeled, cut into thin strips resembling matchsticks

Reserved pear juice, as needed

7. To make the roasted pears: Using a vegetable peeler or small paring knife, remove the peels over a bowl to catch any juice. Reserve the pear juice for a later use. Cut the pear in half lengthwise, then remove the base and stem. Using a melon baller, carefully scoop out the core, then cut into 8 slices. Repeat with the remaining pears.

8. Place a 12×15-inch piece of foil on a rimmed baking sheet. In a medium bowl, toss the pear slices with the sunflower oil and salt. Arrange the pear slices on the foil in a single layer and drizzle with the remaining oil left in the bowl. Measure the reserved pear juice, adding enough water to bring the total liquid volume up to 3 tablespoons, and drizzle this liquid over the pears. Note: This will depend upon the ripeness of the pears. Fold all the edges of the foil in toward the center and crimp the seams to seal to keep the juices inside the packet. Bake in the oven until fork-tender, about 20 minutes, depending on the ripeness of the pears. Remove from the oven and set aside, reserving the roasted pear juice.

9. To make the toasted walnuts: Ten minutes before the pears are done, toast the walnuts. Place the walnuts in a small oven-proof skillet, and toast, stirring occasionally, until golden brown and fragrant, about 8 minutes. Set aside.

10. To make the salad: Cut the celery leaves, parsley leaves, and mint leaves into uniform thin strips. Transfer the herbs to a bowl along with the watercress. Set aside.

11. For the CBD-infused pear vinaigrette: In a blender, blend 12 of the roasted pear slices, 3 tablespoons reserved pear juice, white balsamic vinegar, maple syrup, parsley, salt, and pepper, until smooth. Adjust seasonings with salt and pepper to taste. Add the CBD oil and blend for another 30 seconds.

12. To serve: Arrange the squash and the remaining 12 roasted pear slices shingle-style onto 4 individual plates. Scatter the shallot leaves evenly over the squash and pears. Place 1 serving of the salad greens and 1 tablespoon of the vinaigrette in a small bowl, tossing until evenly coated, adding more to taste. Place on top of one plate of the squash and pear slices. Scatter the top with ¼ cup

of walnuts and ¼ of the raw pear matchsticks. Using a vegetable peeler, shave some of the cheese into long thin strips directly over the salad. Drizzle the top with the reserved pear juice, to taste. Adjust seasonings with salt and pepper to taste. Repeat for the remaining 3 plates. Serve at once.

NOTES

Another medium-size variety of shallot may be substituted for the banana shallots.

The CBD-infused pear vinaigrette makes more than you will need for this recipe. Add the extra vinaigrette to a green bean or chicken salad.

Butternut squash can be used as a substitute for Honeynut squash.

The skin of the Honeynut squash is thin like that of a Delicata squash. There is no need to peel Honeynut squash when baking, broiling, or roasting because the skin is completely edible. Whether you decide to remove the skins or leave them on will depend upon your personal preference.

SUNFLOWER CHOCOLATE CHIP ENERGY BALLS

by CHEF DAVID FERRAGAMO, EUPHORIC FOOD

MAKES approximately 15 energy balls, 20 milligrams per energy ball

> **CHEF DAVID FERRAGAMO.** These snacks were developed for my girlfriend who battles with ulcerative colitis. I wanted to give her a sweet treat that she could feel good about eating. It's hard for us to enjoy the same foods, so it is great to share them with her.

Note: You will need to make the dough 1 day before you intend to serve the energy balls.

½ cup organic old-fashioned oats

⅓ cup brown rice flour

¼ cup tapioca flour

⅓ cup potato starch

⅓ cup chia seeds

⅓ cup flax seeds, ground

½ teaspoon baking soda

½ teaspoon aluminum-free baking powder

¾ cup raw, hulled sunflower seeds

300 milligrams CBD oil, Broad Spectrum, preferably The Healing Rose

⅓ cup organic virgin coconut oil, at room temperature

⅓ cup pure maple syrup, at room temperature

¼ cup organic coconut sugar

¼ cup organic sunflower seed butter, unsweetened

2 teaspoons vanilla bean paste

1 cup good-quality dark chocolate chips (60 to 70% cacao)

Rock salt, such as Pink Himalayan, as needed

1. In a food processor, process the oats until almost fully ground.
2. In a large bowl, mix together the oats, flours, potato starch, chia seeds, flax seeds, baking soda, and baking powder. Set aside.
3. To toast the sunflower seeds: In a small dry nonstick skillet over medium heat, toast the sunflower seeds, shaking or stirring the pan often to prevent burning, until fragrant and light golden brown, about 7 minutes. Transfer the seeds to a paper-towel-lined plate and allow to cool.
4. In a bowl of a stand mixer, add the CBD oil, coconut oil, maple syrup, coconut sugar, sunflower seed butter, and vanilla bean paste, mixing on medium speed, until well-combined and smooth, about 2 minutes.
5. Working in batches, add the dry ingredients into the wet ingredients. Mix on medium speed until a dough begins to form, scraping down the sides of the bowl as needed. Using a wooden spoon, stir in the chocolate chips and sunflower seeds.
6. Place a 12×14-inch piece of plastic wrap on a clean work surface. Turn out the dough in the center of the plastic wrap. Using your hands, roll the dough back and forth to form a tight 12-inch log. Using a toothpick, poke the dough to release any air bubbles. Transfer to a baking sheet and refrigerate for 24 hours.
7. Preheat the oven to 350°F. Generously grease two baking sheets or line with parchment paper and set aside.

8. Weigh the dough on a scale and divide into 15 equal portions.

9. Working in small batches, quickly roll the dough into 2-inch balls and drop them on the prepared baking sheets about 2 inches apart. Sprinkle each energy ball with a light dusting of rock salt. Bake in the center of the middle oven rack for 4 minutes, then rotate the baking sheet, and continue to bake until the energy balls are tender on the inside, and slightly firm on the outside, about 6 minutes. Repeat with the remaining energy balls. Allow the energy balls to cool on the baking sheets for 10 minutes. Transfer to cooling racks to cool completely.

NOTE

Before using the sunflower seed butter, make sure to stir it until well combined. Also, you may notice that the organic sunflower seed butter turns green as the energy balls cool. This is a result of a chemical reaction between the chlorophyll in the sunflower seeds and the baking soda and baking powder when baked, causing the greenish color. This chemical reaction is harmless, and the energy balls are perfectly safe to eat.

ASHLEY REYNOLDS

Cofounder/President, Elmore Mountain Therapeutics

Ashley Reynolds, cofounder and president of Elmore Mountain Therapeutics, had no idea that the birth of her second child would not only change her family life, but also open the door to an exciting new business opportunity. After giving birth, the new mother found that severe postpartum anxiety and depression were affecting the quality of her life. Convinced that pharmaceuticals were not the best solution for the problem, she began researching the medicinal properties of CBD. The relief that she experienced, after taking only a few doses, made Reynolds want to share her story with others who were experiencing similar health issues.

Ashley and her husband Colin cofounded Elmore Mountain Therapeutics in May 2017. The couple named the business after their hometown of Elmore in the Green Mountains of Vermont. The word "Therapeutics" was included as part of the company's name to draw attention to the medical benefits of CBD. All products are exclusively grown and produced in Vermont with THC levels that are under 0.3 percent. Looking to source only the best quality CBD, the company works with a network of small boutique Vermont hemp farms that use organic practices.

Elmore Mountain Therapeutics offers medical-grade, high-concentration CBD oil extract products and topical balms. To deliver the highest standard product, their CBD is extracted utilizing supercritical CO_2 extraction methods. Each batch is tested for potency and purity. The batch is then assigned a number that corresponds to its potency and purity certificates of analysis. The company labels this number on each of their products. The information enables consumers to visit Elmore Mountain Therapeutics' website to learn more about the batch they have chosen. Quality assurance is a top priority for the CBD company. Its owners believe in transparency, which helps to build credibility in their product and the industry itself.

The company's product line can be found in 220 retail locations across the state of Vermont and has expanded to bulk sales. Their CBD extract can be found in chocolates, green beauty products, coffee, massage oils, granola, dog treats, and more. The Reynolds are working hard to break down the stigmas that surround cannabis use and the industry itself. It is

Elmore Mountain Therapeutics' mission "to operate at the intersection of well-being, economic development, social justice, and environmental sustainability."

Ashley Reynolds knows that being a woman cannabis business owner is fraught with challenges. Partnering with other companies owned by women in Vermont has enabled Reynolds to learn from their example and experience. She greatly admires these Vermont women who are working hard to move forward with perseverance and positivity, inspired by the courage it takes to be an advocate for the cannabis industry. Reynolds is proud to be part of a sisterhood of cannapreneurs who hope to break the "grass" ceiling.

CBD-INFUSED FLAX SEED CRACKERS

by CHEF JORDAN WAGMAN & ASHLEY REYNOLDS,
ELMORE MOUNTAIN THERAPEUTICS

MAKES about 20 to 24 crackers,
depending on the desired cracker sizes

> **CHEF JORDAN WAGMAN:** Flax seed crackers are simple to make and are wonderful with any combination of seeds and spices and perfect for breakfast, lunch, or dinner!

2 cups flax seeds

1 cup cold water

1 teaspoon sea salt

¼ cup sesame seeds

2 tablespoons chopped chives

2 tablespoons olive oil

1 tablespoon (15 milligrams) CBD-infused sesame seed oil (see Note on page 19)

1. In a medium bowl, stir together the flax seeds, water, and salt. Cover the bowl with plastic wrap and place in the refrigerator for at least three hours, preferably overnight.

2. Preheat the oven to 275°F. Line a half-sheet-sized baking sheet with parchment paper or a silicone baking mat and set aside.

3. Fold the sesame seeds, chives, and the oils into the flax seed mixture until well combined.

4. Turn the dough out onto the prepared baking sheet. Top with a second sheet of parchment paper and flatten with your hands, then roll the dough out in a free-form manner to ¼ inch thick. Carefully remove the top piece of parchment paper, leaving the bottom piece under the dough. Using a silicone spatula, section the dough out into desired cracker sizes and shapes.

5. Bake until the crackers are crisp and pulling away from the sides of the baking sheet and the edges are browned but not burned, about 60 minutes. Note: It is important to check on the crackers periodically to make sure they are not burning.

6. Remove from the oven and let cool completely on the baking sheet, then snap them off at the break into individual crackers.

7. Serve immediately or store in an airtight container for up to 1 week.

These crackers would be great with fresh herbs and garlic too! Combine 2 tablespoons minced garlic and 1 tablespoon finely chopped thyme and combine with the flax seeds before soaking. Note: The dough is very sticky and pieces will stick to your hands. Using a small metal spatula, scrape the remaining bits of dough off your hands, then carefully press the recovered bits of dough into the holes of the flattened dough.

NOTES

To make the CBD-infused sesame seed oil: In a small bowl vigorously whisk together ½ tablespoon of full-spectrum CBD oil with ½ tablespoon of sesame seed oil until well combined.

The crackers are nice and salty and complement a very thin slice of fresh fruit or cheese.

PHYTOCANNABINOID BOILING POINTS AND WHY THEY MATTER

Phytocannabinoids are cannabinoids that occur naturally in the cannabis plant. Each have their own boiling point when heated. If you don't heat the compounds to their boiling point, the biochemical will not activate. If you go beyond the boiling point, you risk scorching it and not getting the most effectiveness out of your product.

THCV—boiling point: 428°F (220°C) (very high boiling point)
CBC—boiling point: 428°F (220°C) (very high boiling point)
CBN—boiling point: 365°F (185°C)
CBG—boiling point: 126°F (52°C) (lowest boiling point of all the cannabinoids)
CBDa—boiling point: 266°F (130°C)
THCA—boiling point: 221°F (105°C)
CBD—boiling point: 320–356°F (165–180°C)
THC—boiling point: 315°F (157°C)

EDEN MARCEAU PICONI

Owner, 5 Birds Farm

Eden Marceau Piconi, along with her husband and five children, returned to her childhood home of Woodstock, Vermont, in 2014. While attending college at Penn State, she had studied art, then worked in the hospitality sector for many years before returning to the place where she had grown up. The couple made the decision to buy a small farm a mile from the center of town, finding it to be the perfect place to raise their family. They named their new home 5 Birds Farm, a nod to their five children, who are the Piconis' "little birds." For Eden Piconi, building the new farm was about sustaining both her family and the land.

The property started out as a small batch lavender and garlic farm that now also specializes in growing hemp. Piconi was drawn to hemp, fascinated by its incredible versatility and the fact that every part of the plant has a use, with nothing going to waste. Because of the farm's size, the decision was made to grow only one variety of hemp, the Midwest strain. The strain, which comes from Oregon, grows well on 5 Birds' hilltop location. Piconi loves that its nature is true to original hemp, not masked behind a fruity exterior.

The farm employs old-school extraction techniques that use small-batch decarboxylation and oil infusion that uses the whole plant. Those who have tried the farm's CBD products have seen positive outcomes with some of their health problems. Folks have experienced a noticeable difference in their muscle, joint, and arthritis pain and found that their sleep habits are much improved. Piconi feels that, "The enhanced healing effects of our body balms are a combination of the phytonutrients and chlorophyll that the plant gives us, not a manufactured high ratio of isolated CBD." It is her belief that our bodies do better metabolizing plants in their natural form.

Organic, hemp-based CBD wellness products are whole plant, full spectrum, and made on site. They include items such as hemp-infused lavender balm, MCT oil tinctures, and lavender hemp sugar scrub. Piconi stresses that there is no psychotropic effect to CBD. She loves that hemp brings a new flavor to our palates, as well as rich nutrients to our bodies. The busy entrepreneur hopes to eventually work with local chefs who will offer cooking demonstrations at the farm, creating exciting recipes that use hemp as the central ingredient.

In 2017, the farm's owners bought an 1820s English barn and brought it back to their property. They had the structure redone with modern stylings, large windows, and cathedral ceilings. This beautiful venue is now the site of farm wellness retreats, harvest dinners, and a variety of other happy celebrations, made even more memorable by the tranquil charm of the surrounding countryside. A visit to 5 Birds Farm offers visitors the opportunity to experience the delights of the great outdoors, knowing that a stop at the quintessential town of Woodstock with its historical buildings, rustic inns, and quaint shops is a mere five minutes away.

HEIRLOOM TOMATO
AND FRESH MOZZARELLA SALAD
with CBD & Lavender-Infused Grapeseed Oil

by EDEN MARCEAU PICONI, 5 BIRDS FARM   **MAKES** 3 to 4 servings

> Lavender and cannabis are both rich in the terpene linalool. The scent is floral with a hint of spiciness. Linalool has a powerful sedative effect and is commonly known for promoting relaxation.

CBD & LAVENDER-INFUSED GRAPESEED OIL

Makes 1 cup

Note: You will need to make the oil 1 day before you intend to use it. This recipe makes more oil than you will need; save the extra oil for drizzling over roasted vegetables or bruschetta.

1 cup grapeseed oil

¾ ounce decarbed hemp flower or early-season leaves

¼ cup (¼ ounce) dried lavender

TOMATO AND FRESH MOZZARELLA SALAD

3 medium-large (about 1 pound) heirloom tomatoes, such as Pruden's Purple, Cherokee Purple, or Valencia, cut into ¼-inch-thick slices

12 ounces fresh mozzarella, cut into ¼-inch-thick slices

20 large basil leaves, cut into thin ribbons (about ¾ cup lightly packed)

¼ teaspoon sea salt flakes, or to taste

¼ teaspoon freshly ground pepper, or to taste

1. To make the CBD & lavender-infused grapeseed oil: Place all the ingredients in a slow cooker and stir until the flower is completely soaked. Turn the slow cooker setting to warm and heat for 3 hours.

2. Strain the infused oil through a cheesecloth-lined fine-mesh strainer into a clean heat-resistant glass jar. When cool enough to handle, gather the corners of the cheesecloth and gently squeeze out any excess oil into the jar, discarding or composting all plant matter. Allow the oil to cool completely before tightly sealing it with a lid. Label the jar with the date and contents. Store in a cool dark place for up to 1 month.

3. To make the tomato and fresh mozzarella salad: Starting in the center of a decorative platter, arrange the tomato and mozzarella slices in a spiral, overlapping them slightly. Scatter the basil on top and drizzle with ¼ cup of the CBD & lavender-infused grapeseed oil, adding more as desired. Sprinkle with sea salt flakes and pepper, adding more, if desired. Serve at once.

NOTES

The salad is also delicious served on top of thinly sliced artisanal bread.

For a stronger potency, allow the infused oil to cool for about 6 hours, then repeat the process one more time.

VARIATION

Using a combination of early-season hemp leaves and buds creates a delicious flavor profile.

ATHENA SCHEIDET
& TIM CALLAHAN

Co-owners, The Green Goddess Café

The Green Goddess Café is nestled in the picturesque town of Stowe, Vermont. Husband and wife team Athena Scheidet and Tim Callahan have been the proud owners of this cozy eatery since 2011. Before changing careers, Scheidet was a NYC advertising executive and Callahan a wildlife fishing guide and licensed massage therapist. Their café is a labor of love, a means of connecting with folks through the joy that good food can bring.

The Green Goddess Café offers a breakfast and lunch menu of freshly made dishes that are inspired by its owners' Greek and Italian backgrounds. The food is an eclectic mix of casual global flavors. Athena and her grandmother share the same first name, as does the Greek Goddess of War and Wisdom. Because of this special connection, it was decided to retain the restaurant's unique name.

Scheidet and Callahan try to support local businesses and farmers. Stowe is a small town, making it easy to meet folks from the community and create working relationships. The café has its own garden that supplies some of the fresh produce that they use. Everything is made in-house including the restaurant's delicious build-your-own scrambles, handcrafted coffees and smoothies, and a wide variety of sandwiches, salads, and vegetarian fare.

Callahan has been taking CBD for a few years to help with the aftereffects of the Lyme disease that he contracted as a child. He finds that it helps to relieve his joint pain. Scheidet and their son also take a CBD supplement to assist with health issues. Feeling that the substance has greatly improved their family's quality of life, the couple began experimenting to see how different preparations, at various temperatures, affect CBD. Their goal was to be comfortable working with the product before offering it to their customers. By doing so, they have gained the skills to craft menu items that contain exact and appropriate dosages of CBD.

In 2017, the café became even greener when it began to add CBD to some of its menu choices. The very popular "Green Goddess Jamaican Me Shake" is a cannabis oil green shake that contains tropical fruit, spinach, avocado, organic apple juice, and whipped cream. A selection of smoothies, lattes, and baked goods also contain CBD. The Green Goddess grilled cheese sandwich with CBD is a favorite. Customers have the option of adding 10 milligrams of CBD to some of the café's smoothies and coffee drinks. Names like Jolly Green, Chilled Out Chai, and Chronic always seem to pique people's interest. The café's owners want to give visitors an awareness of the healing properties of these beverages.

Callahan and Scheidet buy their product from Sunsoil in Hardwick, Vermont, a producer of certified organic full-spectrum hemp CBD oil. The café also sells the company's full-spectrum CBD capsules and edible salve CBD oil. The folks at the Green Goddess Café are trying to spread the word about the health benefits of CBD and its positive impact, using their own lives as a prime example.

GREEN GODDESS CAFÉ JAMAICAN ME SHAKE

by GREEN GODDESS CAFÉ

MAKES one 15-ounce drink

This refreshing, creamy drinkable treat is best enjoyed right away.

8 ounces organic apple juice

¼ cup fresh pineapple chunks

¼ cup mango chunks, fresh or frozen

¼ cup organic coconut milk

½ Hass avocado, pitted and peeled

¼ cup fresh local baby spinach, packed

20 milligrams of CBD oil, preferably Sunsoil

Whipped cream, optional

GARNISHES

1 cannabis leaf, optional

1 cantaloupe slice, optional

1. Place all the ingredients in a blender and process until smooth. Pour into a chilled 15-ounce glass. Top with whipped cream and garnish with a cannabis leaf and a cantaloupe slice, if desired. Serve at once.

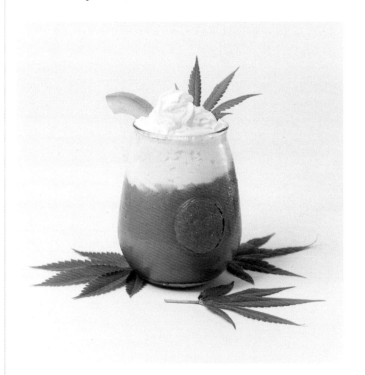

GODDESS GRILLED CHEESE

by GREEN GODDESS CAFÉ

MAKES 1 sandwich

This grilled cheese is a nice departure from the traditional sandwich. It is the perfect sandwich for a delicious lunch or dinner. Serve alone or with a fresh green salad and a hearty soup, if desired. The CBD Herbes de Provence butter uses clarified butter (see page 29), which must be made at least 30 minutes before, so prepare accordingly.

CBD HERBES DE PROVENCE BUTTER

2 tablespoons clarified butter, homemade (page 29) or store-bought

1 teaspoon Herbes de Provence

20 milligrams CBD oil, preferably Sunsoil

PESTO AIOLI

1 tablespoon pesto, homemade or store-bought

1 tablespoon organic mayonnaise

Salt and freshly ground black pepper

GODDESS GRILLED CHEESE

2 tablespoons Herbes de Provence butter, divided

2 slices ½-inch-thick Pullman or other white bread

4 thin slices fresh local mozzarella cheese

½ ripe Hass avocado, pitted, peeled, and sliced

2 slices tomato, such as Roma or heirloom

½ cup fresh local baby spinach

2 tablespoons pesto aioli (see recipe above)

1. To make the CBD Herbes de Provence butter: In a small bowl, whisk together the clarified butter, Herbes de Provence, and CBD oil until well combined. Set aside.

2. To make the pesto aioli: In a small bowl, whisk together the pesto and mayonnaise until smooth. Adjust seasonings with salt and pepper to taste. Set aside.

3. To make the sandwich: Preheat a small skillet over medium heat. Add 1 tablespoon of the CBD Herbes de Provence butter to the preheated skillet. Spread the remaining 1 tablespoon of butter over the top side of each bread slice. When the butter melts, place 1 slice of bread, butter-side down, in skillet. Layer with 2 slices of cheese, avocado, tomato, spinach, and finally the remaining 2 slices of cheese. Spread the inside of the second slice of bread with pesto aioli and place on top, butter-side up.

4. When the cheese has melted and the underside is golden brown (about 4 minutes), use a spatula to carefully flip the sandwich over. Continue to cook, gently pressing down on the sandwich occasionally, until the second side is golden brown, about 3 minutes. Cut the sandwich in half and serve at once.

Recipe continues on page 29

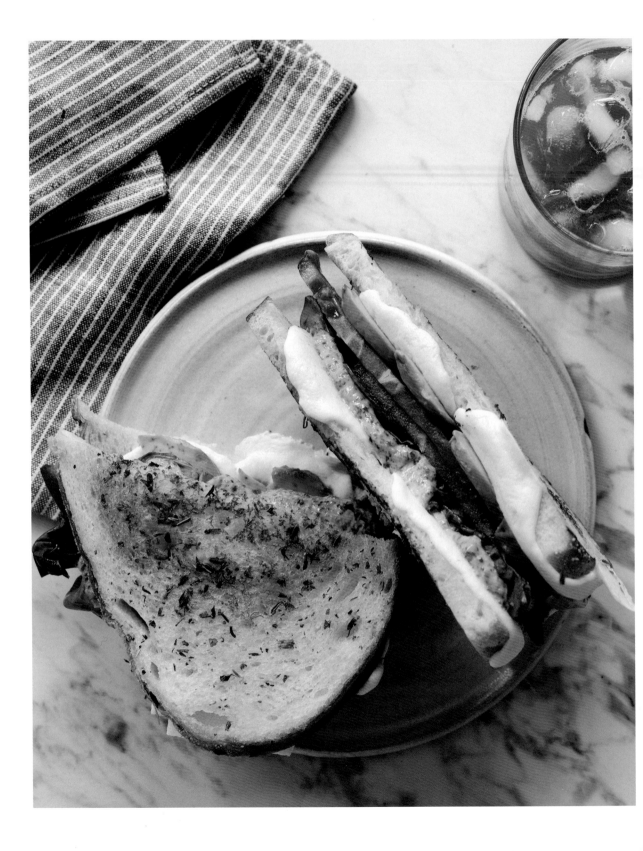

NOTE

You will need to clarify the butter at least 30 minutes before you intend to use it.

HOW TO MAKE CLARIFIED BUTTER, "THE LIQUID GOLD"

MAKES about ½ cup

This recipe makes more clarified butter than you will need for the sandwich. The extra butter can be used for cooking eggs or whisked into a hollandaise sauce.

1. Melt 1 stick of unsalted butter in a small saucepan over low heat. Simmer, do not stir, until all of the whey proteins have risen to the surface and whitened into a foam.
2. Remove from the heat and allow to cool for about 20 minutes.
3. Using a spoon, gently skim off the top layer of foam (known as the whey proteins) and carefully strain through a fine sieve lined with a cheesecloth and into a heatproof jar.
4. Use at once or cover and refrigerate for several months.

Note: While making the clarified butter, be careful not to overcook or it will become bitter tasting.

JENNIFER ARGIE

Founder, Jenny's BAKED at home

For Jennifer Argie, food is more than sustenance—it represents family, tradition, love, and memories. When she was growing up, cooking was one of her favorite pastimes. Her paternal grandparents, who came from Greece and Poland, showed her how to prepare the authentic cuisine of their respective countries. She would spend a great deal of her free time cooking with her grandmother and the older ladies from her church. They taught young Jennifer a great deal about the importance of good healthy food, as did her mother who also had a passion for the culinary arts. These experiences left a lasting impression that remains with Jennifer to this day, the awareness that food can represent medicine, healing, and the source of life.

After completing graduate school in Philadelphia, Jennifer moved to Brooklyn, New York, in September 2011. For many years she worked in the field of design, learning how to develop and market ideas. Jennifer found that designing products was truly something she loved and had a passion and talent for.

In 2016, Jennifer was diagnosed with breast cancer. The busy working mother of three wanted to find an edible that would help her to feel better as she went through her course of treatment. She searched for appropriate edibles that would be suitable for her situation but was disappointed to find that there was nothing that she deemed to be healthy and safe. With this goal in mind, Jennifer set out to create her own CBD gluten-free mix which could help her through this rough patch in her life. Not having used cannabis since high school, her biggest hurdle was learning how to microdose.

As her illness progressed, doctors advised Jennifer to begin taking cancer medications following her traditional treatment. Instead, she chose to study the research being done in Israel and Canada that dealt with reducing cancer cells by using a high-CBD diet. After discovering the benefits of full-spectrum hemp, Jennifer began experimenting with CBD in her cooking, developing a versatile canna-oil based baking mix in the process.

It became clear to Jennifer that as CBD became more and more popular, and the products were easier to come by, finding those that were organic and of high quality presented a problem. Consumers were becoming more aware of the toxins and chemicals found in food, medication, personal products, and the environment and were demanding higher standards in the way that they were produced. After extensive research and hard work, Jennifer was granted one of the first New York licenses to produce, extract, manufacture, and distribute CBD hemp. Having learned the science behind the plant's therapeutic effects, she is now committed to sharing this knowledge with others. Jennifer is dedicated to producing whole hemp oil products that are good for the body and soul. Her company, "Jenny's BAKED at home," is a lifestyle brand that educates and empowers its clients about the use of cannabinoids, seeking to increase health and wellness in their daily lives.

"Jenny's BAKED at home" follows the strictest standards from seed to sale. The company uses only organic hemp that is pesticide free and USA grown. Hemp oil is extracted using a clean CO_2 method of extraction that yields a full-spectrum, high-quality product. The hemp oil is then tested for potency by a third-party lab. The finished product contains all the hemp plant's various nutrients, including hemp terpenes. Raising the bar when it comes to hemp, the company offers some of the best CBD products on the market. All are carefully dosed and compatible with gluten-free, kosher, paleo, and vegetarian diets.

The company provides a wide variety of products that are infused with full-spectrum hemp. These range from organic CBD-infused olive and coconut oils, ginger tinctures, CBD coffee, gluten-free CBD brownie mix, curated gift sets, and a continually expanding line of hemp-infused offerings. Jennifer has even used the infused olive oil to bake into her pizza crust and drizzle on top of the pie. She is always up for trying something different with a product, expanding her line and horizons with shampoos, lotions, conditioners, salves, and body washes. "Jenny's BAKED at home" can be found at local New York wellness centers, cafés, and restaurants, and in CBD stores throughout the United States, and is also available on Amazon.

Jennifer Argie's company is about more than products. Its website is home to a community of folks who are taking control of their lives. People from all backgrounds share their stories and struggles. It gives them hope to hear how others have found the path back to health through the power of hemp. Learning from her own life's experience, Jennifer has discovered how important it is for people to know that they are not alone. Her online community gives participants the opportunity to exchange stories and feel supported, a place to go where others will listen and understand.

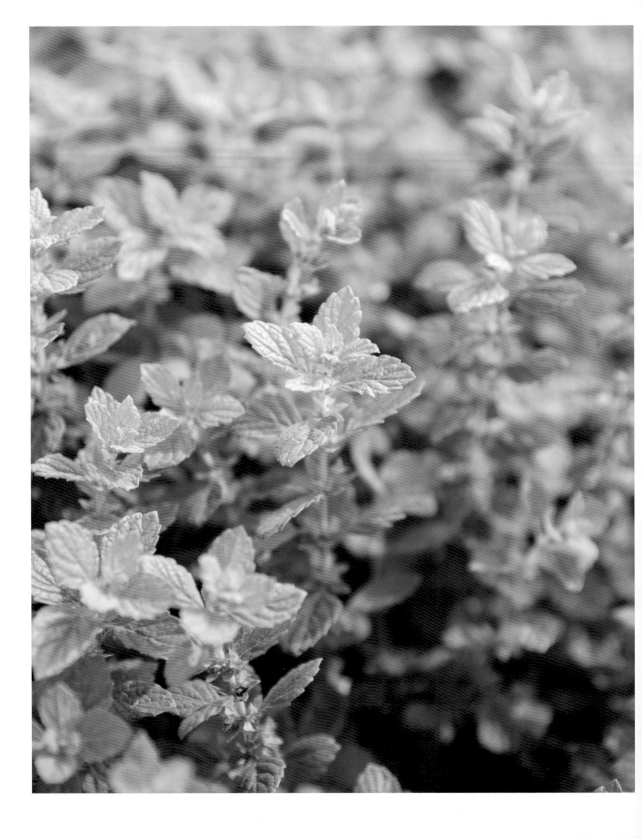

JENNY'S PAPA'S COUSCOUS SALAD
with Feta and Mint

JENNIFER ARGIE, Jenny's BAKED at home

MAKES 4 to 6 servings

JENNY ARGIE: Imagine yourself soaking in the warm Grecian rays on Perissa Beach in Santorini while feasting on fresh Mediterranean cuisine. You can imagine this scene, or you can enjoy this couscous salad with all the bold flavors of the Mediterranean. It will instantly transport you there.

Olive oil and lemon is a classic pairing that gives the salad its vibrancy. Feta brings the perfect amount of creaminess and brine to the party. Cucumber, tomato, and mint give a refreshingly cool vibe. It's great for lunch, a side salad, or as an appetizer. It's light yet satisfying, filled with nutrition, packed with flavor, and charged with CBD oil.

COUSCOUS

1¼ cups water

1 cup Greek or Israeli couscous

SMOKED PAPRIKA LEMON DRESSING

4 tablespoons full-spectrum CBD olive oil, preferably Jenny's BAKED kitchen

1 tablespoon fresh lemon zest

2 tablespoons fresh lemon juice

2 teaspoons Dijon mustard

1 medium bulb garlic, grated

1 teaspoon smoked paprika

1 teaspoon kosher salt

¼ teaspoon freshly ground black pepper

1. To make the couscous: Bring 1¼ cups of water to a boil in a 2-quart saucepan over medium heat. Add the couscous and return to a boil. Cover and reduce the heat to a simmer. Let cook until the liquid is absorbed, about 16 minutes, or cook according to package directions. Remove from heat and fluff with a fork. Set aside.

2. While the couscous is cooking, start the smoked paprika lemon dressing. In a bowl large enough to hold the couscous, whisk together the olive oil, lemon zest and juice, mustard, garlic, smoked paprika, salt, and pepper.

3. While the couscous is still warm, add it to the bowl with the dressing, tossing until evenly coated. Place in the refrigerator until the couscous is cool, about 10 minutes. Remove from the refrigerator and fluff with a fork.

4. While the couscous is cooling in the refrigerator, toast the almonds. In a small skillet over medium-low heat, toast the almonds, tossing frequently until fragrant, about 3 minutes. Remove from heat and set aside.

5. When ready to serve, fold in the almonds, arugula, cucumber, tomatoes, cheese, onion, mint, and basil until well combined. Adjust seasonings with additional lemon juice, salt, and pepper to taste, if desired. Serve at room temperature.

Ingredients list continues on next page

SALAD WITH FETA AND MINT

⅓ cup almond slivers or slices

2 cups arugula, tightly packed

1 medium English cucumber, unpeeled, quartered, and sliced into ¼-inch slices (about 2 cups)

2 cups halved cherry tomatoes or assorted colored halved baby heirloom tomatoes

⅔ cup feta cheese, crumbled, or chopped into ½-inch pieces

¼ cup small diced red onion, or to taste

¼ cup fresh mint leaves, lightly packed

⅛ cup fresh basil leaves, thinly sliced, lightly packed

JENNY'S GRANDMOTHER'S WILD RICE SOUP

with CBD-Infused Olive Oil

by JENNIFER ARGIE, Jenny's BAKED at home

MAKES 6 servings

JENNY ARGIE: Now that winter is coming, it's time for watching classic movies, snuggling on the couch with the pooch, and eating hot soup. Ahh, soup. Consuming it in the winter is like a mother's embrace after a bad day. This recipe is time-tested—it's been passed down from one generation to the next. Grandma's Wild Rice Soup is the much-needed shelter in a winter storm. Adding Jenny's Baked at Home CBD-infused olive oil is the antidote to your unpleasant ailments. The combination of nutritious wild rice, beneficial CBD-infused olive oil, and soothing broth will make you want Grandma's soup all year long.

Did you know wild rice isn't considered rice? It's actually from four species of semiaquatic grasses. The earthy, nutty, toasted undertones are perfect for cold nights. It is an excellent source of fiber, folate, magnesium, phosphorus, manganese, zinc, vitamin B6, and niacin. It's also considered a complete protein.

This soup is easy to make. Don't even think about grabbing that bland can of soup that's been lounging in your cupboard. In less time than the length of your favorite TV show, you'll have nutrient-rich soup with the benefits of CBD oil.

¾ cup wild rice

1 pound boneless, skinless chicken breast, cut into large pieces

8 ounces shiitake mushrooms, stems removed and reserved for another use

2 tablespoons full-spectrum CBD olive oil, preferably Jenny's BAKED kitchen

1½ teaspoons salt, divided, or to taste

¼ teaspoon freshly ground black pepper, divided, or to taste

3 tablespoons unsalted butter

2½ cups finely diced onions

1 cup finely diced celery

1. Preheat the oven to 425°F. Line a baking sheet with parchment paper and set aside.

2. While the oven is preheating, start soaking the rice. Place the wild rice in a fine-mesh strainer, then put the strainer over a bowl. Fill the bowl with cold water and let the rice soak for 5 minutes. Repeat this process 2 more times, draining off any excess water with each soak.

3. While the rice is soaking, start roasting the chicken and mushrooms. Place the chicken and mushrooms on the prepared baking sheet and drizzle both with the infused-olive oil, tossing the mushrooms until evenly coated. Season with 1 teaspoon of salt and ¼ teaspoon of pepper. Transfer to the oven and roast, stirring the mushrooms halfway through cooking. Roast until the chicken is cooked through and mushrooms are golden and just crisp on the

Ingredients list continues on page 37

Recipe continues on page 37

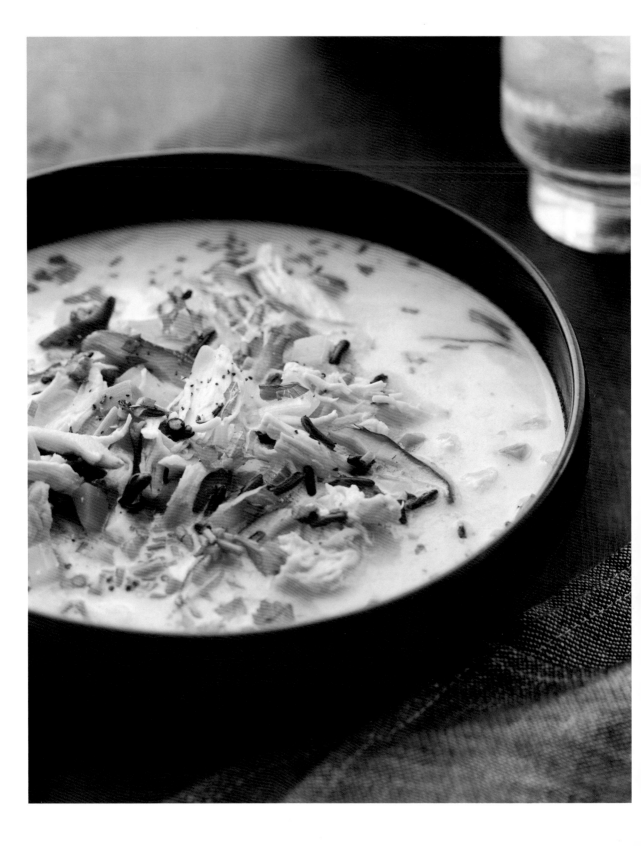

1 cup finely diced carrots

2 medium cloves garlic, minced

¼ cup all-purpose flour

2 quarts low-sodium organic chicken broth, warm

¾ cup heavy cream, hot

3–4 tablespoons dry sherry, or to taste

1½ tablespoons fresh chopped rosemary leaves, or to taste

GARNISHES

¼ cup minced chives

3 tablespoons chopped parsley

edges, about 25 minutes. Note: The cooking time will vary, depending on the thickness of the chicken and on the size of the mushrooms used in the dish. Remove from oven and let the chicken rest for 5 minutes.

4. Shred the chicken and coarsely chop the mushrooms, then set aside until ready to use.

5. While the chicken and mushrooms are roasting, start sautéing the vegetables. Melt the butter in a large Dutch oven over medium heat. Add the onions, celery, and carrots, and sauté until the onions are soft and translucent, about 12 minutes. Add the garlic and sauté until fragrant, about 1 minute. Add the flour, and cook, stirring continuously, for 2 minutes.

6. Slowly stir in the broth, scraping up the bits on the bottom of the pan, then add the rice. Bring to a boil, stirring occasionally. Reduce the heat to a low simmer, and cook, stirring occasionally, until the rice is tender and the kernels begin to pop open, about 40 minutes.

7. Stir in the chicken, mushrooms, cream, sherry, rosemary, and the remaining ½ teaspoon of salt and cook until heated through, about 5 minutes. Adjust seasonings with salt and pepper.

8. To serve, ladle into soup bowls and garnish with chives and parsley.

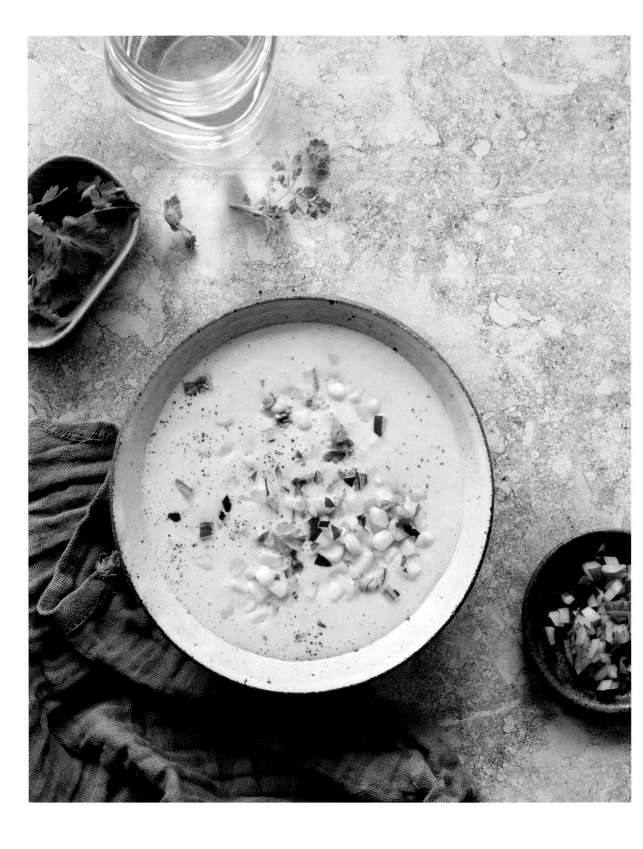

RAW SWEET CORN AND CASHEW CHOWDER

by JENNIFER ARGIE, Jenny's BAKED at home   **MAKES** 4 servings; 1¼ cups per serving

JENNY ARGIE: This raw vegan chowder is perfect for the warmer months. It's a breeze to make and easy on your digestive system. Cashew crema and sweet corn form a silky, buttery, and slightly frothy soup. Unlike standard chowders, this is light; it won't leave you feeling like there is a lead zeppelin in your belly. This recipe is spring falling into summer and forming vibrant cannabinoid blooms. In two shakes of a lamb's tail you'll have gracefully devoured this Raw Sweet Corn and Cashew Chowder and made use of the advantages of CBD oil.

Raw Sweet Corn and Cashew Chowder isn't *just* delicious, it's nutritious too. Cashews are chock-full of vitamins, minerals, and antioxidants such as vitamins E and K, B6, copper, phosphorus, zinc, magnesium, iron, and selenium. Corn has significant fiber content, which aids with digestion. And, of course, CBD oil is said to help with ailments like anxiety, depression, insomnia, pain, and more.

Note: You will need to soak the raw cashews in hot water for at least 15 minutes on the counter, before you intend to use them.

½ cup raw cashews

3¼ cups fresh organic sweet yellow corn kernels (about 4 large ears), or frozen and thawed, divided

2 cups vegetable stock

6 tablespoons full-spectrum CBD olive oil, preferably Jenny's BAKED kitchen

1 tablespoon nutritional yeast

Juice of 1 large lime

2 medium cloves garlic, minced

2 teaspoons kosher salt

¼ teaspoon freshly ground black pepper

GARNISHES

¼ cup red onion, minced

1 tablespoon cilantro leaves, minced

1. To prepare the raw cashews (using the quick-soak method): Place the raw cashews in a small bowl. Fill the bowl with very hot water (just below a boil), making sure the cashews are completely submerged. Soak the cashews for at least 15 minutes. Drain, rinse, and set aside.
2. To prepare the chowder: Working in batches, place the cashews, 2¼ cups of corn, vegetable stock, olive oil, nutritional yeast, lime juice, garlic, and salt and pepper into a blender and blend until smooth. Tip: When blending hot liquids, always fill the blender jar halfway, remove the lid's center insert and place a kitchen towel over the top, holding it securely, then blend. Repeat with the remaining ingredients. This will avoid a soup explosion.
3. To serve: Pour into 4 soup cups, then top with the remaining cup of corn kernels. Garnish with red onion and cilantro.

NOTE

This soup can easily be doubled to feed more. Make sure to add the ingredients in batches when blending.

DIFFERENT CANNABINOIDS AND SOME OF THEIR THERAPEUTIC EFFECTS ON THE BODY

THCA—Tetrahydrocannabinolic acid (nonintoxicating cannabinoid found in raw and live cannabis)—anti-inflammatory effects

THC—Delta 9-THC, Tetrahydrocannabinol (strong psychoactive properties/induces euphoric high)—mild analgesic effect

CBDa—Cannabidiolic acid (predecessor to CBD)—anti-inflammatory effects

CBD—Cannabidiol (nonintoxicating)—anti-inflammatory effects

CBN—Cannabinol (nonintoxicating)—antibacterial agent/effect

CBG—Cannabigerol (non-psychotropic)—antibacterial effects and anti-inflammatory effects

CBC—Cannabichromene (nonintoxicating)—anti-inflammatory effects

THCV—Tetrahydrocannabivarin (strong psychoactive properties/induces euphoric high)—appetite-suppressant effects (abundant in C. sativa landrace strains from Africa)

CBDV—Cannabidivarin (nonintoxicating)—potential treatment in the use in the management of epileptic and other forms of seizures (abundant in C. indica landrace strains from Asia and Africa)

CBGA—Cannabigerolic Acid (a.k.a. "Mothership" cannabinoid)—precursor to three major cannabinoids: THCA, CBDa and CBCA

*It should be noted that the above information is based on preliminary research and anecdotal evidence.

VERMONT MILK PUNCH

by TRACEY MEDEIROS

MAKES 1 cocktail

TRACEY MEDEIROS: The richness of the milk is the perfect complement to the sweetness of the pure Vermont maple syrup. The earthy and piney flavors of the alpha-pinene terpene adds a subtle contrast to the oak and caramel notes of the bourbon.

1 ounce Vermont bourbon, or to taste

¼ ounce Vermont dark rum, or to taste

3 ounces whole milk, cold

½ ounce Vermont maple syrup, or to taste

⅛ ounce pure vanilla extract

1 drop alpha-pinene terpene

Freshly grated nutmeg, for garnish

1 slice applewood-smoked bacon, cooked and crisp, for garnish

1. Combine the bourbon, rum, milk, maple syrup, vanilla extract, and terpene in a cocktail shaker three-quarters filled with ice.
2. Vigorously shake for about 30 seconds. Adjust seasonings to taste. Strain into a small rocks glass. Garnish with a pinch of nutmeg and bacon slice. Serve at once.

Milk punch is a milk-based beverage that commonly uses brandy, or bourbon, as an ingredient, although other spirits may be substituted. Sugar and vanilla extract are added along with a dusting of spice, usually nutmeg. This drink can be served hot or cold. It is thought that milk punch was first created back in the 1600s, reaching the peak of its popularity in the 1700s through mid-1800s. Its mass appeal was attributed to Aphra Behn, a seventeenth-century English writer, who mentioned the punch in one of her plays and was thought to be its creator. The earliest written record of this drink was found in a 1711 cookbook by Mary Rockett. Many famous people were known to be fond of this smooth-tasting libation. Ben Franklin created his own recipe for milk punch, enclosing it in a letter to one of his acquaintances in 1763. His was a rather strong creation that has been softened by today's mixologists, who use only a select number of Franklin's ingredients.

Due to its lasting power, milk punch reached the height of favor in the middle of the eighteenth century. Because it was a bottled drink with a long shelf life, it was very much in demand. Part of the drink's appeal was the fact that it could be made with any spirit, juice, or tea. Queen Victoria loved the beverage so much that she employed a special company to supply the royal family with the drink.

There are two kinds of milk punch. The first, called bourbon or brandy milk punch, was very popular in New Orleans in the eighteenth century. This punch is citrus free and includes milk. The second type is called English milk punch, or clarified milk punch. In this creation the milk is usually hot when added to a mixed cocktail, which curdles the milk. The punch is then strained through a cheesecloth to remove the curds. This process removes most of the color and cloudiness from the drink, clarifying it. If the punch is kept cool, it can be preserved for months or even years. It is said that bottles of milk punch were found in Charles Dickens's wine cellar after he died in 1870.

Now that milk punch has returned to popularity, bartenders are putting their own spin on the drink. The key to the success of dairy cocktails and punch is the freshness of the milk. Be sure to keep an eye on the milk's expiration date, remembering that it is best when served immediately after mixing. Using the milk in your refrigerator is fine, but, with a bit of tweaking, rice, almond, and soy milks can be used. Bartenders like to work with different types of milk including half-and-half and cream. Versatility is the name of the game.

After 150 years, milk punch is back. The fact that it can be made in advance, does not spoil if handled properly, and is easy to serve makes this drink very popular. Garnish with your favorite fruit: Lemons, limes, pineapple, apples, and mangoes are a few that pair well with spices such as cinnamon sticks, nutmeg, ginger, or cloves. Tailor your creation to suit the occasion and serve hot or cold. If warming the milk, heat gently—just until steaming. Milk that is too hot will curdle and may burn your mouth. Matching your glass temperature to the drink proves helpful.

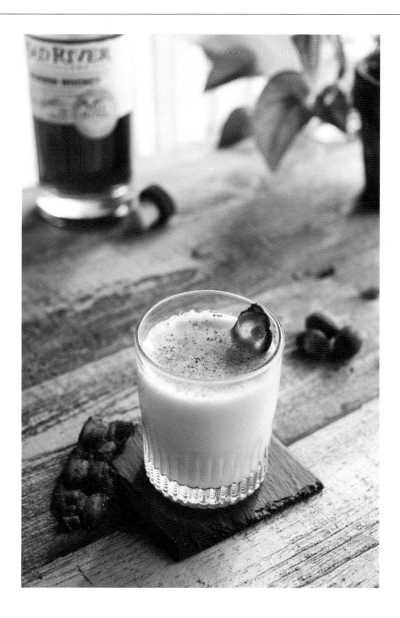

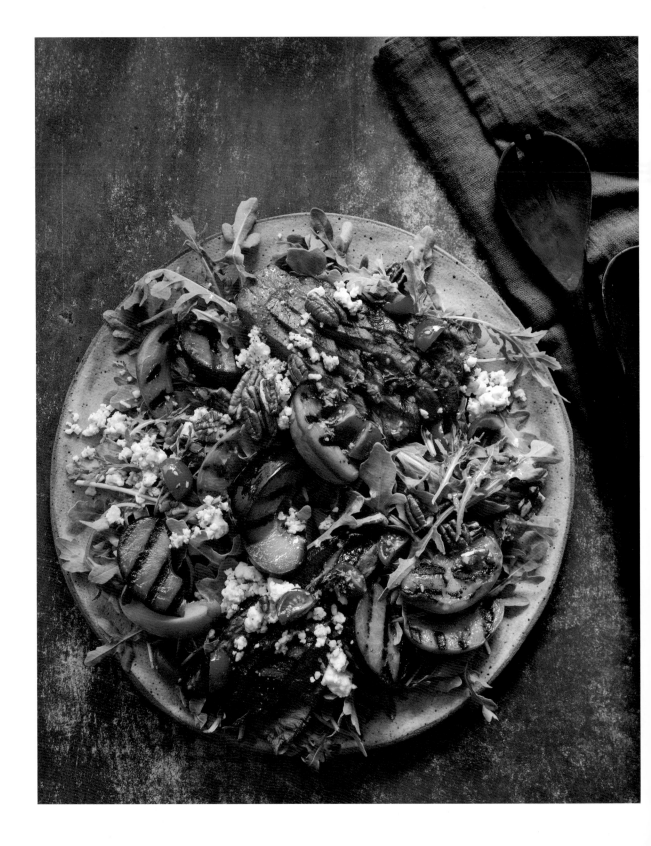

FLAT IRON STEAK &
GRILLED STONE FRUIT SALAD
with CBD-Infused Honey Apple Cider Vinaigrette

by TRACEY MEDEIROS

MAKES 4 servings

TRACEY MEDEIROS: Grilled plums are one of my secret obsessions. During the summer when the farm stands are brimming with these juicy jewel-toned gems, this becomes my go-to summer salad. The flat iron steak is a tender cut of beef that has a rich, beefy flavor that pairs beautifully with stone fruits. For the most tender results, the steak is best cooked to an internal temperature of 130–135°F.

VINAIGRETTE

Note: The CBD-Infused Honey Apple Cider Vinaigrette is found on page 109.

FLAT IRON STEAK

1 tablespoon olive oil for brushing grill grate, or as needed

1 pound grass-fed flat iron steak, 1 inch thick

Kosher salt and freshly ground black pepper

SALAD

3 large ripe stone fruits, pitted and cut into 6 wedges each, such as peaches, plums, or apricots

1 tablespoon extra-virgin olive oil

1 (5 ounce) package baby arugula

½ cup crumbled blue cheese, or to taste

½ cup coarsely chopped pecans

1. Heat a grill to high heat and generously brush the cooking grate with oil.
2. To make the CBD-Infused Honey Apple Cider Vinaigrette, see recipe found on page 109.
3. To make the flat iron steak: Pat the meat dry with paper towels, then season both sides with salt and pepper. Place the steak on the grill and cook for 5 minutes. Turn once and continue to cook until an instant-read thermometer reads between 130–135°F. Reduce the grill temperature to medium-high heat for the stone fruits.
4. Transfer the steak to a cutting board and tent lightly with foil and let rest for 10 minutes. Thinly slice the steak across the grain on a slight diagonal.
5. To grill the stone fruits: While the steak is resting, grill the fruits. Place the fruits in a large bowl and toss with the oil until evenly coated.
6. Place the fruits, cut-side down, on the grill and cook until well charred, about 3 minutes per side, depending on the size and ripeness. Transfer to the plate with the steaks.
7. To assemble the salad: Place the greens, cheese, and pecans in a large bowl. Toss with ¼ cup of vinaigrette, adding more to taste. Fan the meat and fruit slices on top of the salad and drizzle with any accumulated juices. Season with salt and pepper to taste. Serve at once.

SCOTT JENNINGS & PAUL ROSEN

Founders, Pantry Food

Los Angeles–based Pantry Food is a chef-crafted, low-dose CPG (consumer packaged goods) company that makes healthy food products infused with cannabis. Its creation was premised on the belief that the cannabis-infused edible market is underserved and lacking good-tasting quality ingredients. To fill this void, the folks at Pantry have created a unique line of low-dose, high-end food made from premium all-natural components. These products avoid trans fats and high-fructose corn syrup, replacing them with healthier, better-tasting options.

The business is headed by chairman Paul Rosen, a Canadian cannabis entrepreneur, along with Scott Jennings, cofounder and president. Chef Michael Magliano serves as an adviser to the privately held food-branding company. The chef has a formidable culinary background, working for a few years at the Michelin three-star restaurant The French Laundry in Yountville, California, before moving on to open Craft restaurants for Tom Colicchio in Dallas and Los Angeles. His next stint involved working with Michael Tusks at Quince in San Francisco, followed by a time as chef de cuisine at Animal in Los Angeles, later becoming executive chef of Soho House in both New York and Los Angeles.

Chef Magliano now focuses on creative consulting across the manufacturing and new-products segments of the food service and retail industries. He most recently became an adviser for Pantry Food, with a goal to expand the company's product line. With a focus on plant medicine, the team at Pantry is working to research how the properties of CBD pair with the support found in adaptogenic herbs. In an ever-evolving process, they work to tailor effects that are safe, meet consumers' expectations, and set a standard for excellence. At Pantry, the goal is to bridge the world of culinary arts with cannabis. Their unique line now includes keto-friendly chocolate bites, tiramisu ganache, olive oil ganache, and fruit-based gummies, with other tasty delights on the horizon.

Pantry Foods' line of delicious treats can be found in select California dispensaries and include low-dose edibles that are free of preservatives and artificial flavoring. These high-end products appeal to foodies, the wellness community, and cannabis connoisseurs from all walks of life. Although Los Angeles–based, the hope is to soon extend distribution to Nevada dispensaries. The line is being expanded to include folks who are vegans, gluten-free eaters, and those who follow low-sugar, low-carb keto diets. It is Pantry's goal to not only offer its consumers the best-tasting food possible, but a matchless cannabis experience as well.

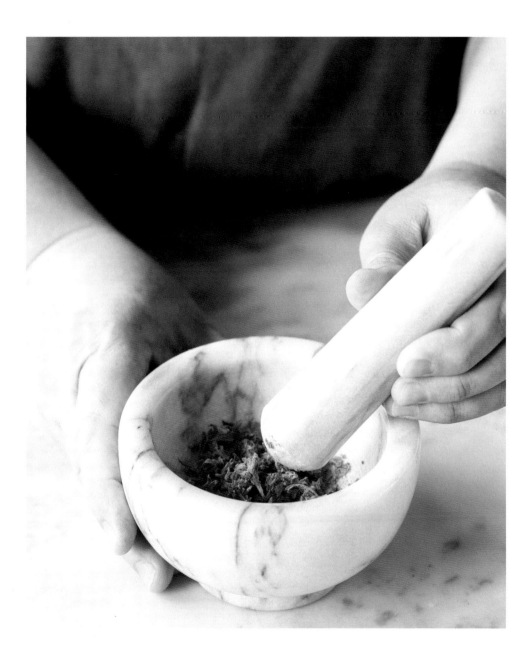

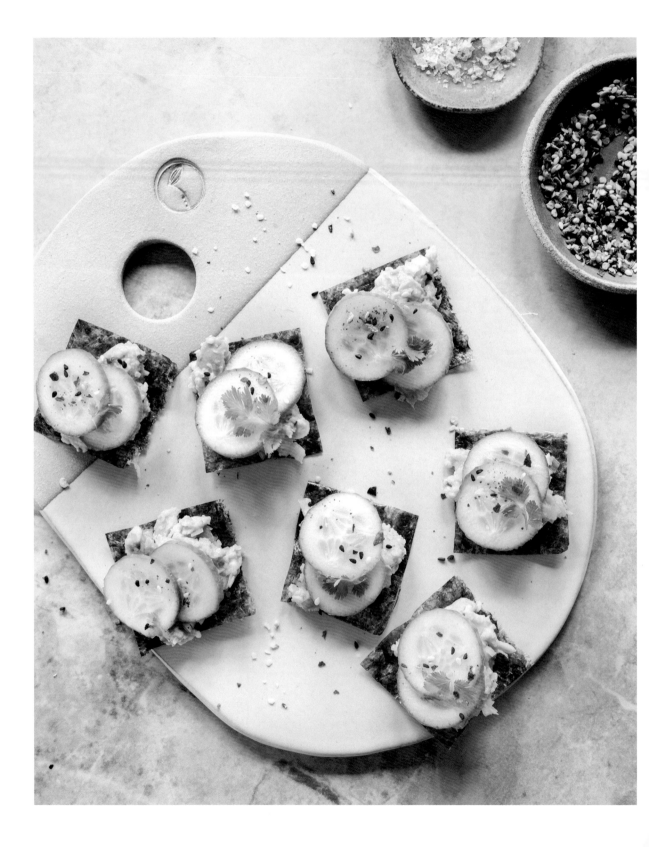

AVOCADO MASH
with Nori and Cucumber

CHEF MICHAEL MAGLIANO, PANTRY FOOD

MAKES 12; Serves 6 (2 per person) as an appetizer, or 12 as an amuse-bouche

Shichimi Togarashi is a popular spicy Japanese seasoning. In this recipe, this blend of seven spices is used as a garnish. Lightly sprinkled over the top, it adds both brightness and heat to the dish. Remember, a pinch goes a long way!

1 large ripe Hass avocado

Zest and juice of 1 lime, divided

¾ teaspoon Maldon salt

1 medium-large scallion, trimmed and minced, about 1½ tablespoons

1 tablespoon hemp seeds

1 tablespoon CBD-infused extra-virgin olive oil, preferably Pantry

2 sheets of nori, about 6×6 inches each

1 (6-inch) Persian "hothouse" cucumber, unpeeled and sliced into ⅛-inch-thick slices

GARNISHES

Fresh cilantro sprigs, cut just below the leaf

Shichimi togarashi spice

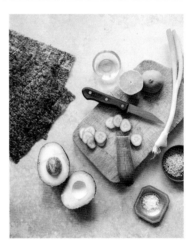

1. Cut the avocado in half and remove the seed. Using a sharp knife, score the flesh of the avocado with ½-inch spacing, creating cross marks.

2. Scoop out the flesh into a bowl, discarding the skin. Set aside.

3. Place 1 teaspoon of lime zest in a small bowl. Add the salt and mix until well combined. Add the lime-salt mixture to the bowl with the avocado. Then fold in the scallion, hemp seeds, and CBD-infused olive oil until just combined.

4. Add 1½ tablespoons of the lime juice, and mix until just combined. Adjust seasonings with additional oil, lime juice, and salt, if desired.

5. Cut the nori sheets into 2×2-inch squares.

6. To serve: Place an equal rounded tablespoon of the avocado mixture in the center of the nori square. Top with 2 slices of cucumber and a sprig of fresh cilantro. Lightly sprinkle shichimi togarashi spice over the top. Repeat until all of the nori squares are filled. Serve at once.

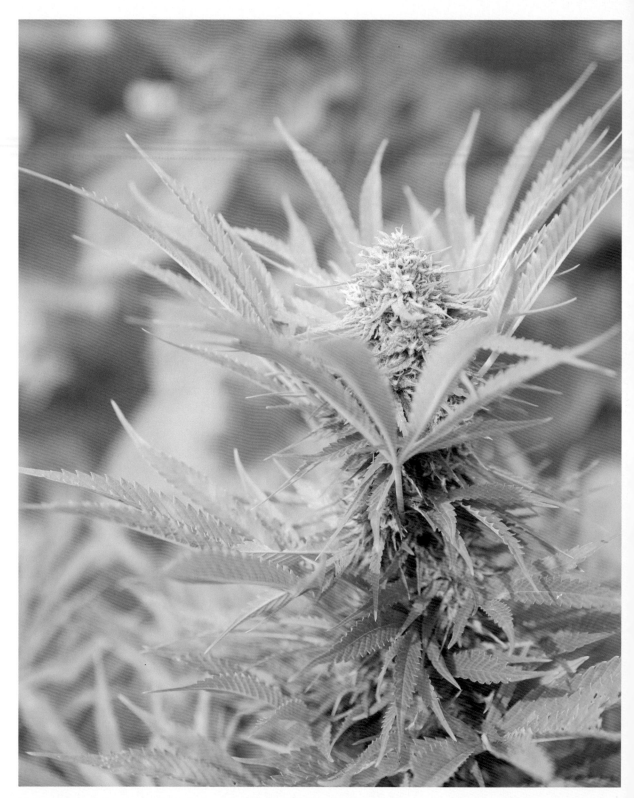

GABE KENNEDY & HUDSON GAINES-ROSS

Chef/Cofounder and Cofounder, Plant People

Gabe Kennedy and Hudson Gaines-Ross, the cofounders of Plant People, first met while hiking at a nature retreat. After sharing their mutual history of back surgery trauma, both were surprised to find that they had come to the same conclusion: Good nutrition, herbalism, and alternative medicines were better at healing the body than pharmaceuticals. Having learned from their own personal health experience, they felt a need to help others by creating highly efficacious products that consumers could not find elsewhere. This dream was realized in 2017 when their company, Plant People, became a reality.

Kennedy and Gaines-Ross want consumers to know that it is their company's mission to help empower people to make alternative and more positive choices when it comes to healing the body and mind. Their manufacturing company, which is based in New York City, focuses on finding unique plant genetics and combining them with herbs and botanicals that have different healing modalities. Plant People is a manufacturer of CBD products, sourcing its raw material from Hudson Hemp, just outside Hudson, New York. A non-GMO, food-grade ethanol extraction process is used for most of the oils, and CO_2 extraction for the high minor oils. All extracts are full spectrum, meaning that CBD is only a small part of the process. Plant People employs a team of alternative medicine doctors and scientists who experiment with herbs and botanicals. They are working to discover effective and innovative formulas. Their goal is to approach not only cannabis but also all other plants holistically, educating folks on the CBD compound and hemp plant.

Classically trained chef Gabe Kennedy has an extensive background in food and the healing properties of nutrition, herbalism, and cannabis. He has blended these parts of his life as a chef and entrepreneur. The busy chef may be found cooking in a professional kitchen where he enjoys using local, seasonal, and natural ingredients in his creations.

Plant People produces high-performance hemp products and herbal supplements for specialty markets such as natural food stores, pharmacies, doctors' offices, boutiques, hotels, and restaurants throughout the United States. The business has also collaborated with the well-known beauty brand Tata Harper to produce a limited edition CBD-based revitalizing beauty oil. The company's products are vegan, gluten-free, cruelty-free, and non-GMO and have a basis in regenerative agriculture. Kennedy and Gaines-Ross want to provide plant-based solutions to modern health problems using a collection of hemp and herbal products, some of which help with the management of stress, sore muscles, and the improvement of sleep and cognition.

The folks at Plant People have partnered with the nonprofit American Forests, the goal of which is to create healthy resilient forests which in turn will benefit our environment, waterways, wildlife, and population. A percentage of every sale is donated to this organization. Kennedy and Gaines-Ross work to produce a product that exemplifies trust, integrity, and responsibility. Plant People is the perfect name for a company that is rooted in wellness.

Plant People

Quality is imperative because cannabis is a remediation plant, which means it will suck up any impurities, heavy metals, or toxins within the soil. Potency does not equate to quality. You want the cannabis flowers to be visually consistent, free of mold or mildew, and have an enticing aroma, not a harsh chemical smell. There should be a nice coat of rosin that contains cannabinoids and terpenes (pleasant smell). To determine quality, think of buying cannabis flowers in the same way you would purchase other fresh flowers or produce.

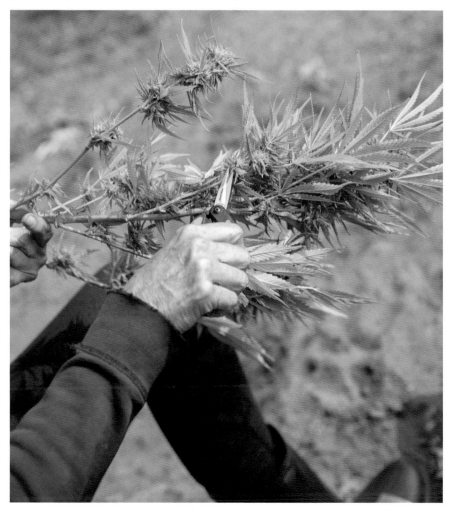

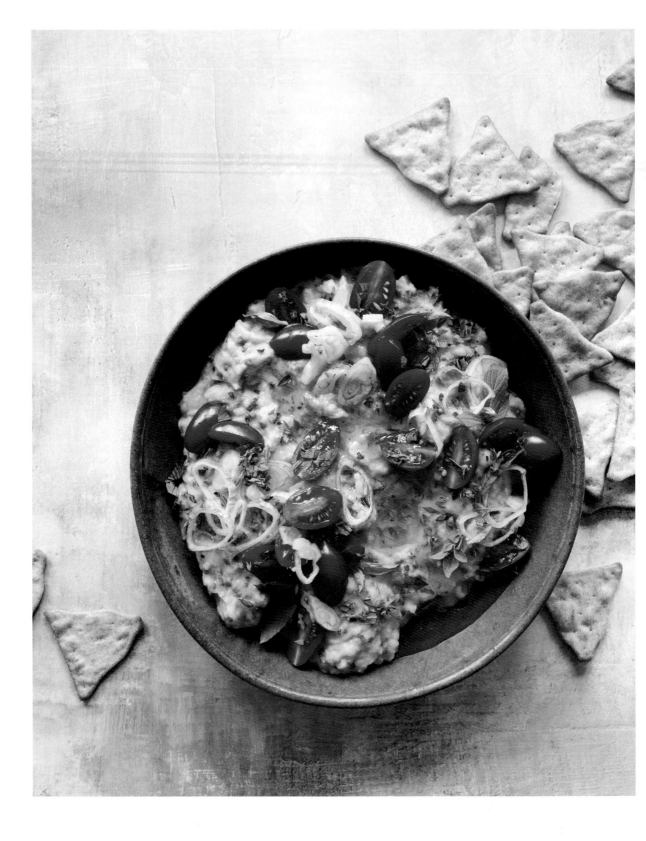

GRILLED SMOKEY EGGPLANT DIP

by GABE KENNEDY, PLANT PEOPLE

MAKES about 2 cups

GABE KENNEDY: My first trip to Israel left me in awe. The commitment to high-quality ingredients and simplicity was especially noticeable when it came to eggplant. The first thing I did when I returned to the United States was cook an eggplant. Upstate, next to a fire, I tossed it to the side, on the coals, and let it blacken. When I cut it open, I discovered sweet and tender, smoky flesh. I dressed it with my memories of the trip—tahini for fat and harissa for heat and then smashed it all up. Topping it with in-season tomatoes, some onion for bite, and fresh herbs from the garden was all that it needed. This is an elegant dish with a playful preparation.

EGGPLANT

1 tablespoon olive oil for brushing grill grate, or as needed

1 medium eggplant (about 1¼ pounds), washed and pricked a few times with a fork to vent

DIP

1 tablespoon tahini paste, plus more to taste

1 teaspoon harissa

Juice of ½ lemon, plus more to taste

1 teaspoon honey

1 tablespoon extra-virgin olive oil, plus more for drizzling

20 milligrams full-spectrum CBD oil, preferably Plant People

Salt and freshly ground black pepper

½ shallot, peeled and sliced into paper-thin rounds

4 cherry tomatoes, cut in half

1 tablespoon fresh chopped mint leaves, or to taste

1. Heat a gas or electric grill to medium heat and generously brush the cooking grate with oil. Put the whole eggplant on the grill, and close the lid. Grill, giving a quarter turn every 5 minutes, until the eggplant is very tender inside, collapsing, and completely charred on all four sides, about 25 minutes.

2. Remove from the grill and set aside to rest, about 30 minutes. Note: The grilled eggplant is very fragile and should be handled very gently. When cool enough to handle, using a sharp knife, carefully slice the eggplant open and scoop out the flesh. Spoon the flesh into a decorative bowl and coarsely mash with a fork.

3. Add the tahini, harissa, lemon juice, honey, olive oil, and CBD oil, stirring until well combined. Season with salt and pepper to taste. Adjust seasonings with tahini and lemon juice, if desired. Drizzle top with olive oil. Scatter with shallot and tomatoes over the top. Garnish with mint, basil, and oregano.

4. To serve: spread the mixture onto bread, pita chips, or crackers, or make the ultimate crudité platter.

Ingredients list continues on page 57

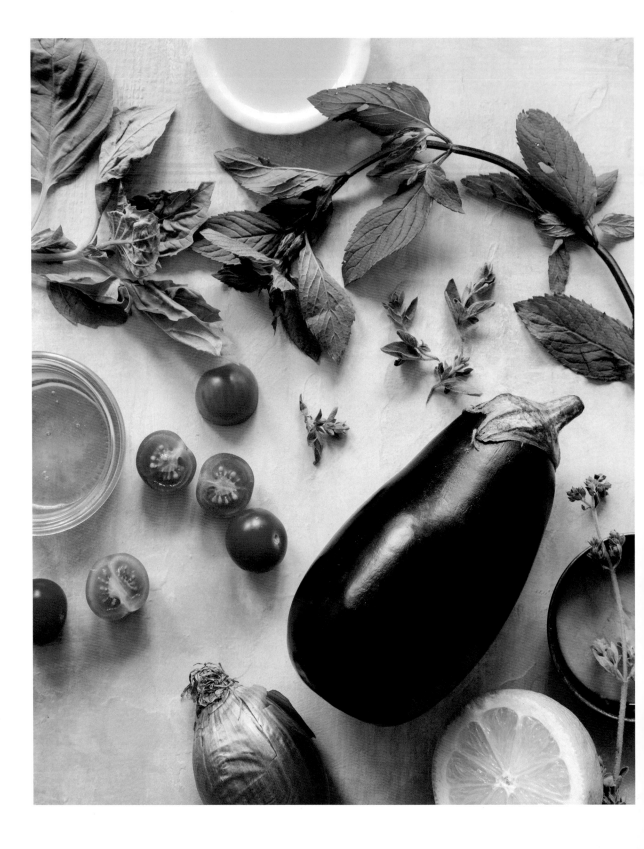

1 tablespoon fresh chopped basil leaves, or to taste

1 tablespoon fresh chopped oregano leaves, or to taste

Bread, pita chips, crackers, or assorted fresh vegetables, for serving

NOTES

Harissa is a North African chile paste available at some specialty supermarkets, grocery stores, and co-ops.

Tahini is a paste made from sesame seeds, which you can find at some specialty supermarkets, grocery stores, and co-ops.

If you don't own a grill, you can roast the eggplant in the oven. Lightly grease a baking sheet and set aside. Arrange a rack in the middle of the oven. Preheat the oven to 400°F. Place the eggplant on the prepared baking sheet. Roast, turning every 7 minutes, until the eggplant is very tender and collapsing, about 30 minutes, depending on the size of the eggplant.

SMOKED BEETS

with Cashew "Cheese," Toasted Hazelnuts, and Fresh Herbs

by GABE KENNEDY, PLANT PEOPLE

MAKES 4 servings

> **GABE KENNEDY:** When I first moved to New York City, I was tasked with cooking for a yoga boot camp. It turned out most of the yogis were vegan. Flustered and in a hurry, I whipped together a dish from what we had on hand: root vegetables, dried nuts, and a few fresh herbs. It may have been beginner's luck, but the recipe is a sure crowd-pleaser.

CASHEW "CHEESE"

Makes 3 cups

Note: You will need to soak the raw cashews in water for about 2 hours on the counter or for up to 12 hours in the refrigerator before you intend to use them.

3 cups raw organic cashews

Water as needed

Juice from 2 lemons

1 tablespoon truffle pâté

100 milligrams full-spectrum CBD oil, preferably Plant People

Kosher salt and freshly ground black pepper

¼ cup minced fresh dill, or to taste

¼ cup minced fresh tarragon leaves, or to taste

¼ cup minced fresh chives, or to taste

ROASTED BEETS

6 medium red and yellow beets, scrubbed

2 tablespoons extra-virgin olive oil, plus extra for drizzling

Kosher salt and freshly ground black pepper

1. To prepare the raw cashews: Place the cashews in a medium bowl. Fill the bowl with water, making sure the cashews are completely submerged. Soak the cashews for at least 2 hours on the counter or for up to 12 hours in the refrigerator. Drain, rinse, and set aside.

2. To make the roasted beets: Preheat the oven to 375°F. Remove the beet greens, reserving them for another purpose. Transfer the beets to a large bowl and toss with the olive oil. Season with salt and pepper. Wrap each beet loosely in foil, then transfer to a baking sheet. Roast until fork-tender, about 60 minutes, depending on the size of the beets. Let the beets rest in the foil until cool enough to handle, about 25 minutes. Remove the skins with a paring knife or rub the skin away with paper towels. Set aside.

3. To toast the hazelnuts: When the beets are cooling, toast the hazelnuts. Keep the oven at 375°F. Arrange the hazelnuts in a single layer on a baking sheet and toast, stirring constantly, until skins are blistered, about 8 minutes. Wrap the nuts in a kitchen towel while hot, and rub to remove the loose skins. Set aside. When cool enough to handle, coarsely chop.

4. To make the cashew "cheese": When the beets are cooling, make the cashew "cheese." Process the cashews in a food processor or blender until finely minced. Add the lemon juice and continue to process until mixture thickens. If you find that the cashew mixture is too thick, add some water until desired consistency is reached. While the food processor is running, add the pâté and CBD oil until well blended, scraping down the sides as needed. Adjust

TOASTED HAZELNUTS

1 cup hazelnuts

¼ cup unsoaked wood chips, such as
   cherrywood

seasonings with salt and pepper to taste. Transfer to a
medium bowl and fold in half of the minced herbs. Set
aside.

5. To smoke the roasted beets: Create a stove-top smoker.
Place a square of heavy-duty aluminum foil on the bottom
of a large heavy-bottomed pot or Dutch oven. The foil
should just fill the bottom of the pot. Scatter the wood
chips in the middle of the aluminum foil square. Place
the beets on a smoker rack or steamer basket, and then
place over the wood chips. Place the pot over high heat
and cover with a tight-fitting lid, slightly ajar. When the
wood chips begin to smoke, about 5 minutes, close the
lid completely and seal the rim with foil. Reduce the
heat to medium-low and smoke the beets for 15 minutes.
Carefully transfer the stove-top smoker to a well-ventilated
area (such as outside) before opening the lid, to avoid
overwhelming your home with smoke.

6. Using tongs, carefully remove the beets and place them
on a cutting board. Cut the beets into bite-size chunks.
Transfer to a large bowl and season with salt and pepper
to taste.

7. To assemble: Spoon approximately ¾ cup per serving of
the cashew "cheese" in the center of individual plates. Top
with beet chunks, about 1 cup per serving. Lightly drizzle
with olive oil over and around the beets. Sprinkle with
hazelnuts and the remaining herbs. Adjust seasonings
with salt and pepper to taste. Serve at once.

NOTE

*When the beets have finished smoking, it is really important
to have the stove-top smoker in a well-ventilated area (such as
outside) before opening the lid. This avoids overwhelming your
home with smoke.*

DARON GOLDSTEIN & JOY KEMPF

Chef/Co-owner and Co-owner, Provender Kitchen + Bar

As you walk along Main Street in downtown Ellsworth, Maine, you will find Provender Kitchen + Bar, a charming culinary treasure. Husband and wife team Daron Goldstein and Joy Kempf are the proud proprietors of this modern bistro known for its historic appeal. Daron hails from Massachusetts and has worked in kitchens from California to Boston. He is a graduate of the College of Culinary Arts at Johnson & Wales University in Providence, Rhode Island. Joy, a native of Maine, is responsible for coining the restaurant's unique name. While researching the word "provisions," she came upon the old English version, *provender*, which she thought to be the perfect name for the couple's fine-dining establishment.

The folks at Provender are passionate about serving fresh artisanal food, putting lots of time and effort into their ever-changing menu. Goldstein's cooking style has many influences, but his ingredients are consistently Maine. His goal is to buy local whenever possible, knowing that you can taste the difference when food is served farm fresh. The menu's footnote, "We make all the cool stuff in-house," often draws smiles of anticipation from Provender's guests. The bistro also offers vegan and gluten-free choices.

The restaurant's far-from-ordinary cocktail menu contains a variety of craft drinks, including CBD-infused creations. Provender was the first restaurant in Maine to introduce CBD cocktails. Their popular Margaweeda cocktail contains CBD-infused pomegranate juice. Always wanting to support the local community, the bistro uses CBD provided by Maine Street Glass in Ellsworth, Maine. The bistro's helpful staff are always ready to answer questions from visitors who are not familiar with CBD. They want folks to know that the wellness points of CBD are stress relief, mood enhancement, and natural inflammation reduction. They are quick to debunk the biggest misconception that CBD drinks will get you high. Delicious food and innovative cocktails, served in relaxed and welcoming surroundings, encourage guests to look forward to their next visit.

MARGAWEEDA

DARON GOLDSTEIN, PROVENDER KITCHEN + BAR   **MAKES** 4 cocktails

> **DARON GOLDSTEIN:** Get your daily dose of greens in more ways than one! The oaky flavors from the tequila and the sweet and slightly tart CBD-infused pomegranate juice complement the pine-like flavor of the sage-infused simple syrup.

CBD-INFUSED POMEGRANATE JUICE

Makes 1 cup

8 ounces organic pomegranate juice

15 milligrams full-spectrum CBD oil

SAGE-INFUSED SIMPLE SYRUP

Makes 1½ cups

Note: This makes more simple syrup than you will need for the cocktail recipe, but it will keep up to 1 month in the refrigerator.

1 cup organic cane sugar

1 cup water

6 sage leaves, muddled

MANGO-PINEAPPLE PURÉE

Makes about 1 cup

3 ounces mango chunks, preferably red

3 ounces fresh pineapple chunks

¼ cup water, or as needed

Rimming lime-salt-sugar cocktail mixture, store-bought or homemade (see Note on page 63)

1 lime, cut into wedges

3 ounces tequila

2 ounces fresh lime juice

Sage sprigs, for garnish

1. Chill 4 rocks glasses in the refrigerator.
2. To make the CBD-infused pomegranate juice: Pour the pomegranate juice and CBD oil into a small container and stir until well combined. Store in the refrigerator until ready to use.
3. To make the sage-infused simple syrup: Pour the sugar and water into a small saucepan. Add the sage leaves and bring to a simmer over medium heat, stirring occasionally, until the sugar has dissolved. Remove from heat and allow to cool completely. Strain the syrup through a fine-mesh strainer into a clean container, discarding or composting the sage. Store the syrup in the refrigerator until ready to use.
4. To make the mango-pineapple purée: While the pomegranate juice and simple syrup are cooling in the refrigerator, make the purée. Purée the mango and pineapple in a blender until smooth, adding 1 tablespoon of water at a time, until desired consistency is achieved.
5. Fill a saucer with about ¼ inch of rimming lime-salt-sugar mixture for the cocktail. Moisten the rims of each glass with a lime wedge. Press the top of each glass into the sugar mixture to rim the edges.
6. To make a single cocktail: Combine the tequila, lime juice, .25 ounces of CBD-infused pomegranate juice, 1 ounce of sage-infused simple syrup, and 2 ounces of mango-pineapple purée in a cocktail shaker filled with ice. Cover and shake for about 30 seconds. Strain into the prepared glass and garnish with a sage sprig. Repeat to make additional cocktails, if desired. Serve at once.

Recipe continues on page 63

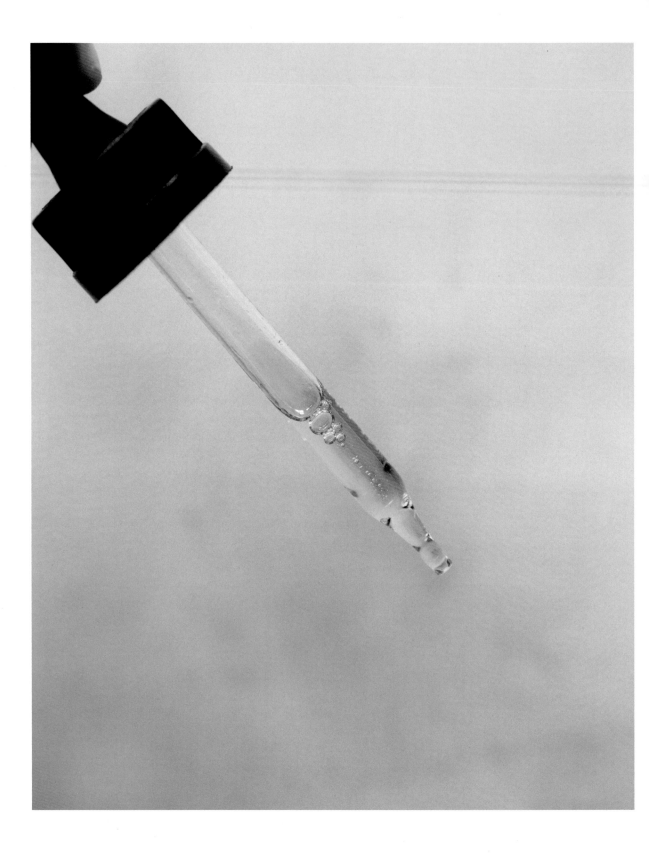

NOTES

Given the quantities of the CBD-infused pomegranate juice, sage-infused simple syrup, and mango-pineapple purée, you can easily make 4 cocktails. Just make sure to have enough tequila, lime juice, and fresh sage on hand.

You will need to make the CBD-infused pomegranate juice, sage-infused simple syrup, and mango-pineapple purée at least 30 minutes before you intend to use it.

Making your own rimming lime-salt-sugar cocktail mixture is simple. Preheat the oven to 300°F. Line a baking sheet with parchment paper. Set aside. Zest 2 limes and bake on the prepared baking sheet until just dried, about 3 minutes. Allow to cool completely. In a small bowl, mix together equal parts lime zest, kosher salt, and sugar until well combined. Store in an airtight container until ready to use. Yield: about 2 tablespoons.

Muddling the fresh sage leaves before adding them to the simple syrup helps to release some of their essential oils, providing a subtle pine-like flavor and aroma to the cocktail.

GIN AND "CHRONIC"

by DARON GOLDSTEIN, PROVENDER KITCHEN + BAR   **MAKES** 1 Cocktail

> **DARON GOLDSTEIN:** This Gin and "Chronic" recipe is a twist on the classic gin and tonic cocktail. The combination of the Maine-grown aromatics and CBD-infused honey complements the citrusy notes from the lime, the sweet yet spicy herbaceous flavors from the Green Chartreuse liqueur, and the distinctive flavor of pine from the gin.

2 ounces dry gin, such as Hendrick's

1 ounce dry vermouth

½ ounce Green Chartreuse liqueur

½ ounce fresh lime juice

15 milligrams CBD-infused honey, or to taste

1. Chill 1 martini glass in the refrigerator.
2. Combine the gin, vermouth, Green Chartreuse liqueur, lime juice, and CBD-infused honey in a shaker three-quarters filled with ice. Vigorously shake for about 30 seconds. Strain into a martini glass. Serve at once.

ARI FISHMAN & NOAH FISHMAN

Co-owners, Zenbarn

When Ari Fishman and his family moved back to Waterbury, Vermont, the community where he had spent his childhood years, he was truly over-joyed to be in such familiar, welcoming surroundings. Much to his surprise, Fishman found out that Tanglewoods Restaurant, the very first place his brother Noah had ever worked, was for sale. Always wanting to own his own business, Ari consulted with Noah and they devised a plan to purchase the iconic 1920s Vermont dairy barn that housed the restaurant.

Ari and Noah had a goal to "build community" in the space that they now owned. They wanted to nurture the agricultural heritage of their new place, providing respite from our busy and sometimes harsh world. The brothers decided to rename their business Zenbarn, feeling that it better suited the vision that they had for the new enterprise. The establishment is aptly named—a peaceful haven where folks can relax and enjoy themselves, their experience enhanced by good food and drink, great music, and calming yoga.

Most of 2016 was spent renovating the barn, tearing the structure down to its bare bones. With the Fishmans' mother in charge of design, the newly constructed barn was transformed into a warm, welcoming venue. The facility offers a little something for everyone—amenities for weddings, conferences, and group functions; a restaurant that serves fresh locally grown food; regionally made craft beers served in the cozy, rustic bar; a stage that showcases popular bands and music groups; and the tranquil yoga and wellness center tucked away in the barn's loft area.

In addition, the Fishman brothers have developed Zenbarn Farms, where they grow a variety of fresh products while also producing CBD for use in their restaurant. They work with other farms and have hosted events that use CBD products from around the state. Each spring, they hold a "420 Fest" during which Zenbarn's chef, Mike Giffune, presents a variety of CBD-infused dishes. Giffune, the restaurant's executive chef, enjoys cooking creatively with CBD. This element of the menu has been a fun and well-received part of the restaurant's offerings.

On any given night at Zenbarn, you can relax and sip on CBD cocktails, craft beer, and CBD-infused foods alongside globally inspired locally sourced cuisine, often with world-class live music.

The restaurant offers a farm-to-table menu that also includes vegetarian, gluten-free, and CBD-infused options. "EAT. DRINK. BE." is the motto at Zenbarn. Eat a delicious dinner in their dining room. Sip a CBD cocktail at the rustic bar. Relax while practicing calming yoga in the cozy loft or spend quality time with family and friends listening to live music.

Food has the power to bring people together. The brothers strongly believe that food supports our ecosystem, educates us about cultures, and connects us to one another. Building community is what Zenbarn is all about.

BABY KALE SALAD

with Sunchoke Purée, Toasted Sunflower Seeds,
and CBD-Infused Honey Vinaigrette

by CHEF MICHAEL GIFFUNE, ZENBARN

MAKES 4 servings

The Sunchoke, also called the Jerusalem artichoke, sunroot, earth apple, or topinambour, is usually available year-round in specialty supermarkets, grocery stores, and co-ops. Peak seasons are fall and early spring. Select those that are firm to the touch and free of black spots and blemishes. Look for sunchokes with fewer knobs to avoid waste when peeling. Stored in the produce drawer, the tubers should last for 2–3 weeks.

This vinaigrette recipe makes more than you will need for the salad. Use the leftover portion for a homemade vinaigrette coleslaw.

ROASTED SUNCHOKE PURÉE

Makes approximately ¾ cup

½ pound sunchokes, scrubbed, peeled, and cut into ½-inch cubes

½ tablespoon sunflower oil

Salt and freshly ground black pepper

¼ cup heavy cream

1 tablespoon local honey

CBD-INFUSED HONEY VINAIGRETTE

Makes approximately 2 cups

½ cup champagne vinegar

1 tablespoon Dijon mustard

3 ounces CBD-infused honey, homemade or store-bought

1 cup sunflower oil

Salt and freshly ground black pepper

¼ cup raw, hulled sunflower seeds

8 ounces baby kale (2 ounces of kale per person)

1. To make the roasted sunchoke purée: Preheat the oven to 350°F. Lightly grease a baking sheet and set aside. In a medium bowl, combine the sunchokes and oil and toss until well combined. Place the sunchokes on the prepared baking sheet in a single layer. Season with salt and pepper to taste. Bake in the oven, stirring every 5 to 7 minutes until crispy and golden brown, about 30 minutes.

2. Place the sunchokes, cream, and the honey in the bowl of a food processor and purée until smooth. Adjust seasonings with salt and pepper to taste. Cover with plastic wrap and let cool in the refrigerator before serving.

3. While the purée is cooling in the refrigerator, make the vinaigrette. In a blender, combine the vinegar, mustard, and and the CBD-infused honey. While the blender is running on high speed, add the oil in a slow and steady stream, and combine until emulsified. Season with salt and pepper to taste.

4. While the purée continues to cool in the refrigerator, toast the sunflower seeds. In a small dry nonstick skillet over medium heat, toast the sunflower seeds, shaking the pan

Recipe continues on next page

often to prevent burning, until fragrant and light golden brown, about 5 minutes. Transfer the seeds to a paper-towel–lined plate and allow to cool. Sprinkle with salt, if desired.

5. To assemble: In a medium bowl, toss the baby kale with about 2½ tablespoons of the vinaigrette, adding more to taste. Using the back of a spoon, smear about 2 tablespoons of the sunchoke purée on a plate, or to taste. Place the tossed salad on top of the sunchoke purée and sprinkle with toasted sunflower seeds. Season with salt and pepper to taste. Serve at once.

NEW YORK STRIP STEAKS

with CBD-Infused Butter Rosettes and "Herbed" Baked Potato Wedges

by CHEF MICHAEL GIFFUNE, ZENBARN

MAKES 6 servings

> **CHEF MICHAEL GIFFUNE:** This is our take on the traditional steak frites recipe. It's buttery and savory and melt-in-your-mouth delicious. In this recipe we use some delicious hearty baked potato wedges instead of the traditional Belgian-style fries for a stick-to-your-ribs meal. The butter is the true star of the dish, adding an unctuous fat and pervasive flavor that coats all of the elements and brings the dish together.

CBD-INFUSED BUTTER ROSETTES

Makes about 9 to 11 rosettes, depending on the size

½ cup (1 stick) unsalted grass-fed organic butter, softened

½ fluid ounce (15 milligrams or 1 tablespoon) CBD MCT oil

1 tablespoon minced fresh thyme

1 tablespoon minced fresh rosemary

¼ teaspoon kosher salt, or to taste

"HERBED" BAKED POTATO WEDGES

6 (about 2.5 pounds) organic russet potatoes, scrubbed and unpeeled

¼ cup extra-virgin olive oil

1 teaspoon salt

Freshly ground black pepper, to taste

1.5 grams organic CBD flower, finely ground (about ½ tablespoon ground)

NEW YORK STRIP STEAKS

Six (8-ounce) New York strip steaks

Salt and freshly ground black pepper

2 tablespoons olive oil, or as needed

1. To make the CBD-infused butter rosettes: Line a baking sheet with parchment paper. In a small bowl, mix together all the ingredients until well combined. Spoon the butter into a pastry bag fitted with a star tip. On the prepared baking sheet, pipe out 9 to 11 equal-size rosettes, depending on the size of the star tip. Place in the refrigerator and chill for at least 2 hours before using, or until firm to the touch.

2. To make the "herbed" baked potato wedges: Preheat the oven to 350°F. Line a baking sheet with parchment paper. Place the potatoes on the prepared baking sheet, prick them a few times with a fork to vent, and bake for 45 minutes. Remove from the oven and set aside to cool.

3. Increase the oven temperature to 400°F. Line the same baking sheet with a new sheet of parchment paper, discarding the old paper. When the potatoes are cool enough to handle, about 10 minutes, cut into 8 wedges per potato. Place the potatoes, olive oil, salt, and pepper in a large bowl and toss until well combined. Spread the potato wedges out in a single layer on the prepared baking sheet and bake for 7 minutes. Using tongs, carefully flip the wedges over and bake for 8 minutes. Reduce the oven temperature to 300°F. Sprinkle the ground hemp flower evenly over the potatoes and bake until the wedges are crispy on the outside and tender on

Recipe continues on next page

the inside, about 15 minutes. Adjust seasonings with salt and pepper to taste.

4. To make the New York strip steaks: While the potatoes are cooling, allow the steaks to come to room temperature for 20 minutes on the counter before cooking. While the steaks are resting, season them on both sides with salt and pepper to taste. While the hemp flower is baking on the fries, heat 2 tablespoons of the oil in a large heavy skillet over medium-high heat until hot but not smoking. Cooking in batches, place the steaks in the skillet and cook for 4 minutes. Turn once and cook for about 4 minutes, depending on the size of the steaks, or until desired doneness is achieved. While the steaks are resting, repeat with remaining steaks.

5. To serve: Place a steak on top of about 8 potato wedges and top with 1 to 2 butter rosettes. Repeat with the remaining steaks, wedges, and butter rosettes.

NOTES

You will need to make the CBD-infused butter rosettes at least 2 hours before you intend to use them.

You do not need to decarboxylate the flower, as the heat from the oven, while baking on the potato wedges, will activate the hemp.

BITTERSWEET CHOCOLATE POTS DE CRÈME
with Salted Caramel

by CHEF MICHAEL GIFFUNE, ZENBARN

MAKES eight 4-ounce mason jars

CHEF MICHAEL GIFFUNE: What would a meal be without dessert? What would dessert be without chocolate, and chocolate without cream? Add a little CBD and find yourself relaxing and having some great after-dinner conversations as you drift off, ready to curl up after an incredible night's experience with your friends. This dessert is best served at room temperature to bring out each of its unique flavors and allow you to enjoy all of its decadent, creamy chocolate textures.

BITTERSWEET CHOCOLATE POTS DE CRÈME

½ vanilla bean

2 cups heavy cream

¼ cup organic cane sugar

¼ teaspoon kosher salt

4 ounces good-quality bittersweet chocolate (60 to 70% cacao) finely chopped

5 large egg yolks, at room temperature, reserving the egg whites for another use

80 milligrams full-spectrum CBD MCT oil

SALTED CARAMEL
Makes about 1 cup

1 cup organic cane sugar

¼ cup water

½ cup heavy cream, room temperature

½ teaspoon kosher salt

GARNISHES

Sea salt, flakes, such as Maldon Salt Company or Jacobsen Salt Company

8 pretzel sticks

1. Arrange a rack in the middle of the oven. Preheat the oven to 325°F.

2. To make the bittersweet chocolate pots de crème: Place the vanilla bean on a work surface and split it in half lengthwise using a small sharp knife. Scrape half the seeds into a medium heavy-bottomed saucepan. Add the vanilla bean pod to the saucepan. Note: Since this recipe calls for only part of a vanilla bean, place the leftover portion into a bottle of Vermont maple syrup and let it steep in the refrigerator for a month before using. Pour the cream, sugar, and salt into the saucepan, whisking until well combined. Bring to a simmer, whisking occasionally, over medium heat, about 8 minutes. Remove from the heat, then using a fork, remove and discard the vanilla bean pod. Add the chocolate to the cream mixture, and whisk until smooth and melted, about 4 minutes.

3. In a 4-cup, heatproof glass measuring cup with pouring lip, whisk together the egg yolks and CBD MCT oil. In a slow and steady stream, whisk 1 cup of the hot chocolate mixture into the egg mixture. Slowly whisk in the remaining chocolate mixture.

4. Pour the mixture directly into eight 4-ounce ovenproof mason jars. Gently tap the jars on the counter to remove any air bubbles.

Recipe continues on next page

5. Set the mason jars in a 9×13-inch baking dish. Carefully pour enough boiling water in the baking dish to come halfway up the sides of the jars. Cover the pan tightly with foil and bake until the pots de crème are set around the edges but still slightly jiggle when you gently shake the pan (lifting the foil to check), about 35 minutes.

6. Carefully remove the jars from the water bath and place them on a cooling rack for about 1 hour.

7. To make the salted caramel: Combine the sugar and water in a heavy-bottomed medium saucepan. Bring to a boil over medium heat. When the caramel is in the simmering phase, whisk just enough so that it does not clump or stick to the bottom of the saucepan. Note: As the mixture starts to reach a boil, the caramel will turn clear and glassy. Do not whisk at this point; allow the caramel to continue to boil without disturbing it. Note: With too much agitation, the liquid will start to crystallize, and there is a risk of scorching the caramel. As soon as the caramel starts to turn a light amber color, immediately remove from the heat, as the hot sugar will continue to caramelize off the heat and will become darker quickly. Whisk until the color is evenly distributed before adding the cream.

8. In a slow and steady stream, carefully add the heavy cream, whisking vigorously until thoroughly combined. Note: The mixture may form lumps when adding the cream; whisk until smooth. Let cool to room temperature before using. Once cooled to room temperature, about 30 minutes, whisk in the salt. Transfer to a heatproof glass measuring cup with pouring lip.

9. To serve: Pour a ⅛-inch layer of salted caramel on top of each of the pots de crème, sprinkle with a pinch of sea salt flakes, and serve with a pretzel stick.

NOTE

Pots de crème are best enjoyed fresh at room temperature or warm.

MIDWEST

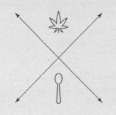

BEAU KELLY-FONTANO

Beverage Director, Entente

Beau Kelly-Fontano is the Beverage Director at the Michelin-starred, James Beard Award–winning Entente restaurant in Chicago, Illinois. He has worked at the casual urban establishment since 2019. Fontano was always inventive when he was younger, but really found his niche when he started working in the restaurant industry. Seeing and tasting the cocktails concocted by award-winning bartenders opened his eyes to the creative side of food and beverage that he had never seen before. He started his career at Eat Street Social in Minneapolis the year that their bar team was named to *Food & Wine*'s Top 40. After the team received the prestigious award, Fontano was invited to barback and then tend bar, which gave him the golden opportunity to keep learning the art of bartending. The position allowed him to express himself professionally in ways that he had never imagined.

When Beau moved on to Entente in 2019, he felt more than prepared for the task at hand. Entente has an open-kitchen, open-room layout with marble and wood accents. Its huge windows offer a nice view of the neighborhood as well as an intriguing snippet of the city's skyline. The bar portion seats nine with a restaurant area that can accommodate approximately fifty guests. Visitors are pleased to find that this Michelin-starred restaurant's prices are much more affordable than others in the same category.

Cannabis has always been something that Fontano believes in, finding it to be a source of fun and joy. With CBD becoming more and more a part of today's social scene, he is pleased that his position allows him an opportunity to create an experience that highlights an evening to remember. Inventive cocktails are the perfect medium for showcasing his creatively inspired CBD or spirit-free beverages.

Entente purchases its CBD oil from Colorado-based purveyor Hapi Innovations. Fontano has found their product to be high quality, clean, and professional. He enjoys using the company's CBD to make cocktails that are innovative and nicely balanced. Suffering from shoulder, elbow, and wrist pain, which are often associated with his profession, Fontano has found that CBD has greatly helped this problem. It has also improved his sleep patterns and quality of daily life, although the busy Beverage Director is quick to note that it is not a cure-all, end-all.

One of Fontano's bestselling beverages is his CBD-laced 700 Club, a popular spirit-free cocktail with delightful floral notes. This purple-hued drink gives non-imbibers of spirits the opportunity to wind down, making them feel as though they are having something more than a substitute for a real cocktail. Besides the CBD, the drink contains freshly squeezed lime juice, cucumber and mint lemonade, butterfly pea flower tea, French violet-flavored syrup, and cucumber citrate. Opalescent in the bottom three quarters (of an old-fashioned glass), deep purple on the top, The 700 Club is a sight to behold! Entente offers its guests the option to add CBD to each of their cocktails or spirit-free choices. Beau Kelly-Fontano thinks about the farmers who are growing cannabis with the intention of helping people, carefully watching their CBD find its way into the restaurant industry. As Entente's talented Beverage Director explains, "From seed to final product, CBD is being used to make people happy and that is what life should be all about: happiness."

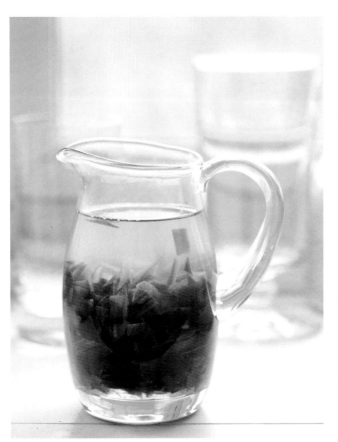
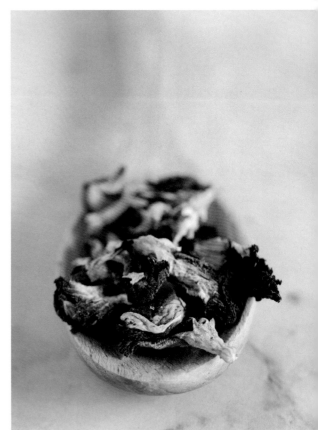

THE 700 CLUB

by BEAU KELLY-FONTANO, ENTENTE

MAKES 1 cocktail

This is a "plan-ahead" sort of cocktail. Given the quantities of the cucumber citrate and butterfly pea flower tea, you can easily make more than 1 cocktail (maximum of 7); just make sure to have enough cucumber and mint lemonade and fresh limes (1 lime per cocktail) on hand.

CUCUMBER CITRATE

Makes 1½ cups

Note: The cucumber citrate will need to be made at least 5 hours before you intend to use it. To save time, prepare the cucumber citrate 1 day before making the cocktail. Store it in an airtight container in the refrigerator.

½ cup coarsely chopped organic Persian cucumber skins (from 7 cucumbers)

⅔ cup granulated sugar

½ tablespoon citric acid

¾ cup boiling water

BUTTERFLY PEA FLOWER TEA

Makes just under a cup

Note: This drink is best served cold, and the tea should chill in the refrigerator at least 2 hours before you intend to use it.

1½ teaspoons (loose dried flowers) organic butterfly pea flower tea

1 cup filtered water

1. To make the cucumber citrate: In a heat-resistant bowl or large mason jar with a lid, combine the cucumber skins, sugar, and citric acid. Cover and let steep at room temperature for 2½ hours. Add the boiling water, stirring until well combined, and let steep on the counter, covered, until it comes to room temperature, about 40 minutes.

2. Place a fine-mesh strainer over a bowl and strain the cucumber citrate, pressing down on the cucumber skins with the back of a large spoon. Discard or compost the cucumber peels. Allow the syrup to chill in the refrigerator for at least 1½ hours. The cucumber citrate should be cold before you intend to use it.

3. To make the butterfly pea flower tea: Place the tea into a stainless-steel mesh tea ball or tea strainer with a handle. Set aside. Place the water in a small saucepan and bring to a temperature of 208°F, just below boiling, over medium heat. Remove from the heat and steep the tea in the water for 5 minutes or according to the directions on the tea package. The tea will have a deep blue hue. Remove the tea ball and allow the tea to cool to room temperature. Pour into a measuring cup and allow the tea to chill in the refrigerator for at least 1½ hours. The tea should be cold before you intend to use it. Note: To get the right temperature of 208°F, the water needs to be watched carefully in an open saucepan.

4. To make the cocktail: Combine the lemonade, cucumber citrate, lime juice, and French violet-flavored syrup, in

Ingredients list continues on page 79

Recipe continues on page 79

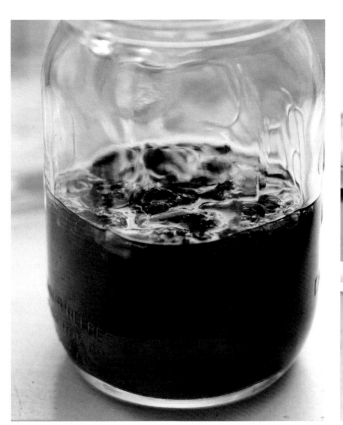
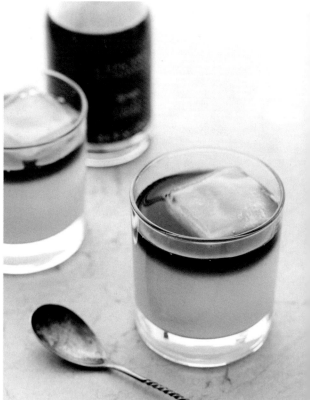

COCKTAIL

Makes 1 cocktail

2¼ ounces organic cucumber and mint lemonade, homemade (page 81) or store-bought such as Belvoir Fruit Farms, or Flow

¾ ounce cucumber citrate, or depending on desired sweetness

¾ ounce freshly squeezed lime juice, or to taste

¼ ounce French violet-flavored syrup, such as L'Epicerie de Provence

2×2-inch ice cube

GARNISH

1 milligram CBD tincture, preferably Hapi Innovations, per cocktail

an old-fashioned glass. Using a bar spoon, gently stir the cocktail until well combined. Top with a 2×2-inch ice cube.

5. Slowly pour 1 ounce of the tea over the exposed ice cube. This will gently disperse the tea over the surface of the cocktail. Do not stir in the tea; it should be its own separate layer. Garnish with the CBD tincture over and around the cocktail. Serve at once.

NOTE

It is important to build this cocktail in an old-fashioned glass over an ice cube. Stir everything, except the butterfly pea flower tea and CBD tincture. The drinker is encouraged to adjust the flavors and sweetness to suit their palate before adding the tea. In order to balance the flavors of the cocktail, the amount of syrups used may need to be adjusted to account for the sweetness of the lemonade.

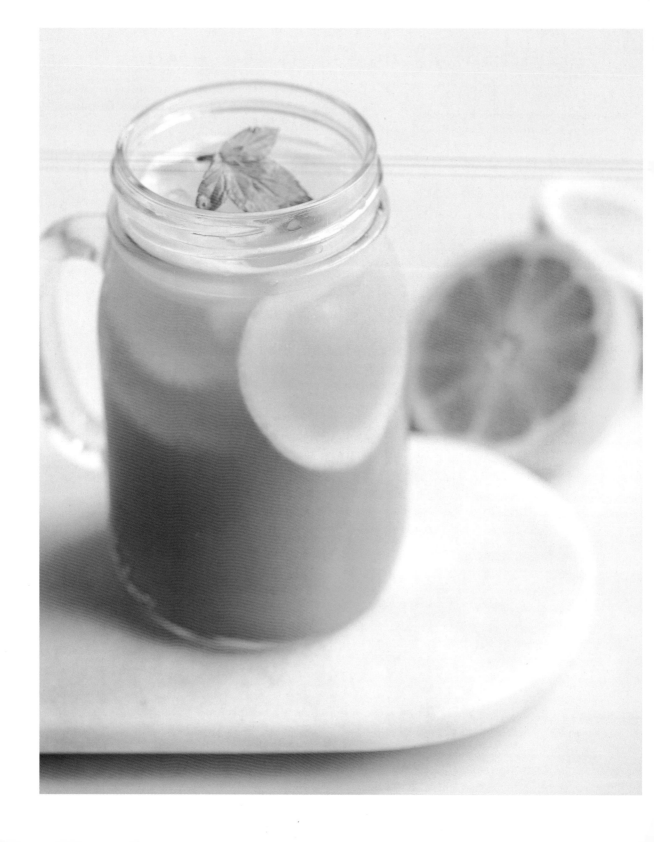

CUCUMBER AND MINT LEMONADE

SARAH STRAUSS

MAKES just under 1 quart

SARAH STRAUSS: To save time, prepare the cucumber and mint lemonade 1 day before you intend to use it. Shake or stir the lemonade vigorously before adding to The 700 Club cocktail (page 77).

¼ cup sugar

2 cups water, divided

1 cup Persian cucumbers, peeled and sliced (3 to 4 cucumbers)

1 cup mint leaves

1 cup freshly squeezed lemon juice

1. To make the simple syrup: Bring the sugar and ¼ cup of water to a boil in a small saucepan over medium heat, whisking occasionally, until the sugar dissolves, about 5 minutes. Remove from heat and allow to cool for 15 minutes.

2. To make the cucumber and mint lemonade: Place the cucumbers, mint leaves, lemon juice, and simple syrup in a blender and blend on medium speed until completely smooth, about 1 minute.

3. Strain the cucumber mixture through a cheesecloth-lined fine-mesh strainer into a clean container with a spout. Gather the corners of the cheesecloth and gently squeeze out any excess juice into the container. Stir in the remaining 1¾ cups of water. Transfer to the refrigerator and let chill completely before using.

WE'RE ALL MAD HERE

by BEAU KELLY-FONTANO, ENTENTE   **MAKES** 2 cocktails

Given the quantities of the rhubarb juice, black peppercorn simple syrup, and celery bubbles, you can easily make more than 2 cocktails (maximum of 8); just make sure to have enough alcohol and fresh lemons (½ large lemon per cocktail) on hand.

RHUBARB JUICE

Makes about 2⅓ cups

Note: The fresh rhubarb juice will need to be made at least 3 hours before you intend to make the cocktail. This recipe makes more rhubarb juice than you will need. Save the extra and enjoy as a refreshing drink or use to create more cocktails.

½ pound fresh rhubarb

2 cups water

BLACK PEPPERCORN SIMPLE SYRUP

Makes about 1½ cups

6 tablespoons coarsely cracked black peppercorns

1½ cups water

¾ cup sugar

CELERY JUICE

Makes 1½ cups

1 pound of celery, trimmed and cut into 1-inch pieces (about 4 cups)

¼ cup water

1. To make the rhubarb juice: Cut the rhubarb into 1-inch pieces. Bring the rhubarb and water to a boil in a medium saucepan over medium-high heat, about 7 minutes. Cover, then reduce the heat to a simmer, and cook until most of the pieces have fallen apart, about 15 minutes. Strain the rhubarb mixture through a cheesecloth-lined fine-mesh strainer into a clean container with a spout. When the fruit mash is cool enough to handle, gather the corners of the cheesecloth and gently squeeze out any excess juice into the container with the juice. After about 20 minutes, the juice will begin to separate. Decant the clear pink liquid into a clean container with a spout, discarding the sludge left behind. Refrigerate for at least 2 hours.

2. To make the black peppercorn simple syrup: Crush the peppercorns in a mortar and pestle and set aside. In a small saucepan, combine the water and sugar and bring to a boil over medium-high heat, whisking occasionally, until the sugar dissolves, about 5 minutes. Remove from the heat, then add the peppercorns and steep for 20 minutes. Strain the syrup through a cheesecloth-lined fine-mesh strainer, pressing on the peppercorns, into a clean container with a spout. When cool enough to handle, gather the corners of the cheesecloth and gently squeeze out any excess syrup into the container with the syrup. Cover and refrigerate until ready to use.

3. To make the celery juice: Place the celery and water in a blender and blend until smooth, about 3 minutes. Strain the celery mixture through a cheesecloth-lined fine-

CELERY BUBBLE MIXTURE

Makes 2 cups

Note: This recipe makes more bubbles than you will need for the cocktail. Save the leftovers and serve over seared scallops or prawns.

½ cup fresh organic celery juice, homemade (page 82) or store-bought

⅔ cup black peppercorn simple syrup

¼ cup water

¼ heaping teaspoon Versawhip

⅛ heaping teaspoon xanthan gum

COCKTAILS

1 ounce Cocchi Americano

1 ounce Hovding Aquavit

1 ounce Bol Genever or gin

½ ounce Strega liqueur

2½ ounces rhubarb juice

1½ ounces fresh lemon juice (or from 1 large lemon)

1 ounce black peppercorn simple syrup

2 eyedroppers Bittercube Bolivar Bitters

GARNISH

2 milligrams CBD tincture, preferably Hapi Innovations, divided

mesh strainer into a clean container with a spout, about 5 minutes. Gather the corners of the cheesecloth and gently squeeze out any excess juice into the container with the juice.

4. To make the celery bubble mixture: Set up the air pump for aquariums and clean plastic tubing according to the manufacturer's instructions. Set aside. Place the celery juice, black peppercorn simple syrup and water into a blender and blend on high for 20 seconds, then add the Versawhip and blend on high for 20 seconds. Add the xanthan gum and continue to blend on high until well combined, about 20 seconds. Set aside.

5. To make the cocktails: Combine Cocchi Americano, Hovding Aquavit, Bol Genever, Strega liqueur, rhubarb juice, lemon juice, black peppercorn simple syrup, and bitters in a shaker three-quarters filled with ice. Vigorously shake for about 30 seconds. Double strain into two coupe glasses. Set aside.

6. To make the celery bubbles: Pour half of the celery bubble mixture into a large bowl and aerate with the other end of aquarium pump by gently moving the end of the tubing around just below the surface of the liquid until enough bubbles form for the cocktails. Repeat with the remaining celery bubble mixture.

7. Carefully scoop some of the bubbles over the finished cocktails. Garnish with CBD tincture. Serve at once.

Recipe continues on next page

NOTE

In order to make the celery bubbles you will need an aquarium air pump and plastic tubing. Tetra Whisper Easy to Use Air Pump for Aquariums is a great inexpensive pump. Just remember to buy some standard airline tubing.

TIP

To ensure the success of the bubble making, it is necessary for the end of the tubing to be moving around continually and gently under the surface of the celery bubble mixture. If the hose stays in one place, the larger bubbles will not be made. The celery foam bubbles are very fragile and can pop easily. Make sure when transferring them to the cocktails that you scoop them up very delicately.

CRÉMANT DU JURA AND CBD FOAM

by BEAU KELLY-FONTANO, ENTENTE

MAKES 1 pint and 5 tablespoons

> **BEAU KELLY-FONTANO:** Crémant du Jura is the appellation for sparkling wines from the Jura region of France. The Crémant du Jura and CBD foam can be used to top a large assortment of cocktails. Some of my favorite uses for this recipe are a French 75, sidecar, and our house cocktail, "I Wish I Was a Little Bit Faller" (page 86).

1½ sheets of gelatin, cut or broken into 1-inch strips

¼ cup ice water, or just enough to cover gelatin strips

CRÉMANT DU JURA SYRUP

5 ounces simple syrup

15 ounces Crémant du Jura

⅛ teaspoon (1,000 milligrams) preferably Hapi Innovations CBD Isolate

1. Place the gelatin strips in a bowl, then place 3 ice cubes on top of them, then carefully pour the water over them. Note: The ice cubes will keep the strips from floating. Let stand at room temperature until they are soft, clear, and bloomed, about 8 minutes.

2. To make the Crémant du Jura syrup: While the gelatin is blooming, in a saucepan, bring the simple syrup to a simmer over medium heat. Slowly whisk in the Crémant du Jura.

3. Using your fingers or a small slotted spoon, carefully remove the gelatin and gently place them into the syrup. Once all the gelatin has been removed and transferred to the syrup, whisk until completely dissolved. Remove from the heat and let cool to room temperature, about 50 minutes. Once cooled to room temperature, whisk in the CBD Isolate.

4. Pour the syrup-gelatin liquid into a 1-pint or 1-quart whipping siphon with two N2O cartridges. Charge with one canister of nitrous oxide and shake 4 to 5 times for pint-size siphon or 10 times for quart-size siphon, or process according to manufacturer's instructions. Note: This recipe makes 1 pint, plus 5 tablespoons of syrup-gelatin liquid. If you decide to use a pint size whipping siphon, 5 tablespoons of the syrup-gelatin will need to be discarded, before added to the siphon.

5. Charge with the second cartridge of nitrous oxide and repeat once more. It is now ready to use. If not using right away, store your whipping siphon in the refrigerator to keep it cold. Note: The final product will be mildly structured but still foamy and creamy. Label, date, and store for up to 1 week in the refrigerator.

I WISH I WAS A LITTLE BIT FALLER

by BEAU KELLY-FONTANO, ENTENTE

MAKES 1 cocktail

1½ ounces cognac

½ ounce apricot liqueur

¼ ounce blackstrap rum

¾ ounce fresh lemon juice

¾ ounce peach syrup

1 eyedropper Bittercube Cherry Bark
   Vanilla Bitters

GARNISH

Freshly grated cinnamon

1. Combine all the ingredients in a shaker three-quarters filled with ice. Vigorously shake for about 30 seconds. Double strain into a coupe glass. Top cocktail with Crémant du Jura and CBD foam (page 85). Garnish with a light sprinkle of cinnamon.

TIP

To keep the foam from splashing, spray on a small dish first, then top the cocktail with it.

WEST

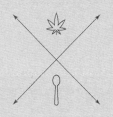

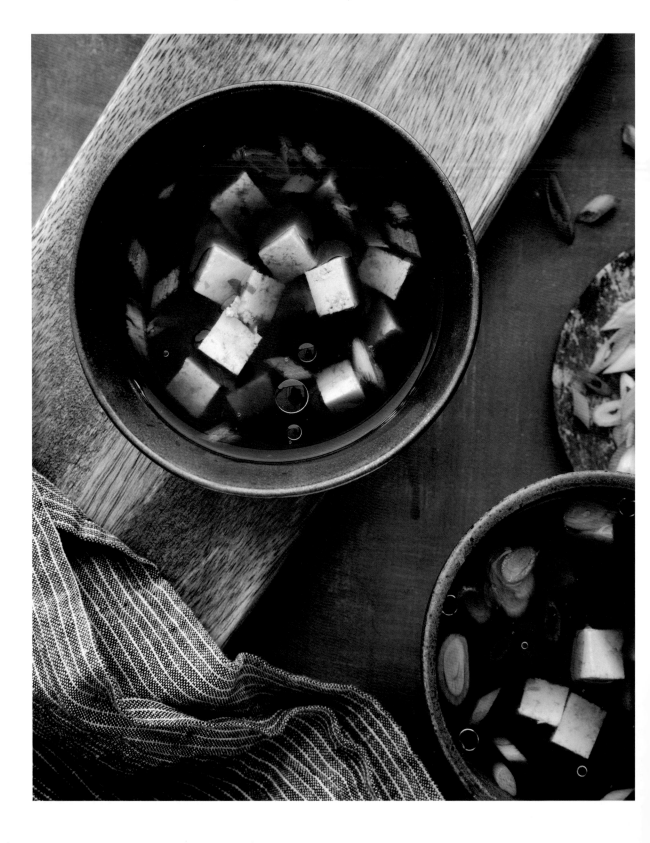

CBD-INFUSED VEGAN GLUTEN-FREE MISO BROTH

by JESSICA CATALANO

MAKES 5 cups; 4 servings (1¼ cups each)

JESSICA CATALANO: Miso soup is a lifesaver when it comes to colds during any season. It supplies your body with salt, protein, and essential nutrients. Miso is rich in B vitamins, vitamin K, vitamin E, and folic acid. And because it is fermented, it provides food that promotes the growth of good gut bacteria—something we all need! "Warm," "comfort," "savory," and "wholesome" are all thoughts that come to mind when I enjoy a nice bowl of homemade miso broth.

4 cups filtered water

1 sheet nori, cut into 1–1½-inch rectangles

4 tablespoons organic red miso paste

½ cup firm tofu, drained and cut into ¼-inch cubes

½ cup thinly sliced scallion rings, cut on the bias, white and green parts

2 tablespoons extra-virgin olive oil

100 milligrams full-spectrum CBD oil, preferably F L O R A + B A S T Age Adapting Sleep Tincture

1. To make the broth: Place 4 cups of filtered water into a 2-quart saucepan and bring to a simmer over medium-high heat. Add the nori and continue to simmer for 5 minutes.

2. While the nori is simmering, prepare the miso paste. Place the miso paste and ¼ cup of the simmering broth in a small bowl and whisk until the miso paste is completely dissolved and smooth. Set aside.

3. Add the tofu, scallions, and olive oil to the pot with the nori and maintain a simmer, and cook until tofu is heated through, about 2 minutes. Remove from heat and stir in the miso paste until well combined. Stir in the CBD tincture until well combined. Adjust seasonings with additional miso paste if desired. Divide between 4 soup bowls. Serve immediately.

JESSICA CATALANO'S NOTE

Miso can be found in the refrigerator section of some grocery stores and in Asian markets.

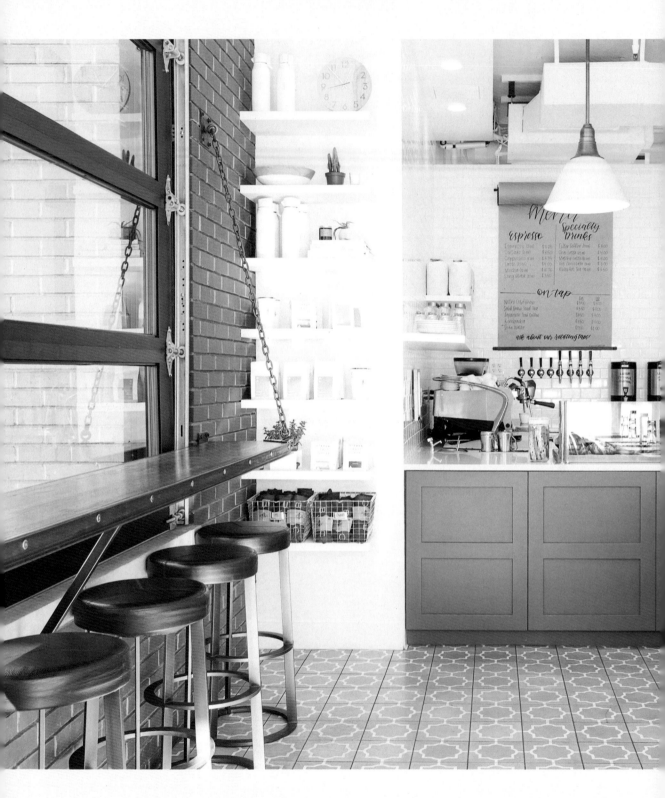

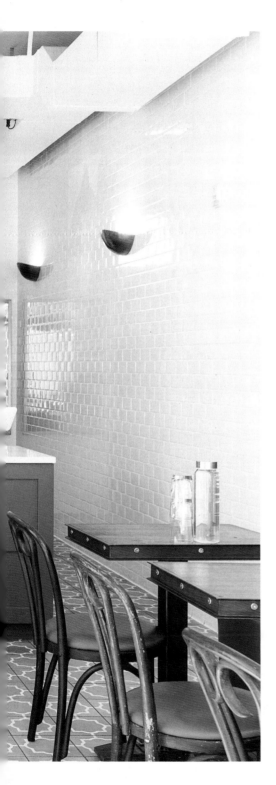

JEFFREY KNOTT

Owner, Blue Sparrow Coffee

Jeffrey Knott has traveled the world, eager to discover its hidden wonders. He lived in California, Pennsylvania, Japan, and New York before deciding that Denver was the perfect place to call home. For Knott, the city's biggest draw was its ideal balance of weather, people, culture, and food.

The New Mexico native developed a love of coffee during his college days. There was not a day that went by that he did not have a cup of his favorite brew. After graduation, his connection to the beverage remained so strong that he eventually decided to change careers, switching from the field of finance to that of coffee entrepreneur. Over time, Knott worked as a barista at a variety of coffee shops. Those that were in the formative stages frequently offered him an opportunity to help with their design. This experience proved invaluable when the time came to launch a business of his own.

Knott's dream became a reality when he opened Blue Sparrow Coffee in 2017. The shop is conveniently located in the Backyard Blake, a small collection of Denver businesses that surround a picturesque courtyard dotted with trees, grass, and fountains. The popular coffee shop is a welcome addition to the residential neighborhood. Blue Sparrow Coffee is the perfect name for the quaint 480-square-foot shop, which is minuscule, just like its tiny namesake. The interior's beautiful blue counters and high-backed banquette lend a cozy, European feel to the bright welcoming space. For those who enjoy a breath of fresh air, patrons may choose between the shop's relaxing outdoor patio, or peaceful rooftop area with its lovely view.

For Knott, quality is everything, from equipment to the coffee itself—only the best will do! Patrons are quick to notice that Blue Sparrow Coffee features roasters from around the world. Its owner loves to see how different roasters use contrasting methods to develop the same coffee. When traveling, Knott may explore as many as five coffee shops a day to sample their craft coffees. Every few weeks the Blue Sparrow introduces a new coffee roaster, always making sure that they have been carefully vetted.

The coffee aficionado came across Strava Craft Coffee during the period that he was preparing to open the Blue Sparrow. Knott had been sampling the same roasters for years, but this one completely blew him away. He quickly committed to carrying Strava's non-CBD coffee before being introduced to their CBD variety. To his delight, it was love at first sip. Blue Sparrow not only carries a highly curated selection of coffee, it is also one of Denver's only providers of ready-to-drink CBD coffee. The business always has Strava beans on its retail shelf alongside Nespresso pods, and K cups. They also always have CBD on tap in the form of a nitro iced coffee.

Among their other selections, the shop also serves hot teas, iced black tea on tap, organic matcha tea lattes, espresso, Japanese iced coffee, kombucha on tap, and house-made tea sodas. When Knott finds other topnotch roasters from around the world, he integrates and rotates them into the mix. To complement the shop's variety of beverages, Knott has partnered with popular local food producers to offer patrons a variety of delicious locally made bites. The owner of Blue Sparrow Coffee is dedicated to quality, sustainability, and community. His business is committed to the shop's neighbors and the people who live and work in the Denver area. A second location, Blue Sparrow Coffee Platte, which opened in 2020, offers the same unique menu. Not much bigger than the first shop, they too believe that less is more.

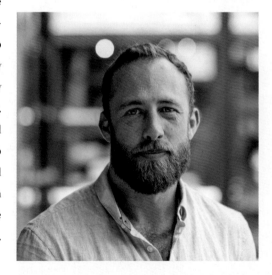

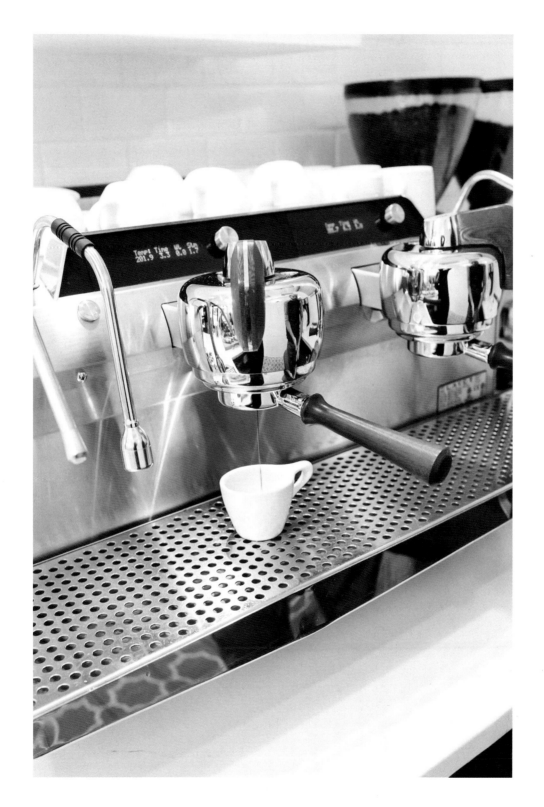

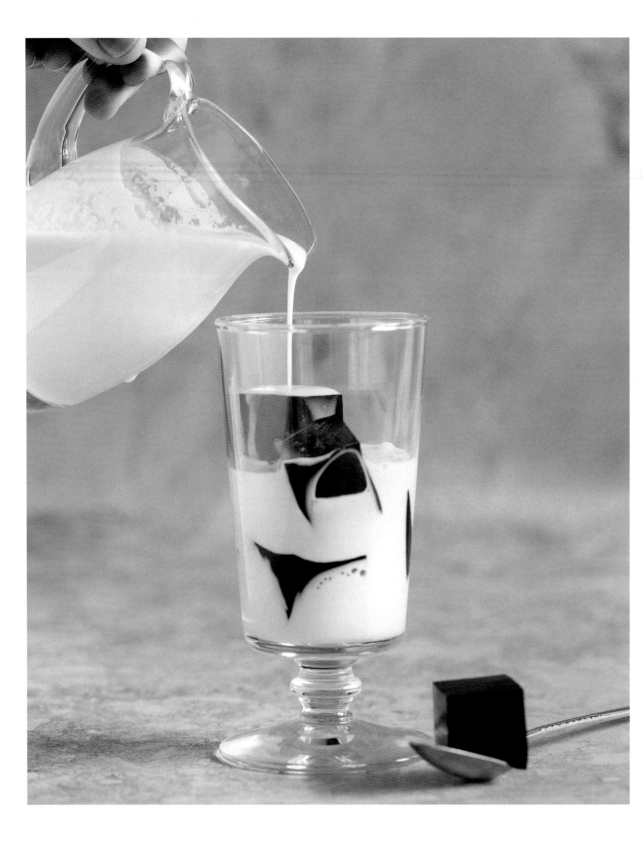

CBD-INFUSED COFFEE JELLY

JEFFRY KNOTT, BLUE SPARROW COFFEE

MAKES approximately 32 (1-inch square) cubes; 5 servings with 6 cubes in each glass

JEFFREY KNOTT: Living in Japan changed the way I think about food. I appreciate the desire to keep flavors true to their inherent nature—but I can also appreciate experiencing these flavors in wildly different ways by playing with texture and color. Simple flavors, wild textures! This minimal treat is a great example. Flavors we all *think* we know, morphed into an entirely new experience. I highly recommend the "Black" variant of this recipe to really elevate this drink.

COFFEE JELLY

2 cups plus 1 ounce freshly brewed hot CBD-infused coffee, dark roast, preferably Strava Craft Coffee

⅓ cup (75 grams) sugar

15 grams (about 1 heaping tablespoon) powdered unflavored gelatin (2 gelatin envelopes; Knox brand)

3 tablespoons cool filtered water

SWEET MILK

Makes 1 quart

1 cup heavy cream

1 (14-ounce) can sweetened condensed milk

1 (12-ounce) can evaporated milk

1. In a small saucepan, combine the 2 cups of coffee and sugar and bring to a boil, stirring occasionally, over medium heat, about 6 minutes. Remove from the stove top and set aside.

2. In a small bowl, combine the gelatin and water. Let stand at room temperature until bloomed, less than 1 minute, then quickly but gently stir into the coffee, until completely dissolved and smooth.

3. Pour into an 8x4-inch loaf pan. Note: If you don't own a loaf pan, make sure to use a pan that can hold 2 cups of liquid so that the coffee is only 1 inch deep. Allow the coffee to cool to room temperature, about 25 minutes, then transfer to the refrigerator and chill until very firm, about 2 hours.

4. As the coffee gelatin is firming up in the refrigerator, make the sweet milk. In a clean container with a pour spout, whisk together the remaining 1 ounce coffee, cream, and milks, then chill in the refrigerator for 1 hour.

5. To serve: Cut the coffee jelly into 1-inch cubes and spoon 6 cubes into each glass. Pour ¾ cup of sweet milk into each glass, over the cubes, or to taste. Serve immediately with bubble tea straws and spoons.

Recipe continues on next page

VARIATION

Refrigerate 1 ounce of the coffee until ready to use. Whisk in 1 gram (1 teaspoon) activated charcoal powder with the remaining 2 cups of hot coffee until completely dissolved, about 1 minute. Let sit at room temperature for 10 minutes. Strain through an ultra-fine mesh coffee strainer or coffee filter, into a clean container, to remove the charcoal sediments. Once the charcoal sediments have been removed, then proceed to Step 1 in recipe.

KOREAN-STYLE CBD-INFUSED SHORT RIBS

by JEFFREY KNOTT, BLUE SPARROW COFFEE   **MAKES** 4 servings; 2 short ribs per person

JEFFREY KNOTT: I don't often eat meat, but when I do it's all about the meat-to-flavor ratio—the more flavor per ounce of meat the better. I'd take a pepperoni pizza over a ribeye steak any day. I think Korean-style short ribs just might be the flavor-to-meat champ! While everyone's paying premiums for Wagyu and Angus, skip the premium price, and go straight to premium flavor. Take your time choosing your ribs carefully, look for the ones with very fine lines of fat, and lots of them! Think a delicate densely woven spider web. Your patience and diligence will be rewarded.

MARINADE

1 cup brown sugar, packed

½ cup hot CBD-infused coffee, dark roast, preferably Strava Craft Coffee

½ cup reduced-sodium soy sauce

¼ cup mirin (Japanese rice wine)

4 medium cloves garlic, minced

SHORT RIBS

8 Korean-style beef short ribs (2½ pounds)

Oil, as needed for grill grates

GARNISHES

3 to 4 scallions, trimmed, thinly sliced on the bias into rings, white and green parts

1½ tablespoons organic sesame seeds, white

Steamed rice, optional

1. To make the marinade: In a medium bowl, combine the sugar, coffee, soy sauce, mirin, and garlic, whisking until the sugar dissolves.

2. Rinse the short ribs under cold running water to remove any bone fragments, then pat dry with paper towels. Transfer the short ribs to an extra-large ziplock plastic bag, then add the marinade. Refrigerate for 24 hours, occasionally turning the bag.

3. To make the sauce: Remove the ribs from the marinade and transfer them to a plate. Set aside. Pour all of the marinade into a small saucepan and bring to a simmer, whisking often, over medium-low heat, until the sauce becomes syrupy and coats the back of a spoon, about 40 minutes.

4. While the sauce is simmering, preheat the grill to medium-high heat and generously brush the cooking grates with oil.

5. To make the short ribs: Grill the short ribs on one side until nicely browned but still tender, about 3 minutes. Using grilling tongs, carefully flip the short ribs over and cook for another 3 minutes, or until desired doneness is achieved.

Recipe continues on page 99

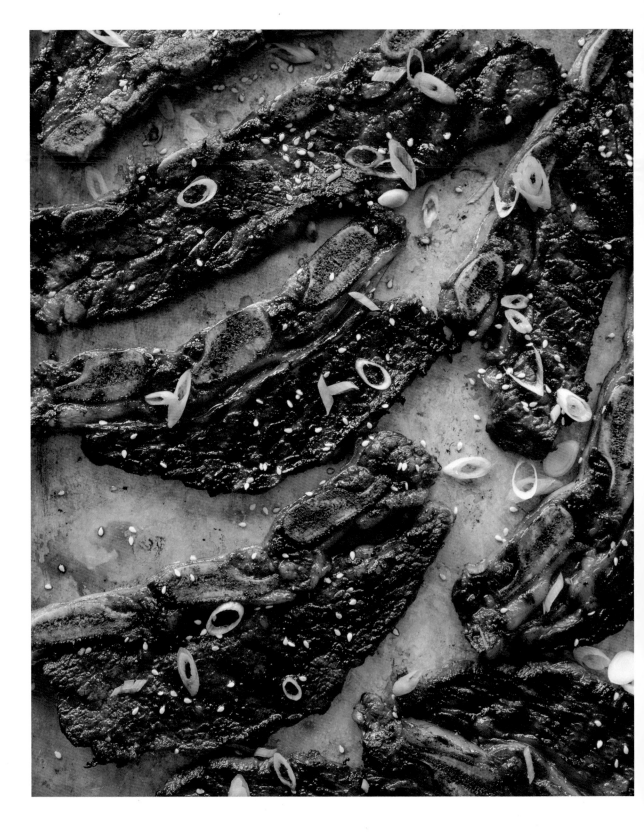

6. To serve: Arrange the short ribs on a platter and drizzle some of the sauce over and around the meat. Scatter the scallion rings and sesame seeds over the short ribs. Serve, passing the remaining sauce at the table along with steamed rice on the side, if desired.

N O T E

Korean-style short ribs (also referred to as "flanken-style") can be found at most Asian markets.

"TURKISH-STYLE" CBD-INFUSED COFFEE MOUSSE

by JEFFREY KNOTT, BLUE SPARROW COFFEE   **MAKES** 6 servings; about 1 cup each

> JEFFREY KNOTT: Chocolate mousse has been a staple dessert in my home for as long as I can remember. Few desserts feel so luxurious, yet are so easy to make! Layering the dark chocolate, coffee, cardamom, and orange takes an already luxurious dessert and adds an unbeatable level of sophistication. These flavors always bring me right back to my time traveling throughout the Middle East—I hope to share a bit of that feeling with you the second your spoon plunges into this silky, smooth treat.

2 heaping tablespoons CBD-infused coffee beans, dark roast, preferably Strava Craft Coffee (see Note on page 101), ground into a fine powder

2 green cardamom pods, husks on, ground finely (see Note on page 101)

3 ounces water

1¾ cups heavy cream, very cold

5 ounces good-quality dark chocolate (60 to 72% cacao), roughly chopped

1 ounce orange liqueur, such Cointreau or Grand Marnier

3 large organic egg whites, room temperature, reserving the egg yolks for another use

2 tablespoons sugar

GARNISHES

Sweetened whipped cream

Good-quality bittersweet chocolate (60 to 72% cacao), shaved

1. To make the coffee: Place the coffee, ground cardamom, and 3 ounces of cold filtered water into a small saucepan and bring to a simmer, over medium-low heat, about 5 minutes. Remove from the heat and allow the cardamom to steep in the coffee for 1 hour. Pour the coffee through a fine-mesh strainer, into a clean container with a pour spout, allowing any excess liquid to drip into the container with the strained coffee for about 15 minutes. Discard or compost the coffee grounds.

2. While the coffee is straining, make the whipped cream: Pour the cream into a well-chilled bowl. Using an electric hand mixer, on medium speed, beat the heavy cream until soft peaks form, about 4 minutes. Cover with plastic wrap and refrigerate until ready to use.

3. To make the chocolate mousse: Place the chocolate into the top pan of a double boiler. Pour about 1 inch of the water into the bottom pan and bring to a simmer. Place the top pan with the chocolate on top, making sure the bowl does not touch the simmering water. When half of the chocolate is melted, gently stir until the chocolate has fully melted, about 5 minutes. Turn off the heat and whisk in the coffee and orange liqueur until smooth. Let sit, whisking occasionally.

4. While the chocolate mixture is sitting, start the egg whites. Using an electric hand mixer, beat the egg whites, on medium speed, in a medium bowl until frothy. Increase the mixer speed to high, then add the sugar in a slow and

steady stream, and continue whipping until stiff peaks form, about 4 minutes.

5. Remove the chocolate mixture from the stove top and fold in the egg whites until well combined, then fold in the whipped cream until almost combined.

6. Spoon the mousse into mason jars or white china ramekins and refrigerate until set, about 1 hour. Let sit at room temperature for 10 minutes before serving.

7. Garnish with a dollop of whipped cream and sprinkles of chocolate shavings.

NOTES

For an elegant look, spoon the mousse into wine glasses or brandy snifters for a fancier presentation.

Add the cardamom pods to the coffee beans before grinding, then proceed to Step 1 in the recipe.

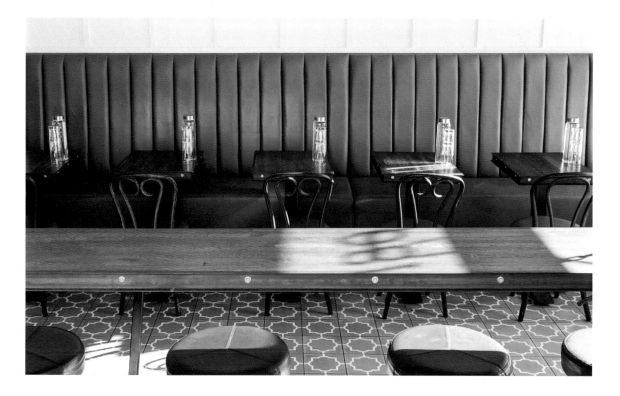

NATHAN HOWARD & AARON HOWARD

Cofounders, East Fork Cultivars

A t the age of seventeen, Aaron Howard took a class to learn how to grow canna-bis, hoping to help his older brother, Wesley, who was suffering from a variety of serious medical issues. As time went on, Aaron and his other brother, Nathan, had one goal in mind: to grow a superior plant-based medicine that would relieve some of Wesley's suffering. The typical THC-dominant cannabis varieties did help their brother but unfortunately were not a complete fit for his medical needs. In 2014–2015, the brothers grew twelve CBD-rich cultivar plants in a blackberry patch near Aaron's cabin in Takilma, Oregon. The positive impact that some of these cultivars had on Wesley's symptoms gave the brothers reason to consider expanding beyond their personal cultivation so that they could provide all Oregonians with the same access to CBD and cannabis therapeutics.

When the acreage next to Aaron's property went up for sale, the brothers were able to pur-chase the East Fork Ranch with the support of friends, family, and community. Mason Walker came onboard as a co-owner and CEO in March 2017, lending his expertise to the workings of the company. A graduate of Portland State University's School of Business, he had worked for seven years for the *Portland Business Journal* before joining the team at East Fork Cultivars. His years in the field of journalism gave him the expertise for disseminating information in a knowledgeable and understandable fashion, a decided advantage for his new position.

Originally a llama ranch, the East Fork property took its name from its location near the East Fork of the Illinois River. Aaron and Nathan retained the property's original name, clev-erly creating a llama logo to signify the history of the place. The property is comprised of thirty-four beautiful acres in the small town of Takilma in the Illinois River Valley of southern Oregon. Located between the sparkling waters of the East Fork of the Illinois River and the Siskiyou Wilderness, the region is one of the world's best environments for cultivating sun-grown cannabis, the perfect spot for the Howards' new company, East Fork Cultivars.

The Oregon adult-use cannabis market has allowed the organic production farm to breed cultivars rich in both CBD and THC. With the growing of craft hemp, the farm is expanding their mission beyond Oregon's state boundaries. It is important to note that hemp can be sold nationally, whereas cannabis can only be legally sold statewide. By offering hemp products nationwide, it furthers the farm's mission to increase everyone's access to superior plant therapeutics.

Because of their cultivation of craft hemp, East Fork Cultivar received USDA organic certification in 2018. This designation is not available for cannabis because the federal government has declared it illegal. East Fork is one of the first hemp farms in the United States to receive this special distinction. It was one of only seven farms to be awarded 100 percent organic certification and the first to be given 100 percent organic certification for their clones, seeds, and flower. USDA organic operations are closely monitored and must demonstrate that they are protecting natural resources, conserving biodiversity, and using only approved substances.

Organic and regenerative cultivation is of the utmost importance because all cannabis plants are bio-accumulators. If the soil they are grown in has any toxins, these contaminants are pulled into the plant, passed through in the CBD extraction and into the final product. By choosing products using cannabis or craft hemp, the risk of being exposed to these contaminants is lowered. Craft cannabis signifies a product made with an artisanal approach. Even though it is still grown on a commercial level, craft cannabis is produced on a smaller scale with a focus on creating the highest-quality product, which generally involves more labor-intensive and costly methods.

At East Fork Cultivars, they strive to be stewards of the native soil by using less-invasive forms of tilling. Soil building consists of cover crops to nourish the soil. Cover seed is applied in the fall, before and during the harvest of the cannabis crop. These "fix" nutrients, improve soil structure, prevent erosion, and provide the soil with biodiversity that offers protection during the long cold winter. The owners of East Fork Cultivars believe that by choosing to grow in their native soil, they reduce their impact on the environment and deepen the connection with place, which helps to create chemically complex cultivars. Experience has taught them that growing in the native soil of the Illinois River Valley allows a unique expression of terroir in their cannabis.

Because the folks at East Fork Cultivars are passionate about what they do, partnering with dedicated, talented product makers who will turn their cannabis flower into high-quality, exciting products is of foremost importance. House of Spain EVOO, Grön Chocolate, Empower BodyCare, and Gaia Herbs are a few of the outstanding companies that work closely with East Fork, collaborating on educational efforts while promoting each other's products.

At East Fork Cultivars, there is an unwavering commitment to environmental responsibility, science-based education, and social justice. The company's statewide educational program is managed by Anna Symonds, who joined the East Fork team in July 2017. She was placed in charge of developing an educational program directed at dispensaries to better inform them about CBD. The hour-long presentation, called "CBD Certified," is offered free of charge to any licensed dispensary in Oregon to make it as easy as possible to access information that will enable participants to understand CBD more fully.

Symonds has given more than 100 presentations to dispensaries, more than thirty to processors, and more than twenty to the general public. Providing the program for free is an investment on East Fork's part, but it is something they strongly believe in. Realizing that many people use cannabis as medicine, the folks at East Fork Cultivars want to give them the informational resources they need to take care of themselves. For the business, the guiding principle is about the value being created and provided; the reward is in the feeling that what they do every day is making a positive difference in someone's life.

PETER GILLIES & AMANDA GILLIES

Co-owners, House of Spain EVOO

Together, Peter and Amanda Gillies have a combined background of forty years' experience working in the food and service industry. Wanting to try another line of work, the couple weighed the pros and cons of starting their own business. During this challenging time, it was Amanda's father who suggested that they consider the idea of importing olive oil. Her dad had emigrated to the United States from Spain at age twenty-eight and started his own furniture business. The furniture that he sold was imported from Spain, which gave him connections to sources, suppliers, and mills throughout that country. For a short while, he had tried his hand at the olive oil business, but soon realized that without prior experience in the area of food production, it would not be prudent to pursue such a project.

Because of their professional backgrounds and close family connections in Spain, Amanda and Peter thought that the olive oil suggestion had exciting possibilities. After much investigating and preparation, they decided to take a leap of faith and imported their first half pallet of olive oil in 2017. Coincidentally, the couple were also using CBD during this time with positive results. The Gillies knew that CBD required a lipid (fat) to bind to in order to make it bioavailable (the percentage that is absorbed into the bloodstream), giving them cause to experience an *aha* moment. They began researching the effects of combining CBD and olive oil, which is largely composed of fatty acids, and were delighted to find that not only could the two be blended, but olive oil was the ideal carrier for CBD. Now their mission was to personally seek out and source the best olive oil that Spain had to offer. They knew that they had created a dynamic duo.

Looking for an opportunity to showcase their product, the couple signed up for a food service show. They did not have a website, Facebook page, or even a name for their new venture. In order to be part of the show, it was required that they be a registered company with a business name; thankfully, Amanda's father generously gave them permission to use his—"House of Spain." When the show was over, Peter and Amanda were inundated with inquires and requests for more product information, which made changing the company's borrowed name seem like a rash decision. To remedy the situation, the two entrepreneurs added EVOO (extra-virgin olive oil) to the tail end of the designated name and prepared to launch their new CBD-infused line of products.

House of Spain EVOO is based in Portland, Oregon. The company produces high-quality CBD-infused extra-virgin olive oil as well as lifestyle and wellness products. The Gillies have personally researched each of the Spanish olive oil producers that they utilize, seeking to ensure premium quality source and product. The company uses only the finest Oregon-grown, USDA-certified organic hemp-derived CBD. They have partnered with East Fork Cultivars, the mission, ethics, and values of which align with Peter and Amanda's philosophy. In addition to East Fork, the Gillies also have relationships with other farms in Oregon and Washington that practice organic farming techniques.

The owners of House of Spain EVOO are working to become a nationally recognized brand that is known for health, quality, and superior service. They source locally—from bottles to labels, boxes, and equipment. Their mission includes supporting those folks that make what they do possible. Peter and Amanda Gillies have a team of six, in addition to a group of advisers and consultants who have worked tirelessly to make the business the success that it is. Together, they strive to promote CBD awareness and move the industry forward, dedicated to "weaving health into the fabric of people's lives."

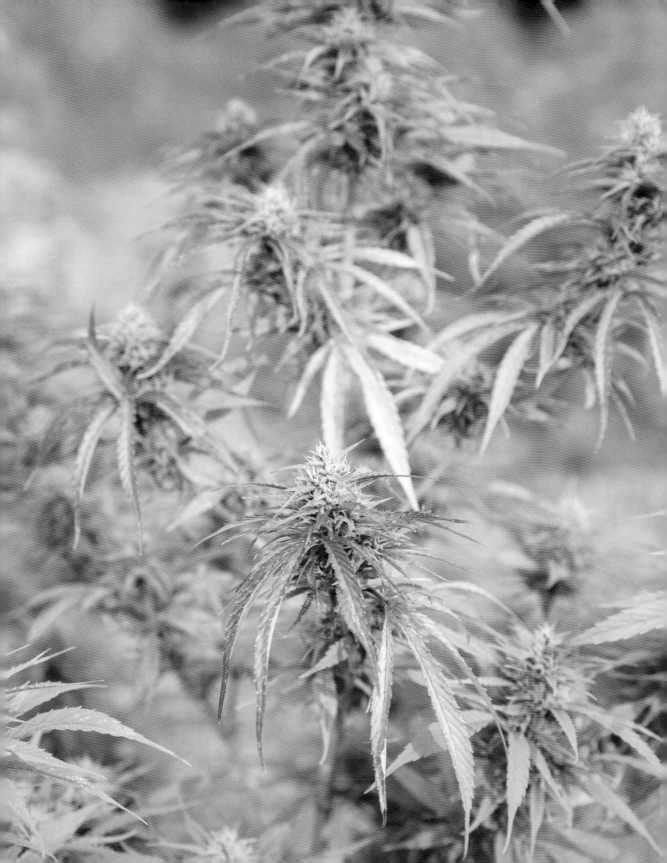

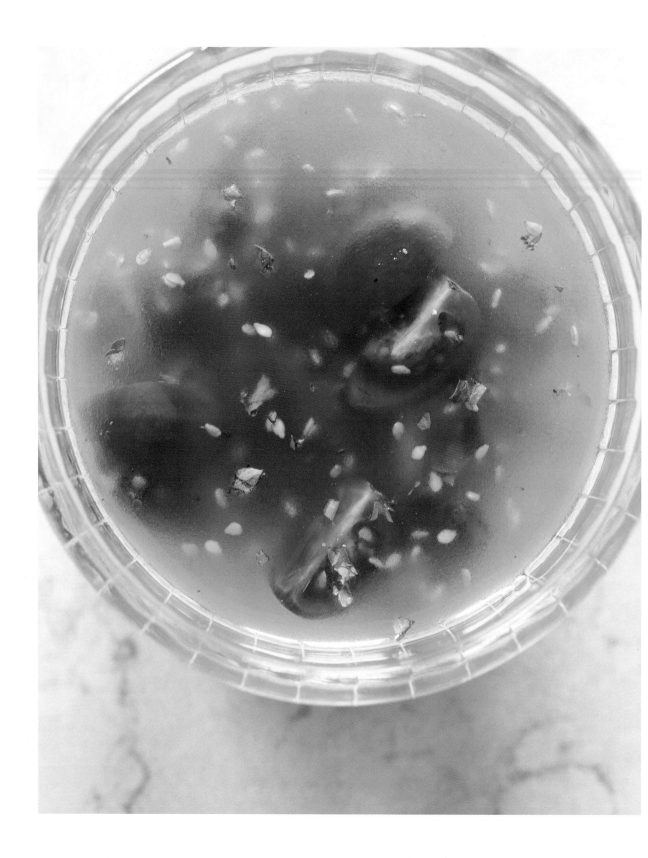

CBD-INFUSED HONEY APPLE CIDER VINAIGRETTE

by HOUSE OF SPAIN EVOO IN COLLABORATION WITH EAST FORK CULTIVARS

MAKES ⅔ CUP

Not just for salads—drizzle this vibrant vinaigrette over asparagus, roasted potatoes, green beans, or the Flat Iron Steak & Grilled Stone Fruit Salad (page 45).

VINAIGRETTE

½ teaspoon sesame seeds

3 tablespoons apple cider vinegar, preferably FIRE BREW apple cider vinegar citrus

2 tablespoons honey, preferably The Queen's Bounty Raw Blackberry Honey

1 tablespoon minced parsley

½ teaspoon chopped oregano

½ teaspoon fine-grain sea salt, or to taste

½ teaspoon freshly ground black pepper, or to taste

½ cup House of Spain CBD-infused EVOO Original Blend

6 quartered cherry tomatoes

1. To toast the sesame seeds: Place the sesame seeds in a small dry skillet, and toast, over medium heat, shaking and stirring continuously, until they start to get fragrant, about 3 minutes. Remove from heat and set aside.

2. In a small bowl, combine the sesame seeds, vinegar, honey, parsley, oregano, salt, and pepper. In a steady stream, whisk in the olive oil until the vinaigrette is emulsified. Adjust seasonings with salt and pepper to taste. Set aside.

3. Add the tomatoes to the vinaigrette 15 minutes before you intend to use.

4. Serve with the Flat Iron Steak & Grilled Stone Fruit Salad (page 45).

CBD-INFUSED OLIVE OIL BITTERSWEET CHOCOLATE MOUSSE

by HOUSE OF SPAIN EVOO IN COLLABORATION WITH EAST FORK CULTIVARS

MAKES 6 servings;
about ½ cup each

This recipe is a great alternative for people who are lactose intolerant looking for dairy-free dessert options—just remember to omit the dollop of whipped cream. The olive oil adds a decadent richness to the mousse.

6 ounces good-quality bittersweet chocolate (60–72% cacao), roughly chopped

1 vanilla bean

⅓ cup CBD-infused extra-virgin olive oil, preferably House of Spain EVOO

4 large organic eggs, separated, at room temperature

¼ cup plus 1 tablespoon confectioners' sugar, divided

¹⁄₁₆ teaspoon (a pinch) plus ¼ teaspoon kosher salt, divided

GARNISHES
Sweetened whipped cream

Orange zest

1. Place the chopped chocolate into the top pan of a double boiler. Set aside.
2. Pour about 1 inch of water into the bottom pan and bring to a simmer. Place the top pan with the chocolate on top, making sure the bowl does not touch the simmering water. When half of the chocolate is melted, gently stir until the chocolate has fully melted, about 5 minutes. Remove from the heat and let sit, whisking occasionally, for 10 minutes.
3. Place the vanilla bean on a work surface and split it in half lengthwise using a paring knife. Scrape the seeds into the bowl with the chocolate. Whisk in the olive oil until well combined. Set aside, stirring occasionally.
4. While the chocolate mixture is cooling, start the egg white peaks. Using a stand mixer, beat the egg whites with 1 tablespoon of confectioners' sugar and ¹⁄₁₆ teaspoon of salt, on medium speed, until stiff peaks form, about 4 minutes.
5. In a separate large bowl, beat the egg yolks with the remaining ¼ cup of sugar and the remaining ¼ teaspoon of salt until pale yellow.
6. In a slow and steady stream, fold the chocolate-oil mixture into the yolk mixture, until completely combined and slightly thickened.
7. Fold the egg whites into the yolk mixture in 3 additions, until mousse is streak-free.
8. Divide the mousse between six 4-ounce ramekins or jelly jars. Cover with plastic wrap and refrigerate until the mousse is set, about 30 minutes. Remove the mousse from the refrigerator and let sit at room temperature for 15 minutes before serving.
9. Garnish with a dollop of whipped cream and orange zest.

DAVE WHITTON

Co-owner, Prank Bar

From the get-go, the owners of Prank Bar had a vision for their new Los Angeles establishment. The business's ideal location set the stage for its unique walk-up bar concept. Situated on a corner, the building's floor-to-ceiling retractable glass doors allow visitors to easily access Prank from the street. The stylish two-story design accommodates seating for up to two hundred people, offering a quieter second floor for those who desire a more intimate dining experience. There is even a dog-friendly patio for guests who do not want to leave the family pet at home. Co-owner Dave Whitton and partners have worked hard to make Prank a casual, comfortable place that folks love to visit. Dave has been in the cocktail industry for over eighteen years. His cocktails are made with non-GMO, organic, and locally sourced ingredients. Along with craft choices, the bar is also known for its inventive terpene cocktails. Terpenes are compounds found in the essential oil from cannabis plants. They give these cocktails the anti-inflammatory and other medicinal properties of cannabis without any psychotropic effects. Whitton stresses that Prank uses only high-quality terpenes purchased from US vendors and approved by the USDA. They must be naturally and organically extracted using CO_2 without chemical processing.

To ensure that this is done properly, the owners have a team of physicians and scientists from their partners at BotanaVista, located in Hollywood, California, and Nevada Botanical Science in Reno, Nevada who advise them on sourcing. They are experts in medicine as well as cannabis extractions and have been treating patients using medical cannabis, including terpenes, since 2014. The priority at Prank is always safety and quality. They want folks to know that terpenes do not have a psychotropic effect like THC does and will *not* get you high.

Prank's chef, Ricardo Sanchez, takes a healthy approach when creating the menu, working with local farmers who value the high quality of the food they produce. His dishes are prepared using organic ingredients, and he offers vegan, vegetarian, gluten-free, and hormone- and antibiotic-free options. Burgers and sandwiches are always very popular menu choices. The busy chef's philosophy is not only to create dishes that please, but to do so in an exciting and innovative way. The result is a healthy non-GMO, hormone- and antibiotic-free menu of delicious bar food.

What's with the unusual name? Prank Bar owner, Dave Whitton, recounts the story of how, "My sister Jamie 'tricked' my grandfather into eating healthy by having him turn his entire backyard into a non-GMO, organic soil and hydroponic garden. He started making everything from scratch, creating healthy meals using the fruits of his labor. She had to trick him to eat the 'whole' foods he needed, much like you would do with a two-year-old. Miraculously, he started to feel better!" At Prank Bar, the goal is to also have guests eat healthy. "Our 'Prank' is for you to eat well without knowing it," says Dave with a smile in his voice.

TERPENES
PRANK BAR

Dave Whitton: Terpenes in pure concentrated form are very powerful. Each terpene has a specific health benefit such as anti-inflammatory, bronchodilator, memory enhancer, etc. It is important to know the effects of each as well as the ratios when combining for desired outcome. We call this the "entourage effect," and it is important because terpenes have an effect on each other; for example, some terpenes assist each other and intensify effect, while others work against each other and counteract desired effects.

Terpenes are responsible for the taste and smell of the plant, as well as protecting it from predators and attracting pollinators. In natural form they are potent, so when we concentrate them they become *extremely* potent, which makes them challenging to incorporate into recipes. They easily overpower other ingredients and flavors and can ruin your food or drink in an instant. We pair our terpene doctors with our chefs, confectioners, and bartenders to ensure the perfect flavor and health benefit in every drink, dish, and chocolate. We let our doctors be doctors and our bartenders be bartenders because we feel that when you let the experts combine their knowledge in collaboration, you come up with a perfect product.

REBELLIOUS

by DAVE WHITTON, PRANK BAR **MAKES** 1 (approximately 7.5-ounce) drink

DAVE WHITTON: If you decide you'd like your anti-inflammatory spiked, our spirit of choice is a blanco tequila, which is the only stimulant in the alcohol family and makes for a fun and skinny night.

2 ounces blanco tequila

1 ounce fresh pineapple juice

¾ ounce ginger syrup

2 drops limonene terpenes

2 dashes ANGOSTURA aromatic bitters

4 ounces sparkling water, or to taste

Cayenne pepper

1. Combine the tequila, pineapple juice, ginger syrup, terpenes, and bitters in a shaker three-quarters filled with ice. Vigorously shake for about 30 seconds. Strain into a tumbler and top with sparkling water. Garnish with a pinch of cayenne pepper. Serve at once.

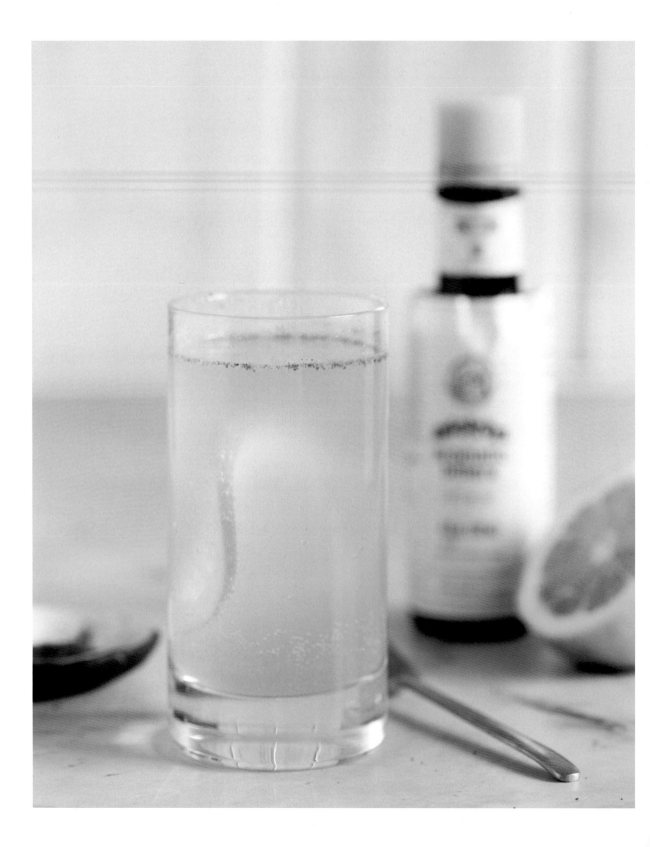

ANTI-INFLAMMATORY COCKTAIL

DAVE WHITTON, PRANK BAR

MAKES 1 drink

DAVE WHITTON: The anti-inflammatory mocktail is a delicious drink of refreshment. Each ingredient was carefully selected not only for its flavor but to combat everyone's hated nemesis . . . bloating. The pineapple juice is a diuretic, and the ginger root, cayenne, and bitters help with your metabolism, digestion, and stomach issues. The terpenes help to boost mood and energy and to reduce inflammation.

2 ounces fresh pineapple juice

¾ ounce simple ginger syrup (recipe below)

¾ ounce fresh lemon juice

2 drops limonene terpenes

2 dashes ANGOSTURA aromatic bitters

6 ounces sparkling water, or to taste

Cayenne pepper

Lemon slice, for garnish, optional

1. Combine the pineapple juice, ginger syrup, lemon juice, terpenes, and bitters in a shaker three-quarters filled with ice. Vigorously shake for about 30 seconds. Strain into a Collins glass. Top with sparkling water and garnish with a pinch of cayenne pepper and lemon slice. Serve at once.

SIMPLE GINGER SYRUP

MAKES 2 cups

2 cups water

1 cup raw organic sugar

4-inch piece fresh ginger, cut crosswise into thin coins

1. Bring the water, sugar, and ginger to a boil in a medium saucepan over medium heat, stirring occasionally until the sugar has dissolved. Remove from heat, and allow the ginger to steep for 40 minutes. Strain the syrup through a fine-mesh strainer, into a clean airtight container, discarding or composting the solids. Refrigerate for up to 7 days.

Aromas, Flavors, and Therapeutic Effects

Myrcene (MUR-seen)
The most common terpene in modern commercial cannabis.

Aromas/flavors include: cardamom, cloves, earthy musk, upturned soil, herbal, and
  ripe fruit
Potential therapeutic value: Antioxidant, highly relaxing, and fights inflammation
Also found in: thyme, mango, hops, and lemongrass
Cannabis strains rich in myrcene include: Bubba Kush and Harlequin

Limonene (LIM-o-neen)
Third most common terpene in cannabis. Limonene helps improve the absorption
  of other terpenes.

Aromas/Flavors include: citrus, peppermint, and juniper
Potential therapeutic value: anticancer effects, antidepressant, and alleviating the
  effects of gastric disorders
Also found in: most citrus fruits, rosemary, juniper, and peppermint
Cannabis strains rich in limonene include: Berry White and Banana OG

Caryophyllene (carry-OFF-uh-leen)
This terpene is known for its spiciness.

Aromas/Flavors: spicy, peppery, woody flavor, and oregano
Potential therapeutic value: brain health as well as anti-inflammatory effects
Also found in: black pepper, cloves, cinnamon, echinacea, and Thai basil
Cannabis strains rich in caryophyllene include: The Mint Girl Scout Cookies and
  Platinum OG

Pinene (PIE-neen)
One of the most researched terpenes.

Aromas/Flavors: pine and rosemary
Potential therapeutic value: Promotes mental focus and energy, anti-
  inflammatory, and antibacterial

Also found in: pine needles, rosemary, basil, parsley, dill, and hops
Cannabis strains high in pinene include: Blue Dream and Island Sweet Skunk

Humulene (HYOO-my-leen)
Aromas/Flavors: hops, wood, earthy with spicy herbal notes
Potential therapeutic value: anti-inflammatory, antibacterial, pain reliever, and
    appetite suppressant
Also found in: hops, coriander, cloves, and basil
Cannabis strains high in humulene include: White Walker and Sour Diesel

L'AVVENTURA

by MICHAEL VERBOS, PRANK BAR

MAKES 1 drink

> **MICHAEL VERBOS:** A beautiful nectar-forward cocktail with a light dried fruit Aperitivo Aplomado and a spice-forward Deleon Reposado Tequila. Add in terpenes to push forward the citrus and vibrance along with their mood-lifting and energy-boosting properties. We garnish it with raspberries to bring a balance for a tart finish.

APRICOT SYRUP

¼ cup fresh apricot juice

¼ cup organic cane sugar

1¾ ounces tequila, preferably Deleon Reposado Tequila

¾ ounce fresh lemon juice

¾ ounce apricot syrup

¾ ounce Amaro, preferably Falcon Spirits Distillery Aperitivo Aplomado

1 drop of limonene terpene

2 raspberries, for garnish

1. To make the apricot syrup: Pour the juice and the sugar into a small saucepan. Heat the ingredients over medium heat, whisking occasionally, until the sugar has dissolved, about 8 minutes. Remove from the heat and allow to cool completely. Carefully pour the syrup into an airtight container and store in the refrigerator until ready to use.

2. Combine the tequila, lemon juice, apricot syrup, Amaro, and terpene in a shaker three-quarters filled with ice. Vigorously shake for 30 seconds. Strain into a coupe glass. Thread the raspberries through a bamboo knot skewer and lay them across the rim of the glass. Serve at once.

NOTE

The apricot syrup will keep for up to 1 week in the refrigerator.

AMARO

Amaro, the Italian word for "bitter," is an herbal liqueur with a bittersweet taste. Italy's signature liqueur is made by infusing grape brandy with a proprietary blend of herbs and aromatics, then sweetened and aged in casks or bottles. The spirit is intended to stimulate the stomach and aid in digestion either before or after a meal.

CLAIRE GUILBERT & MASHA ITKIN

Co-owners, Tasty High Chef

When Claire Guilbert's next-door neighbor, Masha Itkin, dropped by one day to admire her well-maintained garden, neither of the women realized that this visit would mark the beginning of a new chapter in both of their lives. During their time together, the two women began talking about cannabis and its many uses, which gave Claire the idea of adding CBD to the cream used for coffee. That one idea and visit led to many more brainstorming sessions. Before too long, Claire's knowledge of science, coupled with Masha's talent for food and event planning, resulted in the creation of an innovative new cannabis catering company called "Tasty High Chef." The business is located in La Jolla, California. The two personal chef caterers chose the company's unusual name to reflect what they are all about, as well as what they use in their food preparation, highlighted by a short abbreviation that is easy to remember: THC.

Claire is a San Diego native, born in La Jolla, and has once again settled there to raise her family. In her former job, she conducted addiction research, developing a passion for weaning people off addictive opioids. Masha is a personal chef and event planner. She and her family immigrated to the United States from St. Petersburg, Russia when she was nine years old. It did not take long for the young girl to fall in love with San Diego's farm-fresh produce and diverse variety of foods.

Both women were drawn to cannabis-infused cooking, fascinated by all the possibilities and profiles that cannabis legalization brought to the culinary world. They believe in eating for health, letting each ingredient have a stage. The mantra at Tasty High Chef is, "Let food be thy medicine." Claire and Masha believe that food is better when infused, finding that cannabis adds fantastic flavors and mouthwatering aromas to dishes.

Making sure that the dosing of CBD is accurate to a science is Claire's responsibility. Masha takes the lead with event organizing. The two create an infused custom menu for each client, prepared fresh on-site using farm-to-table organic food. They tailor ingredients and the amount of cannabis to meet each participant's needs. The chefs are experienced in a variety of cuisines, including vegan and gluten-free. Food is prepared to clients' specifications either at their homes or, for large gatherings, in a rented kitchen. In addition to catering, the company also offers a unique CannaBar experience, replacing the traditional alcohol bar with innovative fresh cocktails made with cannabis. Tasty High Chef serves a variety of different folks, including veterans, seniors, and individuals who are housebound and find it difficult to cook.

Claire and Masha believe that farmers and chefs should have collaborative partnerships, and they have several farmers that they work closely with at different times. This is based on what strains the farms have to offer and the projects that the co-owners are working on. The cannabis community in San Diego has been very supportive. The co-owners of Tasty High Chef realize that it is essential to know your sourcing because, "Great food begins with great ingredients."

POWERHOUSE CBD GREEN SMOOTHIE

by TASTY HIGH CHEF

MAKES about 3 cups

This smoothie is both refreshing and filling—perfect for an energy boost.

1 cup honeydew melon chunks

1 cup pineapple chunks, fresh or frozen

2 cups fresh local baby spinach leaves, lightly packed

½ fresh ripe Hass avocado, cut into chunks

2 tablespoons organic unsweetened coconut milk, or as needed

1 tablespoon honey, or to taste

30 milligrams full-spectrum CBD oil

½ cup ice, or as needed

1 tablespoon chia seeds, for garnish

1. Place all the ingredients, except the chia seeds, in a blender and blend, scraping down the sides of the blender jar as needed, until smooth. Adjust sweetness with honey, if desired. Pour into chilled glasses. Garnish with chia seeds. Serve at once.

CBD-INFUSED OLIVE OIL

by TASTY HIGH CHEF

MAKES 2 cups

> **TASTY HIGH CHEF:** This is a very simple process for creating your own CBD-infused olive oil. The result is a wonderfully versatile product that can be used in any recipe that calls for olive oil. The higher the quality of the ingredients, the better the product will be, so choose the best whenever possible.

Note: You will need to infuse the oil at least 8 hours before you intend to use it.

3.5 grams CBD flower

2 cups extra-virgin olive oil

1. To decarboxylate the cannabis: Preheat the oven to 230°F. Line a baking sheet with parchment paper. Chop or break the CBD flower into pea-size pieces. Spread the cannabis out in a single layer on the prepared baking sheet. Bake until the cannabis flower is completely dry and its color has changed from green to light brown, watching carefully not to burn, approximately 20 to 30 minutes. Allow the cannabis to cool completely on the baking sheet before using, about 15 minutes.

2. To make the CBD-infused olive oil: Place the decarboxylated cannabis, olive oil, and a candy thermometer into the top pan of a double boiler. Pour about 1 inch of water into the bottom pan and bring to a simmer. Place the top pan with the cannabis on top, making sure the bowl does not touch the simmering water. Infuse the oil, making sure to maintain enough water in the bottom pan of the double boiler, for about 4 hours. Stir frequently, maintaining the oil temperature below 250°F. Remove from the heat and allow the oil to cool briefly.

3. To strain and store: Strain the infused oil through a cheesecloth-lined fine-mesh strainer into a clean heat-resistant glass jar. When cool enough to handle, gather the corners of the cheesecloth and gently squeeze out any excess oil into the jar. Allow the oil to cool completely before tightly sealing it with a lid. Label the jar with the date and contents. Store in a cool dark place for up to 1 month.

NOTES

It is important to check on the cannabis periodically to make sure it is not burning.

It is important to maintain the oil temperature below 250°F to avoid cooking off the valuable cannabinoids.

TIP

Using a candy thermometer will help to ensure that the temperature always stays below 250°F.

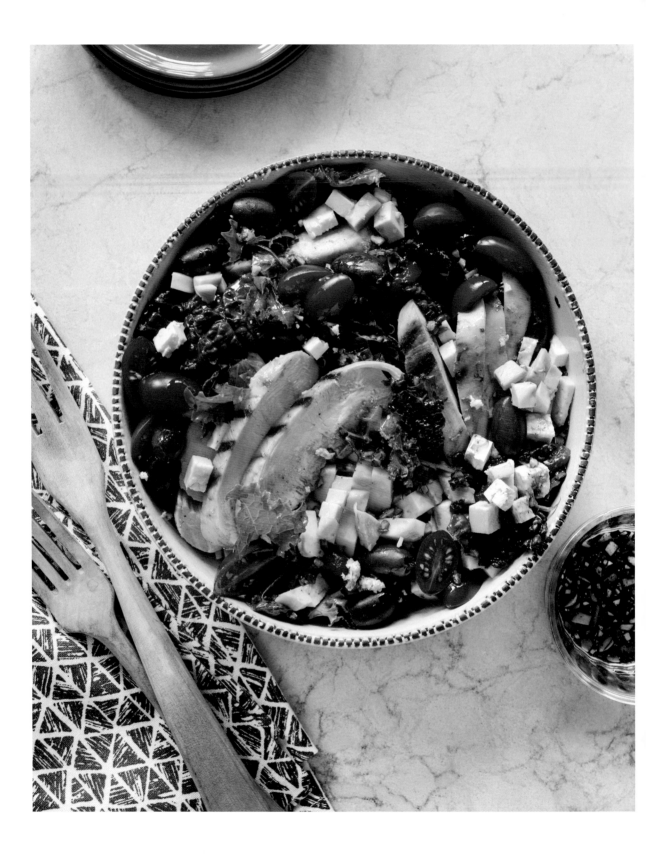

CALIFORNIA GREEK SALAD
with Grilled Chicken

by TASTY HIGH CHEF

SERVES 4 as a main dish, or 6 as a side salad

GRILLED CHICKEN

Nonstick cooking spray, as needed

1 (8-ounce) boneless, skinless chicken breast

Salt and freshly ground black pepper

CBD-INFUSED DRESSING

Makes approximately ½ cup

2 tablespoons balsamic vinegar

2 medium cloves garlic, minced

1 tablespoon lemon juice

2 tablespoons CBD-infused olive oil (page 122)

2 tablespoon extra-virgin olive oil

Kosher salt and freshly ground black pepper

CALIFORNIA GREEK SALAD

4 cups curly green kale, stemmed and cut into bite-sized pieces, tightly packed

½ cup cherry or grape tomatoes, halved

1 small avocado, pitted, peeled, and cubed

1 medium roasted red bell pepper, homemade or store-bought, cut into strips (page 126)

⅓ cup kalamata olives, pitted

¼ pound feta cheese, cut into ¼-inch pieces

1½ tablespoons hulled sunflower seeds

1. To make the grilled chicken: Heat a gas or electric grill to high heat. Lightly oil the grill grate with nonstick cooking spray. Season the chicken with salt and pepper. Place the chicken on the grill, cover, and grill, until the internal temperature reaches 165°F, about 12 minutes per side. Transfer the chicken to a plate and let rest. Cut the chicken against the grain, on a diagonal, into ½ inch–thick slices.

2. To make the CBD-infused dressing: In a small bowl, whisk together the vinegar, garlic, and lemon juice. Slowly whisk in the oils until emulsified. Season with salt and pepper to taste.

3. To make the California Greek salad: In a large bowl, combine the kale and ½ of the dressing. Using tongs, massage the kale until it is bright green and slightly softened, about 5 minutes. Fan the chicken slices out across the top of the salad. Top with tomatoes, avocado, roasted peppers, olives, feta cheese, and sunflower seeds. Drizzle the remaining dressing over and around the salad, or to taste. Serve at once.

NOTE

You will need to make the CBD-infused oil at least 8 hours before you intend to use it in the CBD-infused dressing.

Note: The roasted red bell pepper can be made up to 5 days ahead of time before you intend to serve; just cover and refrigerate.

1 medium red bell pepper
1 teaspoon extra-virgin olive oil

To make the roasted red bell pepper: Move your oven rack to the highest possible position in the oven. Preheat the oven broiler to high. Line a baking sheet with aluminum foil. Set aside.

Place the pepper on the prepared baking sheet and rub with oil. Broil until the skin is charred and bubbly on all sides, turning occasionally with tongs, about 15 minutes. Transfer to a small bowl, cover with plastic wrap, and let sit at room temperature for 20 minutes. Using a sharp knife, remove the stem and cut the pepper into quarters. Remove the skins, ribs, and seeds and discard. Cut the pepper into thin uniform strips.

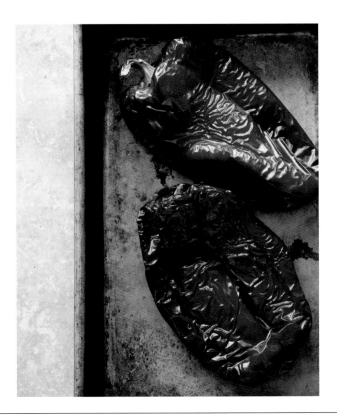

MARIA HINES

Chef/Advocate

Chef Maria Hines was the owner of Tilth Restaurant located in Seattle, Washington. Sadly, the establishment closed its doors in October, 2020 due to the COVID-19 pandemic. After graduating with a degree in culinary arts from Mesa Community College in San Diego, California, Hines has spent over thirty years cooking in kitchens all over the world. The busy chef wears many hats: named one of *Food & Wine Magazine*'s ten best chefs of 2005; James Beard Award Winner for Best Chef of the Northwest, in 2009; winner of an episode of *Iron Chef* for successfully creating five superb Pacific Cod recipes, in 2010; a staunch supporter of sustainable agriculture and farming; dedicated food advocate committed to organics, food labeling, and transparency; and a successful restaurateur.

In 2006, Tilth Restaurant opened in a Craftsman-style house situated in the Seattle neighborhood of Wallingford. The restaurant received organic certification from Oregon Tilth, which promotes sustainability. Although the restaurant and organization shared the same name, they were not affiliated. At that time, Tilth was only the second certified organic restaurant in the country. In 2008, the *New York Times* voted Tilth one of the best restaurants in the country. Hine's restaurant featured American cuisine prepared with certified organic or wild ingredients. She is known as a pioneer of organic and Pacific Northwest cuisine. Using local and seasonal products is the foundation of her cooking philosophy. The busy chef aspires to live a healthy lifestyle eating an organic diet when at home. Hines supports food labeling and transparency, not using antibiotics in livestock and knowing where food comes from. She has always supported locally sourced food and still does, even though Tilth has closed.

The busy chef has also owned two other restaurants: the Golden Beetle, which closed in 2016 and Agrodolce, which was sold to its executive chef, Thomas Litrenta in 2019. Hines felt that the time was right to focus on other endeavors. She is now writing a cookbook as well as launching a retail line of on-the-go organic food.

Hines was drawn to cannabis-infused foods, hoping to decrease the inflammation in her body and relieve some of her dog's health problems. She has found that CBD has helped alleviate her sleep issues, anxiety, and pain. In her spare time, the chef is an avid rock climber who has traveled as far away as Thailand to pursue the sport. CBD has helped to lessen the after-effects of this strenuous sport. Chef Hines strongly believes that "cannabis should be grown, harvested, and prepared with respect to the earth and those who consume it. It has many medicinal properties that can really help some individuals to live a better life."

VEGAN NO-BAKE CASHEW CHEESECAKES

by MARIA HINES

MAKES 16 individual cheesecakes

> **MARIA HINES:** This is a decadent-tasting dessert that is also packed with nutrients. The silky texture and tangy taste create a nice balance of richness and brightness. You can make the cheesecakes and freeze them, so you can have them handy whenever your sweet tooth strikes.

FILLING

Note: You will need to soak the raw cashews in hot water for at least 15 minutes on the counter, before you intend to use them.

3 cups raw cashews

¼ cup fresh lemon juice

1 tablespoon lemon zest

¾ cup pure maple syrup or organic agave syrup

½ cup organic coconut cream, unsweetened

1 tablespoon pure vanilla extract

1 teaspoon ground cinnamon

400 milligrams full-spectrum CBD, or desired dosage

⅛ teaspoon sea salt

4 cups assorted fresh berries

CRUST

2 cups whole cashew nuts, roasted and unsalted

8 fresh Medjool dates, pitted

2 tablespoons coconut oil, melted, plus more for greasing

⅛ teaspoon salt

1. To prepare the raw cashews (using the quick-soak method): Place the 3 cups raw cashews in a medium bowl. Fill the bowl with very hot water (just below a boil), making sure the cashews are completely submerged. Soak the cashews for at least 15 minutes. Drain, rinse, and set aside.

2. While the cashews are soaking, grease 16 muffin cups with coconut oil.

3. To make the crust: In the bowl of a food processor, add the roasted unsalted cashew nuts, dates, coconut oil, and salt and pulse until it partially binds together. The mixture will be chunky and paste-like. Set aside.

4. To make the cheesecakes: Place the prepared raw cashews into a blender. Add the lemon juice and zest, maple syrup, coconut cream, vanilla, cinnamon, CBD oil, and salt and process on high, scraping down the sides of the blender jar as needed, until very smooth, about 8 minutes, depending on the power of the blender.

5. Spoon approximately 2 tablespoons of the crust mixture into the bottom of 16 muffin cups, pressing down firmly and evenly with the bottom of a shot glass or your fingertips. Pour or spoon approximately 3 tablespoons of the filling over the top of each crust, filling the cups evenly. Tap the muffin pans on the counter a few times to flatten and smooth the tops. Cover the muffin pans with plastic wrap and place in the freezer until the cakes are shiny and firm to the touch, about 2 hours.

Recipe continues on page 131

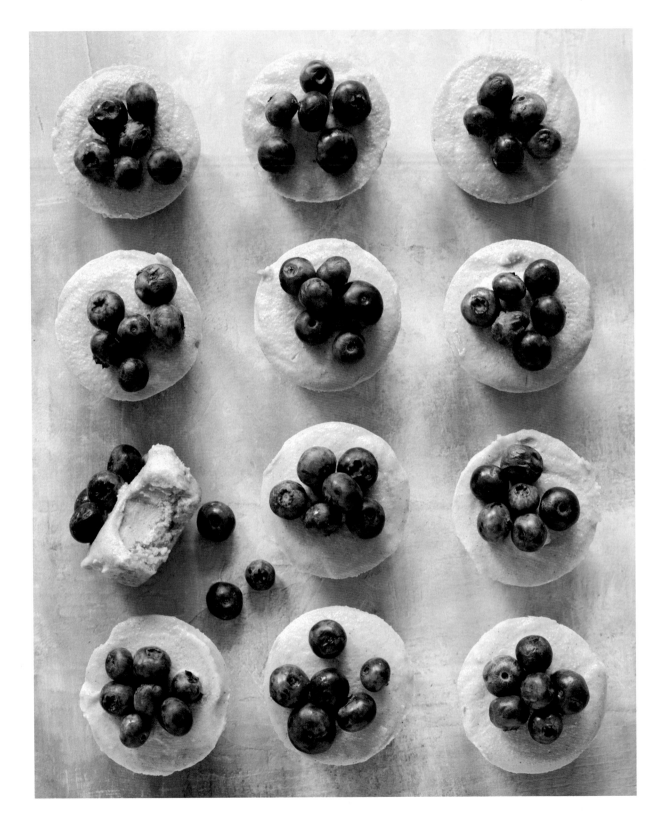

6. To unmold the cheesecakes, place the muffin pans into a shallow basin of hot water for 1 minute. Remove pans, then run a hot, thin, non-serrated knife around the edges of the muffin cups to loosen the cakes, and pop them out. Allow the cakes to thaw and soften at room temperature for about 10 minutes before serving. Top with fresh berries and serve. Leftover cheesecakes can be stored in the freezer for up to 2 months.

MARIA HINES'S TIP

I like to make the Vegan No-Bake Cashew Cheesecakes in silicone muffin pans, but you can also use a traditional cake pan.

AÇAI FRUIT BOWL

by MARIA HINES

MAKES 2 servings

> **MARIA HINES:** Starting out the day with a healthy breakfast can make the biggest difference in energy level. Açai is loaded with antioxidants that help boost your immune system. The CBD works as a wonderful anti-inflammatory, to help your body recover from physical and mental stressors.

AÇAI SMOOTHIE

Makes 3½ cups

1 cup frozen açai berry purée

1 cup assorted fresh organic berries, frozen

1 large ripe organic banana, peeled and sliced

1 cup grass-fed vanilla yogurt, whole milk

1 teaspoon ground cinnamon

1 teaspoon honey

2 teaspoons chia seeds

50 milligrams full-spectrum CBD oil, or desired dosage

Sea salt flakes, to taste

TOPPINGS

1 tablespoon almond slivers

1 tablespoon organic pumpkin seeds, raw and shelled

⅓ cup banana chips

⅓ cup assorted fresh organic berries

1. Run hot water over the package of frozen açai purée to thaw it just enough to break into large chunks.
2. Blend together the açai berry purée, berries, banana, yogurt, cinnamon, honey, chia seeds, and CBD oil, scraping down the sides of the blender jar, as necessary, until smooth. Adjust seasonings with salt. Note: The açai fruit bowls will be thicker than a standard smoothie. Pour into two deep cereal bowls and place them in the refrigerator to chill for about 15 minutes.
3. To serve: Arrange the toppings evenly between both bowls, in neat rows on top of the açai, and serve at once.

NOTES

Açai berry purée is available in the freezer section with frozen fruits and can be found at supermarkets.

For those desiring a looser consistency, feel free to add some almond milk in small increments when blending.

DONALD LEMPERLE & TRAVIS SCHWANTES

Chef/Owner and General Manager, VegeNation

VegeNation, located in Las Vegas, Nevada, opened its doors in 2015. A second location was later started in Henderson, Nevada. Chef/Owner Donald Lemperle dubbed both of his eateries VegeNation, with the thought that they would be the start of a dynasty of plant-based restaurants scattered across our nation. During his career, Chef Donald has worked at a number of high-end restaurants and is well versed in numerous cooking styles and cuisines. After facing a serious health problem, the chef adopted a plant-based diet for himself which he strongly believes is the reason for his return to good health. Convinced that this diet has a positive impact on people's health, as well as the environment, he has created a 100 percent plant-based menu for both of his restaurants.

Chef Donald's goal is to give back to the local community by supporting small businesses and farmers. The restaurants' very popular CBD tea exemplifies this community connection. The tea comes from Bloomin' Desert Herb Farm, which is also in Henderson. This tea is a tropical Ceylon blend infused with CBD oil. VegeNation's very popular Changemaker cocktail uses this CBD tea along with distilled liquor from the Las Vegas Distillery.

General manager Travis Schwantes oversees the everyday workings of the business and its philosophy of serving 100 percent plant-based food. The menu features foods from across the globe, striving to use local fruits and vegetables whenever possible. Visitors are amazed to learn that the meats, cheeses, and even the ice cream are all plant-based. VegeNation wants folks to know that everyone is welcome; you don't have to be vegan to enjoy the variety of delicious global dishes. As the folks from VegeNation explain, "It's good food that's good for you!"

THE CHANGEMAKER COCKTAIL

by VEGENATION

MAKES 1 drink

The Changemaker is a refreshing infused whiskey tea made with local distilled liquor from the Las Vegas Distillery and a proprietary tropical Ceylon tea blend from Bloomin' Desert Herb Farm in Henderson, Nevada. The sweet CBD tea is a brew of rosemary, ginger, holy basil, red clover, nettle, peppermint, clove, raw CBD oil, and purified water.

1.5 ounces whiskey, preferably from Las Vegas Distillery

4 ounces sweet CBD tea, preferably from Bloomin' Desert Herb Farm

1 orange slice

1. Fill an 8-ounce lowball cocktail glass with ice. Pour the whiskey and tea into the glass; stir to combine. Garnish with orange slice. Serve at once.

SOUTH

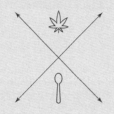

FALLON KEPLINGER

Founder, Rose Glow Tea Room

For as long as Fallon Keplinger can remember, tea has been an integral part of her life. Her mother, an avid tea drinker, always keeps different varieties of the beverage in the house. When Fallon and her twin sister were young, they received a tea set for a gift and spent many a fun afternoon sipping an imaginary cup. Tea was most certainly an important part of the Keplinger's family routine.

Carrying her love for the beverage to the next level, Fallon became a tea sommelier with the International Tea Masters Association. The title means that she is a trained and knowledgeable tea professional who can make recommendations for a beverage program at a restaurant or café. She has been schooled in different types of teas, tisanes, and processing methods and studied what food pairs best with contrasting varieties. To further hone her skills, Fallon traveled to Kyoto, Japan, to spend three weeks there interning with a tea master.

Back in the 1920s and 1930s, the Rose Glow Tea Room was a popular destination in Washington, D.C. While thumbing through an old magazine, Fallon came across an article about the place and found its concept intriguing. When she and her friends started their CBD-infused tea business in 2015, they decided to name it after this historic venue. With a lack of woman- and minority-owned businesses in the cannabidiol industry, the group's mission was to be part of the female movement that was breaking down barriers. They believed that the more people were educated in the area of cannabis, the more this knowledge would spread, lessening the stigma surrounding the plant and its use. The group of friends began offering well-attended CBD tea pop-ups in the D.C. area building a loyal clientele, but then, as it so often does, life happened. After a year, Fallon found herself the sole member of the Rose Glow Tea Room group, her friends having left for other pursuits.

Now the head of the CBD-infused tea business, Fallon matches cannabis terpene flavor profiles to the natural tastes of each tea blend. When sampling a new tea, she uses a tea evaluation form to remember its aroma, taste, and viscosity. If unable to determine what she is tasting or smelling, she will use an aroma wheel and then contact the Woman-owned cannabis company that she deals with to have them offer guidance.

Rose Glow's teas are sold on the company's website and at a few independent shops. Its line of CBD-infused products includes BREATHE, a mixture of rooibos and fresh spices steeped into cashew milk that can be served hot or over ice. This drink has anti-inflammatory, antioxidant, and muscle-relaxing properties and is useful in the treatment of bronchitis and asthma. The REVITALIZE blend contains Gyokuro tea, a shaded green tea from Japan that is blended with coconut and pineapple. It is used to boost the immune system, for respiratory health, and to aid digestion and strengthen bones. SUNSET contains Se Chung Oolong, which has characteristics of both green and black tea. Blended with lavender and honey, it is rich in antioxidants and polyphenols. This tea helps with anxiety, insomnia, and restlessness. The tea bags for each variety are infused with 20 mg of water-soluble CBD.

Fallon Keplinger wants folks to know that the ingestion of cannabis helps to stimulate the endocannabinoid system, which works to create balance and promote calmness. With many people in today's world suffering from anxiety, cannabis can be a benefit when used properly. The owner of Rose Glow Tea Room has a dream to one day own a brick-and-mortar venue where visitors can go to relax and enjoy the safe consumption of cannabis and CBD tea.

CBD-INFUSED ICED GREEN TEA TOPPED
with Cheese Milk

by FALLON KEPLINGER, ROSE GLOW TEA

MAKES 4 servings

FALLON KEPLINGER: I tried cheese tea for the first time in Kyoto, Japan. I was really nervous at first because I didn't think the flavors would go together. I was pleasantly surprised that the drink tasted like a slice of green tea–infused cheesecake. I recreated the process at home and it is really easy!

ICED GREEN TEA

Note: The iced green tea will need to be made at least 1 hour before you plan to serve it.

4 cups brewed CBD-infused green tea, such as Rose Glow Revitalized Tea

Honey, to taste

CHEESE MILK

Makes 2 cups

2 ounces cream cheese

½ cup heavy cream

½ cup half-and-half

3 tablespoons sugar

½ teaspoon salt

GARNISH

4 fresh mint sprigs

1. Prepare the green tea according to the tea instructions on the package, then chill in the refrigerator until very cold.

2. To make the cheese milk: In a stand mixer with the whisk beater attachment, whip the cream cheese on medium speed until light and fluffy, about 2 minutes. While the motor is running on medium-high speed, slowly add the cream and half-and-half in a thin stream and whip until smooth, about 4 minutes. Add the sugar and salt and mix on high speed until the mixture reaches a thick viscosity, similar to a milkshake.

3. Fill 4 pint glasses ¾ full of ice, then pour 1 cup of tea into each glass. Adjust sweetness with honey, as desired. Top with a ⅓ cup of the cheese milk, or to taste. Garnish each glass with a sprig of mint. Serve at once.

VARIATION

The cheese milk is delicious served over iced CBD-infused coffee or chai tea.

CANADA

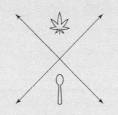

JORDAN WAGMAN

Chef, Cookbook Author, Mental Health and Psoriasis Advocate

Jordan Wagman is a man of many talents—chef, cookbook author, sales leader, youth advocate, musician, father, and husband. Jordan was born and raised in Toronto, Ontario, moving to the United States to start his culinary career at the Art Institute of Fort Lauderdale in Florida, where he majored in culinary arts. During this period of his life he also studied under James Beard Award–nominated chef Oliver Saucy at the East City Grill.

He is one of a select few Canadian chefs to receive the honor of being nominated for "Rising Star of North America" by the James Beard Foundation. Jordan was also part of the celebrated "Great Hotel Chefs of America" series. Working in high-end kitchens throughout the course of his culinary career has taught him how to multitask.

Jordan and his family have moved back to Toronto. He has retired from restaurant life to concentrate on cookbook writing and spend more time with family. His sixth cookbook is soon to be released. He continues to be involved with the world of culinary arts, offering unique, private chef's-table experiences for select clientele. Culinary experiences are a balance of education and entertainment; Jordan strives to make this time both informative and fun. The gourmet chef wants his guests to ask questions and receive answers that they can understand and use when working in their own kitchen.

When Jordan is not in the kitchen, he sits on the board of JFCS, a large children's aid and social services organization which also runs a school he attended in the eleventh grade; Jerome D. Diamond Adolescent Centre, a youth mental health center in Toronto. The school provides services to young people between the ages of eleven and seventeen who are experiencing psychological, behavioral and/or academic challenges. As a trained chef, he has volunteered his culinary expertise to help raise funds for the school's new kitchen. For Jordan Wagman, giving back is an important part of who he is.

A diagnosis of psoriasis at age thirteen has motivated Jordan, as an adult, to change his approach to the food that he eats and its method of preparation. He has eliminated refined sugar, fast foods, dairy, and gluten from his diet. CBD has been a daily part of his dietary regimen for a number of years. The CBD has helped him with psoriasis inflammation and flare-ups, making his recovery time much quicker. Jordan strongly believes that "not all CBD is created equal." Because of this fact, he has formed a relationship with Elmore Mountain Therapeutics in Elmore, Vermont. Trusting in the health benefits of their products, he is in the process of forming a partnership with the company, using only their CBD oil for his personal and cooking needs. Based on his own health experience, Jordan is of the opinion that CBD, when used correctly, can make a difference.

The meals prepared in the Wagmans' kitchen are not only restaurant quality, but accessible in execution and affordability. The way that Jordan cooks reflects how he personally eats. It is his belief that with the right staples in your kitchen you can create quick meals from very little—"If you keep whole natural foods in your kitchen, you will eat good food!"

The busy entrepreneur has an approach to cooking that is very simple—buy the best local and seasonal ingredients available. He only eats organic or "kind food," a term used to describe food from farmers who may not have an organic designation but grow their foodstuff with the same approach as an organic farmer. He always looks for products from producers who care about the environment and have a commitment to sustainability and social responsibility. When you eat cleaner and make better choices about what you are consuming, it can have a positive impact on all aspects of your life.

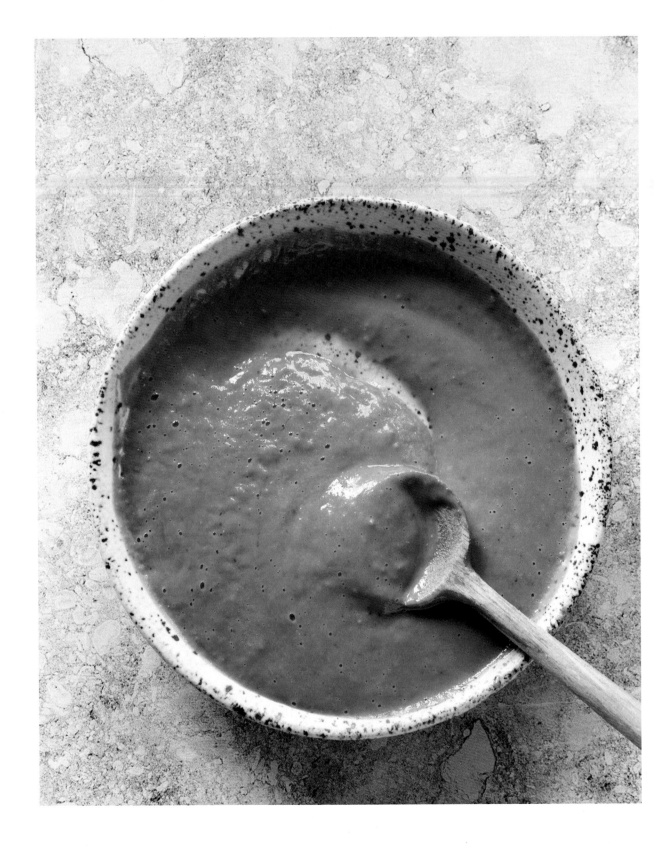

CBD-INFUSED CHERRY TOMATO SAUCE

CHEF JORDAN WAGMAN

MAKES about 2 cups

> **CHEF JORDAN WAGMAN:** Simply the easiest, fastest, and best tomato sauce you will ever make.

2 cups cherry or grape tomatoes

⅓ cup extra-virgin olive oil

¼ teaspoon kosher salt

¼ teaspoon freshly ground black pepper

2 tablespoons (30 milligrams) CBD- or THC-infused olive oil

1. To make the CBD-infused cherry tomato sauce: In a medium heavy-bottomed saucepan, combine the tomatoes, olive oil, salt, and pepper. Bring to a simmer over low heat, about 8 minutes, then continue to cook until the tomato skins begin to split and the juice from the tomatoes has been released, about 25 minutes.

2. Remove from the heat and allow the tomato sauce to cool to 320°F before adding the CBD oil, then carefully transfer to a blender and purée until smooth. Use immediately or cool to room temperature, transfer to an airtight container, and refrigerate for up to 5 days.

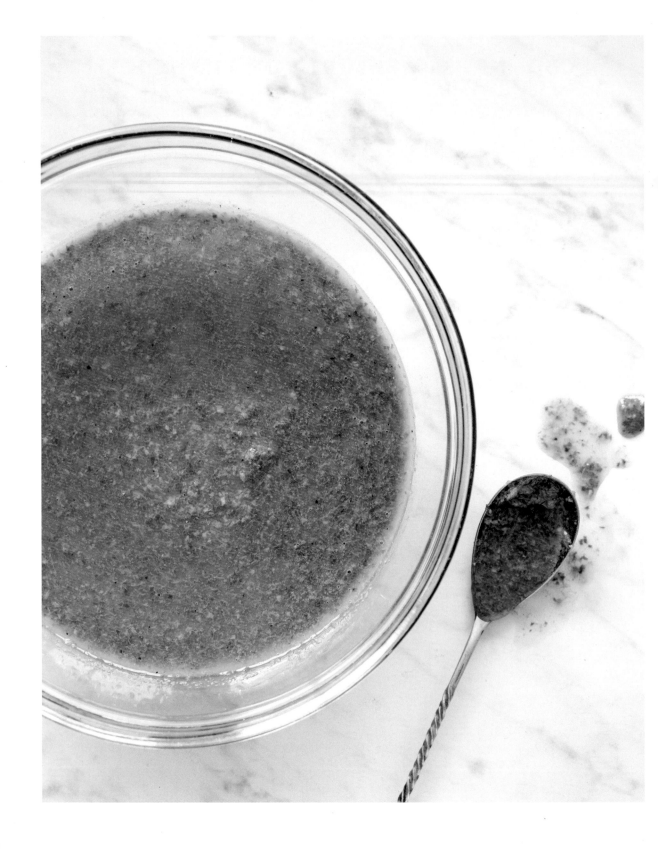

CBD-INFUSED PESTO SAUCE

by CHEF JORDAN WAGMAN

MAKES 1½ cups

> **CHEF JORDAN WAGMAN:** Inspired by a traditional pesto, this nut-free and dairy-free version can be used in vinaigrettes, added to warm vegetables, used as the perfect sauce on pasta or simply to marinate a chicken breast, fish, or meat. Any way you choose to use it, this pesto sauce will add a huge burst of flavor!

2½ cups fresh basil leaves, loosely packed

1 bunch (about 10 stalks) fresh chives

2 scallions, trimmed and coarsely chopped

4 cloves garlic, coarsely chopped

2 tablespoons (30 milligrams) CBD- or THC-infused olive oil

¼ teaspoon sea salt flakes

¼ teaspoon freshly ground black pepper

1 cup extra-virgin olive oil

1. To make the CBD-infused pesto sauce: Process the basil, chives, scallions, garlic, CBD oil (if using), salt, and pepper in a food processor until minced. While the processor is running, slowly add the olive oil in a steady stream until well blended and smooth, scraping down the sides of the bowl as needed. Adjust seasonings with salt and pepper. The pesto sauce will be bright green and have a very loose consistency. Note: The pesto sauce is a cross between a pesto sauce and a pesto oil.

2. Use the pesto sauce immediately or transfer to an airtight container and refrigerate for up to one week.

NOTE

If freezing the pesto, spoon into ice cube trays then freeze until solid. Remove the cubes from the trays and place in a freezer bag. Store in the freezer for up to 3 months.

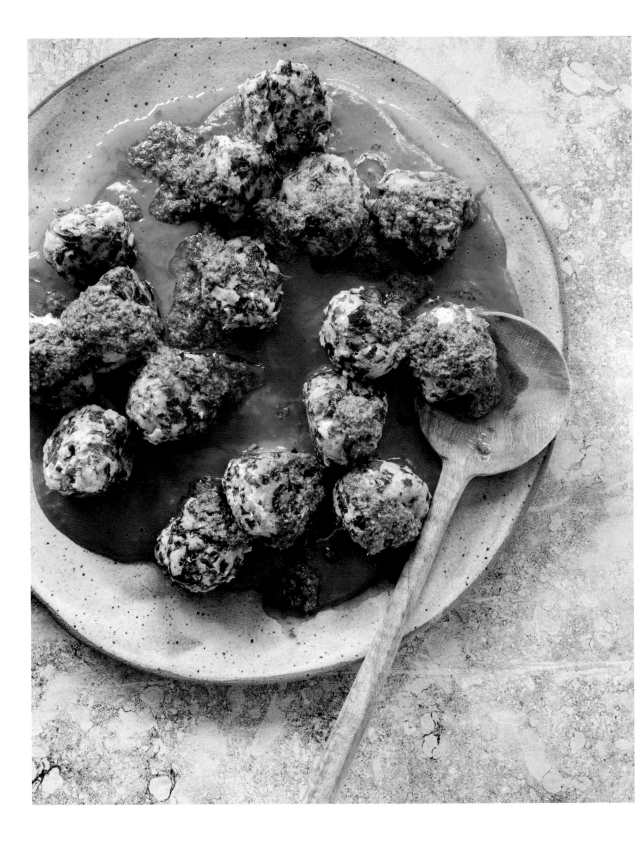

CHICKEN KALE MEATBALLS

with CBD-Infused Cherry Tomato and Pesto Sauces

by CHEF JORDAN WAGMAN

MAKES about 12 meatballs

CHEF JORDAN WAGMAN: These meatballs are stunning and delicious and can be prepared in as little as 25 minutes!

4 cups loosely packed kale leaves, stems and inner ribs removed

1 pound ground chicken

½ teaspoon sea salt flakes

½ teaspoon freshly ground black pepper

2 tablespoons extra-virgin olive oil or avocado oil, or as needed

Basil leaves, for garnish

Crusty bread, optional

1. To make the chicken kale meatballs: In a food processor, chop the kale finely and set aside. In a large bowl, mix the chicken, kale, salt, and pepper until well combined. Using a scale, weigh the meat into 1.5-ounce portions. Using your hands, form into balls. Set aside.

2. Heat 1 tablespoon of the oil in a large skillet over medium-high heat until hot, but not smoking. Reduce the heat to medium and carefully drop the meatballs, in batches, directly into the skillet and cook, turning carefully with a spatula, until browned on all sides, about 2 to 3 minutes per side, then cover and continue to cook until the center of each meatball reaches 165°F. Repeat with the remaining 1 tablespoon of oil and meatballs.

3. To serve: Place 1 cup of the tomato sauce (page 143) in a large serving platter, arrange the meatballs over tomato sauce and drizzle pesto sauce (page 145) over the meatballs to taste. Garnish with basil leaves. Serve at once, passing the remaining sauce at the table along with some crusty bread, if desired.

NOTE *Serve with CBD-Infused Cherry Tomato Sauce (page 143) and CBD-Infused Pesto Sauce (page 145).*

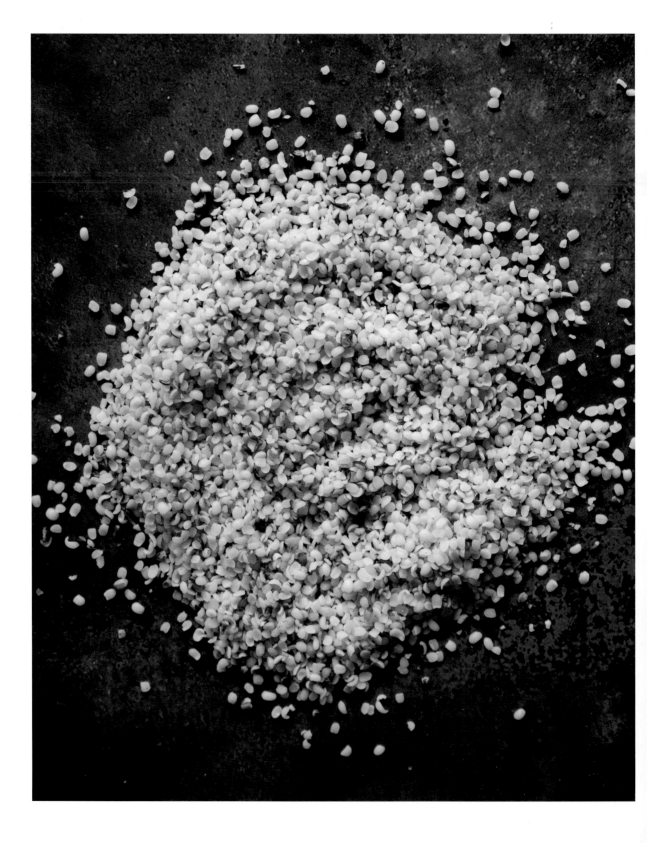

CHAPTER 2

HEMP

Cannabis sativa is the scientific name for the hemp plant. Hemp, the nonpsychoactive form of cannabis, is widely used for clothing, food products, hemp oil, and even fuel. *Cannabis sativa* has two primary strains, hemp and marijuana, which are genetically distinct, distinguished by use, chemical composition, and cultivation methods. Both contain CBD, with a much higher percentage in hemp which also has low levels of THC compared to marijuana. Hemp can hold no more than 0.3 percent THC, while marijuana can carry 30 percent of THC by dry weight.

Hemp seeds are used for oil and are high in essential fatty acids. They are a nutritious source of protein. Hulled hemp seeds are a healthful component of baked goods and can be processed into milk, cheese, ice cream, margarine, and a variety of other foods. As an outstanding nutritional supplement, the seeds add a wonderful flavor to dressings, dips, and spreads. Hemp oil can be combined with or replace olive, walnut, and saffron oils in the creation of various dishes. Hemp seed meal, the derivative of whole hemp seeds after cold pressing, makes a suitable food ingredient and healthy supplement both for people and animals. It has even been used to brew beer.

The oil from the seeds of the hemp plant is rich in omega-3 fatty acids, vitamin E, and protein. Hemp extract oils that come from the flowers and leaves of the hemp plant are the basis of CBD products. CBDa is one of the compounds present in the leaves and flowers of the hemp plant. CBDa turns into CBD after the leaves and flowers have been decarboxylated by a heating process, which is true for THCa as well. When the "a" carboxylic acid that is attached to these compounds is removed, they are converted into an active form.

Refined hemp oil is clear, with little flavor and few nutrients. It is widely used in body care products, lubricants, and paints and for industrial purposes. The oil's antimicrobial properties make it an ideal base for soaps, shampoos, and detergents. Because it is packed with healthy fats that offer moisturizing benefits, it often appears in beauty products.

The fibers and stalks of the hemp plant are used for clothing, construction materials, paper, and more. Canvas, a material made from woven hemp fibers, received its name from cannabis. In 2018 the Farm Bill legalized the cultivation and sale of hemp at the federal level. The bill made it federally legal to grow hemp, allowing consumers who are compliant with their state's rules to grow and produce hemp products, including CBD. It is left up to each state to set their own policies in this area.

NORTHEAST

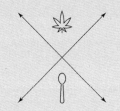

CHRISTOPHER PAUL

In-house product developer, Destino Distribution

Christopher Paul developed a passion for cooking during his early childhood, which was spent on the island of Haiti. Although he was born in Brooklyn, New York, his family decided to move back to Port-au-Prince, Haiti where they were originally from. The young boy spent the first ten years of his life on this tropical island with its sandy beaches and sparkling water views. While living in Haiti, Paul's family always had a garden where they would grow a portion of their food. Each day the ingredients needed for mealtime were freshly picked. It was during this time in his life that Paul developed a love of healthy, sustainably grown local foods.

When Paul was ten, his family moved to Philadelphia, the city that he still calls home. Chef Paul graduated from Drexel University's Culinary Arts Program in 2011. Since then his cooking experience has been evenly split between restaurant, catering, and entrepreneurial ventures.

The chef did not have any involvement with CBD during his college years. It was not until a longtime friend, Patrick Massuci, started a CBD distribution company called Destino Distribution that he had an opportunity to sample some of their CBD products. Chef Paul decided to invest in the business, offering his product development expertise and food safety background to assist the company in building and expanding its in-house manufacturing division.

After using its research and development resources, the company decided to source their bulk hemp flower from southern Oregon. With his years of experience in the food industry, Chef Paul heads all in-house product development at Destino. He curates the best-in-class CBD brands and accessories, distributing these products to quality-focused retailers across the world.

When baking with CBD-infused products, Chef Paul carefully monitors the oven temperature. Experience has taught him that high heat will render the CBD useless; therefore, he tries to bake all CBD-infused products under 300°F, if possible. When infusing oils, the chef always employs a cold method, blending flavors first and adding CBD afterward. He has found that hemp oil and seeds are very flavorful, pairing perfectly with the chef's creations. Even without CBD, hemp oil offers wonderful accents and excellent nutrition.

Chef Paul occasionally hosts cooking classes and demonstrations for various organizations, while also working as an independent contractor for a few catering companies. Sometimes his wife Leigh-Ann will lend a hand when needed, using her expertise as a nutritionist to help craft customized meals. Leigh-Ann was raised in Trinidad and Tobago until moving to the United States at age seven. She graduated from Penn State with a degree in nutrition, most recently receiving her master's degree in public health. Together the two bring a wealth of experience and knowledge to the area of healthy living alternatives.

HUMMUS
with Toasted Hemp Seed "Tahini" and CBD-Infused Sage Oil

by CHRIS PAUL, DESTINO DISTRIBUTION   **MAKES** 5 cups

> **CHRIS PAUL:** Although I did not grow up eating hummus, I've grown to love it over the past few years. I usually try replacing the tahini with other nuts and seeds, as I find them more flavorful. Hemp seeds are a great substitute and when toasted they really add a robust, nutty flavor. I recommend making more hemp "tahini" and using it as a spread, which I guarantee will be a hit.

CBD-INFUSED SAGE OIL
Makes just over ½ cup

½ cup plus 2 tablespoons safflower oil

24 fresh sage leaves

15 milligrams full-spectrum CBD tincture, preferably Super Speciosa (High Potency 750mg CBD Tincture)

HEMP SEED "TAHINI"
Makes about ½ cup

¼ cup safflower oil

8 medium cloves garlic, crushed and peeled

½ cup hemp seeds

Juice from 1 lemon

HUMMUS
4½ cups (three 15.5-ounce cans) cooked chickpeas, drained (reserving ½ cup of liquid) and rinsed

½ cup hemp seed tahini (see recipe above)

Juice from 2 lemons, or to taste

2 teaspoons kosher salt

1 teaspoon freshly ground black pepper

¼ cup CBD-infused sage oil (see recipe above)

1. To make the CBD-infused sage oil: Pour the oil into a small saucepan. Add the sage leaves and muddle them in the oil, then bring to a simmer over medium heat, about 4 minutes. Remove from the heat and set aside, allowing the sage leaves to steep until ready to use.

2. To make the hemp seed "tahini:" Heat the oil in a small skillet over medium-low heat until hot but not smoking, about 3 minutes. Add the garlic and cook, stirring occasionally, until lightly golden brown on all sides, about 3 minutes. Remove from heat, then using a slotted spoon, remove the garlic from the oil and place on a paper towel–lined plate, reserving the garlic oil. Set both aside.

3. Heat a separate small skillet over medium-high heat until hot but not smoking, about 3 minutes. Reduce the heat to medium, then add the hemp seeds and cook, stirring often, until golden brown and toasted, about 3 minutes. Transfer the hemp seeds, reserved garlic, garlic oil, and lemon juice to a food processor, and process, scraping down the sides of the bowl as needed, until the texture resembles a coarse mustard. Let stand in the bowl of the food processor until ready to use.

4. To make the hummus: Add the chickpeas, lemon juice, salt, and pepper to the same food processor with the hemp seed "tahini" and process until smooth. While the motor is running, add ¼ cup of the reserved chickpea juice, adding additional juice as needed, until desired consistency is

achieved. Adjust seasonings with lemon juice, salt, and pepper, to taste. Transfer to a decorative bowl.

5. Strain the sage-infused oil through a fine-mesh strainer into a clean container, reserving the sage. Coarsely chop the reserved sage leaves and set aside.

6. Add the CBD oil to the hummus, stirring until well combined. Drizzle the hummus with ¼ cup of the CBD-infused sage oil, then scatter sage over the top. Serve with crusty bread, assorted vegetables, or crackers.

NOTE

The CBD-infused sage oil makes more than you will need for this recipe. Toss some of the oil with your favorite cold pasta salad.

ALBERT LAVALLEY & SEAN WOODS & JARED FORMAN

Co-owner, Co-owner, and Chef/Co-owner, deadhorse hill

When Albert LaValley, Sean Woods, and Chef Jared Forman chose to open a restaurant on the first floor of the historic 164-year-old Bay State House Hotel in Worcester, Massachusetts, the three friends felt that they were more than ready to meet the challenge. With a limited cash flow, they decided to do most of the construction and renovations themselves. Friends and family aided a bit with finances, contributing whatever time they could to paint, build shelving, and do the various renovation tasks that were needed.

Worcester is known for its seven hills, one of which is aptly named Deadhorse Hill. At the turn of the century, the city hosted an automobile race that drew drivers from across the country. The main objective was to winningly maneuver the racecars up the hill's extraordinarily steep incline. The eatery's new owners located documentation indicating that the headquarters for this popular event was housed in the very space that they now owned. A unanimous decision was made to name the new venture "deadhorse hill" in honor of Worcester's history, revitalization, and growth. For a bit of whimsy, the owners chose to spell the restaurant's name using only small letters, an anomaly they hoped would make it easier to remember.

Each man brought his own special skills to this exciting project. Chef Forman had pursued an associate degree in chemistry and math before he realized that his real passion was food. He then attended Johnson & Wales University in Providence, Rhode Island, which is known for its culinary arts program. His culinary career was officially launched when he landed an internship at the critically acclaimed Per Se in New York City. It was there that he had the golden opportunity to learn the ins and outs of kitchen operations. After honing his cooking skills working with the talented chefs at some of New York's first-class eating establishments, Chef Forman moved on to Boston and then Worcester, Massachusetts to experience that state's restaurant scene. It was through the Boston food connection that he met his future business partner, Sean Woods.

Sean was a former guitarist for an American rock band, Open Hand. He was not just Chef Jared's neighbor; the pair had also worked together in the kitchens of two of the city's finest restaurants. Rounding out the trio was their neighbor Albert LaValley, who happened to live across the street from the two men.

Bert, with a degree in electrical engineering, worked for a large firm after graduation. He eventually founded his own business that specialized in sustainable housing. The company improved multifamily homes by making the buildings more efficient. In 2015, Jared and Sean asked their neighbor to use his engineering expertise to assist with the upgrades needed for their restaurant. They were looking for Bert to use his entrepreneurial skills and passion for reviving storied buildings and local preservation, to do the same for deadhorse hill. Believing that the idea had tremendous potential, Bert agreed and came onboard as the third member of the partnership, assuming the role of CFO.

The team rebuilt deadhorse hill from the ground up, seeking ways to preserve the integrity of the original space and its unique aspects, including breathing new life into the brick walls that had been boarded over and restoring the beautiful black tin parquet ceiling's long-lost luster. When the job was completed, the newly created restaurant was representative of historic Worcester and the revitalization and growth of that city. Having put their heart and soul into the establishment's rejuvenation, the men felt an unspoken connection to this special place.

The restaurant's bar program is run by Sean Woods. In his role as beverage director, Sean works alongside wine director and general manager Julia Auger. Julia provides a selection of wines made by smaller-grow producers from around the world. It is also her job to oversee the hospitality aspect of the business, making sure that patrons feel comfortable and welcome.

Chef Forman's goal is to make fine dining an option for everyone, hoping to inspire patrons to try new ingredients and creative dishes. As a farm-to-table restaurant, the menu changes daily; selections vary depending upon seasonality and availability. At deadhorse hill, the goal is to celebrate the seasons, whether it be with a deftly crafted cocktail made with fresh ingredients or a delicious menu selection created with locally sourced meats, cheeses, and produce.

The restaurant's relationship with Joe and Becca Pimental, from Luce Farm in Stockbridge, Vermont, is a remarkable example of the farm-to-table connection. The co-owners of deadhorse hill know that these hardworking farmers not only grow wonderful produce, but also create the highest-quality hemp and CBD products. When the farm transitioned to hemp, Chef Forman realized that this was something to take notice of and incorporate into the restaurant's menu. Always open to new ideas, in 2018, deadhorse hill hosted the first hemp dinner to be held in Massachusetts. The five-course menu, which included some of Luce Farm's cannabidiol-infused culinary products, such as CBD-infused honey and coconut oil, was a great success. Chef Forman feels that he is extremely fortunate to be able to work with a variety of incredible farms that give him the opportunity to expand his food repertoire and support their exceptional products.

In the kitchen, the staff painstakingly prepare the day's menu delights, all of which have been sourced with the utmost care and attention to detail. Their house-made pasta and ice creams are a small part of the many wonderful culinary creations that make this restaurant so remarkable. With a focus on seasonality, the folks at deadhorse hill are offering their patrons food that is approachable, affordable, and exciting, driven by a mission to make "Everyday, better!"

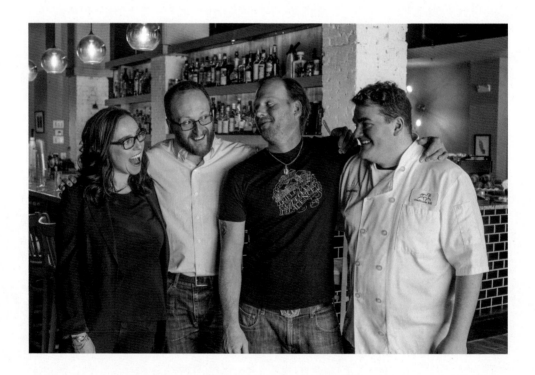

MIXED GREENS SALAD
with a Beet Vinaigrette

by CHEF JARED FORMAN, DEADHORSE HILL

SERVES 4 to 6

CHEF JARED FORMAN: Down a fairly busy road in Putnam, Connecticut, there is a small entrance to what looks like someone's driveway. Driving past the inconspicuous mailbox down a dusty road through the woods, you will come to a clearing. Then your life will be forever changed by a farming couple named Alex and Yoko of Assawaga Farm. They farm this nearly untouched land completely without the use of machines. Their backbreaking labor yields the most beautiful produce, and their constant curiosity brings us varieties of vegetables and greens that are new to our local food scene. When their baby lettuces and greens show up at the restaurant, even I can't resist making a big bowl of salad. This vinaigrette can be stored in the refrigerator to be used at any time, on everything from a smoked piece of summer bluefish, to a grass-fed strip steak, or, yes, even a big bowl of salad.

VINAIGRETTE
Makes just over 2½ cups

Note: This recipe makes more beet vinaigrette than you will need for the salad. Save the the extra and spoon it over smoked bluefish or grass-fed strip steak.

½ pound red beets, scrubbed and trimmed

1 cup water

4 ounces raspberry vinegar, store-bought or homemade (page 165)

½ teaspoon kosher salt, or to taste

¼ teaspoon freshly ground black pepper, or to taste

3 ounces extra-virgin olive oil

1 ounce full-spectrum hemp extract, preferably Luce Farm Wellness

SALAD
12 cups assorted baby lettuces, lightly packed

⅓ cup raw unsalted pistachios

GARNISHES
2 ounces soft fresh goat cheese, coarsely crumbled, or to taste

Zest of 1 lemon, about ¾ tablespoon

1. To make the beets: Cover the beets with water in a heavy-bottomed saucepan and simmer until fork-tender, about 40 minutes. Drain and set aside to cool. When cool enough to handle, remove the skins and cut into ¼-inch pieces.

2. To make the vinaigrette: Place 1 cup of the beets, 1 cup of water, vinegar, ½ teaspoon of salt, and ¼ teaspoon of pepper in a blender and blend until smooth. With the motor running, in a slow and steady stream add the oil and hemp extract and blend until emulsified. Adjust seasonings with salt and pepper to taste, if desired.

3. To make the salad: Combine the lettuces and pistachios in a large bowl and toss with ¼ cup of the vinaigrette, until evenly coated, adding more to taste, if desired. Garnish with goat cheese and lemon zest and serve.

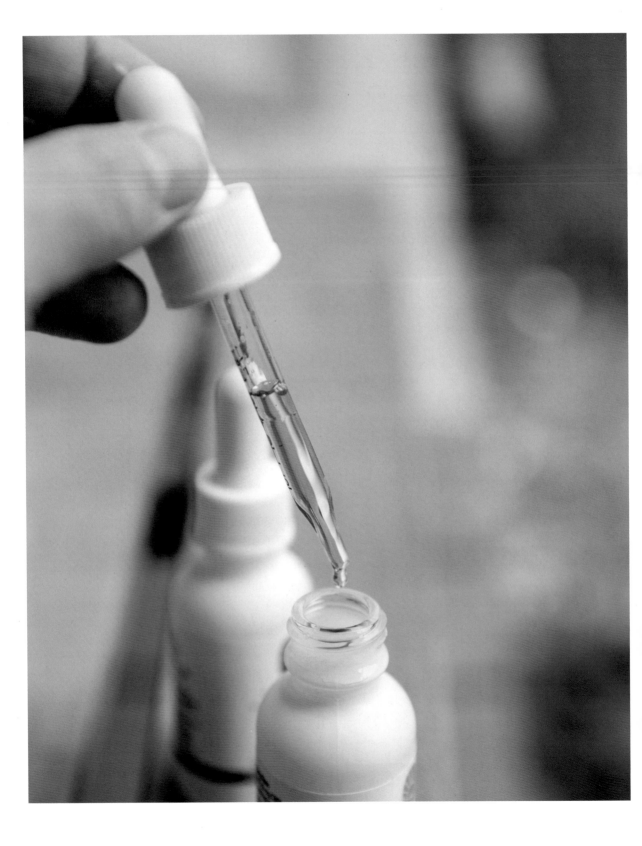

WILD MAINE BLUEBERRY SORBET

by CHEF JARED FORMAN, DEADHORSE HILL   **MAKES** approximately 3 cups

CHEF JARED FORMAN: To me, nothing screams New England more than wild Maine blueberries packed with antioxidants. Julia Auger, our general manager, grew up summering with her dad's family in Southern Maine. We buy big boxes of blueberries from Gile's Family Farm in Alfred, Maine at the end of the summer to make jams and preserves for the coming winter.

1½ cups puréed wild Maine blueberries, fresh or frozen and thawed (about 2⅛ cups or 12 ounces whole blueberries)

½ cup sugar

½ cup water

2½ tablespoons corn syrup

1 tablespoon fresh lemon juice

½ ounce (1 tablespoon) hemp oil, preferably Luce Farm Wellness

Fresh mint leaves

1. To make the sorbet base: Bring the blueberries, sugar, water, and corn syrup to a boil in a heavy-bottomed stainless-steel saucepan, stirring occasionally, over medium-high heat, about 13 minutes. Remove from heat.

2. Stir in the fresh lemon juice, then allow the base to cool to room temperature, about 2 hours.

3. Pour into a clean container, then place in the refrigerator to cool overnight.

4. Right before you plan to make the sorbet, stir in the hemp oil until well combined.

5. Pour into an ice cream maker, no more than three-quarters of the way, and process according to the manufacturer's instructions.

6. Scoop the sorbet into bowls and top each serving with a mint leaf. Serve at once.

NOTE *The corn syrup adds a creamy texture to the sorbet base.*

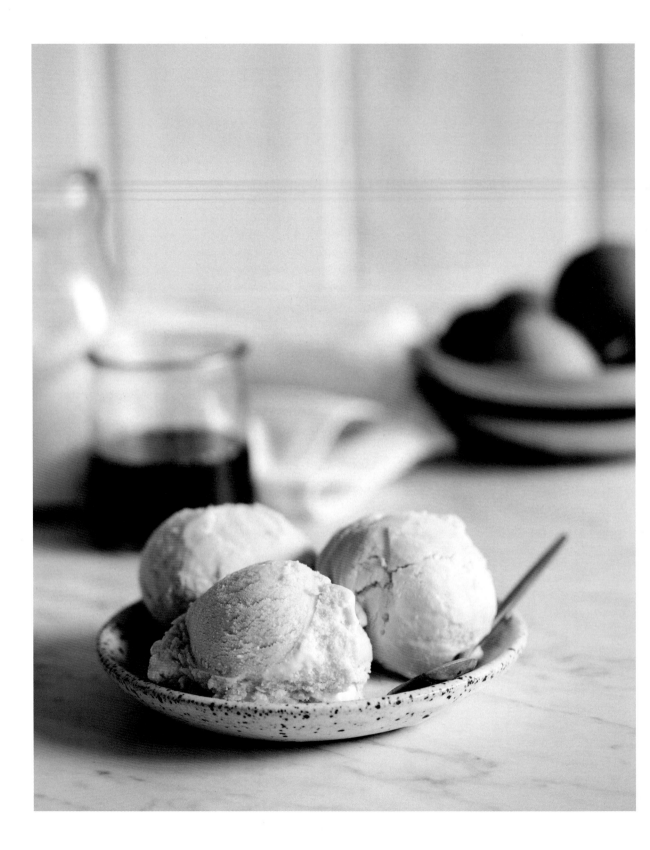

MASS MAPLE ICE CREAM

CHEF JARED FORMAN, DEADHORSE HILL **MAKES** just over 1 quart; nine ½-cup servings

CHEF JARED FORMAN: Our opening sous-chef, Robin Clark, is from Chesterfield, Massachusetts. Her grandparents' sugarhouse produces an outstandingly delicious dark maple syrup. All of the dairy that we use at the restaurant is from Cooper's Hilltop Farm. Their milk is the most flavorful I have ever tasted. We purchase farm-fresh eggs from our friends, Halley and Curtis Stillman, at StillLife Farm in Hardwick, Massachusetts. The yolks are bright orange and shine through in any recipe. The CBD products that we utilize are grown in Stockbridge, Vermont by our friends Joe and Becca Pimentel of Luce Farm Wellness who pour their heart and soul into their work. I feel extremely fortunate to be part of such a talented, hardworking community.

3 cups (14% milk fat) heavy cream, cold

1 cup whole milk

1 cup grade B dark maple syrup

1 teaspoon coarse sea salt

6 large free-range egg yolks, reserving the egg whites for another use

1 ounce full-spectrum hemp extract, preferably Luce Farm Wellness

1. To make the ice cream base: In a 2-quart heavy-bottomed saucepan, bring the heavy cream, milk, maple syrup, and salt just to the boiling point, whisking occasionally, over medium heat, about 18 to 20 minutes.

2. At the same time, in a separate bowl, whisk together the egg yolks until light and frothy.

3. Whisking continuously, add the hot cream mixture to the egg yolks, in a slow and steady stream. Return the mixture back to the saucepan and cook over medium-low heat, whisking constantly until the mixture thickens and coats the back of a wooden spoon, about 5 minutes. Note: Do not allow the ice cream base to boil.

4. Immediately remove the custard from the heat and pour through a fine-mesh strainer into a large shallow pan. The wide base and shallow sides of the pan allow the ice cream base to cool more quickly. Cover with plastic wrap, pressing directly onto the surface of the mixture, and refrigerate overnight.

5. Add the full-spectrum hemp extract and whisk the ice cream base until well combined. Pour into a cold ice cream maker bowl, filling the machine no more than three-quarters of the way, and process according to the manufacturer's instruction.

Recipe continues on next page

NOTE

Since the custard is thick, it will take a while to pass it through the sieve.

TIP

If your custard breaks, whisk the custard in the sieve, so that the clumps dissolve and relax into the custard as the material passes through the sieve.

RASPBERRY VINEGAR

by SARAH STRAUSS

MAKES approximately 1 cup plus 2 tablespoons

Raspberry vinegar is both versatile and refreshing and so easy to make! Pair with a high-quality olive oil to brighten your vinaigrettes or use in the Beet Vinaigrette (page 159).

¾ cup frozen and thawed or fresh white, golden, or red raspberries

1 cup high-quality white wine vinegar

1 tablespoon sugar

1. Place the raspberries in a mason jar and crush them with the back of a spoon to extract the juice.
2. In a small saucepan, bring the vinegar and sugar to a simmer over medium heat, stirring occasionally, until the sugar dissolves.
3. Pour the vinegar over the raspberries and cover tightly with a lid.
4. Let the vinegar rest on the counter, shaking it periodically, for 48 hours.
5. Strain the raspberry mixture through a cheesecloth-lined fine-mesh strainer, pressing on the berries with the back of a large spoon, into a clean mason jar. Gather up the corners of the cheesecloth and gently squeeze out any excess juice into the mason jar with the vinegar.
6. Store in a cool dark place.

BRYAN D'ALESSANDRO, MARK JUSTH & DAN DOLGIN

Cofounders, Eaton Hemp

The cofounders of Eaton Hemp traveled different paths during the course of their lives, until a lucky twist of fate brought the two men together. Mark Justh was raised in a small Pennsylvania farming community where he learned how to farm from his grandfather. Justh put himself through college at Princeton before beginning a career in finance which sent him across the world to live, and work, in Hong Kong for J. P. Morgan. Always wanting to return to his agricultural roots, he prepared for that day by purchasing a consortium of run-down dairy farms in the town of Eaton, in upstate New York. The next few years were spent transitioning the property into a working organic farm on which he raised livestock and grew organic forage.

Dan Dolgin, on the other hand, was raised in a suburb of New York City with no knowledge of the art of farming. He earned a master's degree in international relations from the Fletcher School of Law and Diplomacy, spending most of his career in national security. Dolgin worked at the National Counterterrorism Center until 2010, when he left government work for related projects in the private sector. In 2015, both men found themselves working together on a medical marijuana license project that unfortunately did not come to fruition. Having enjoyed the time that they worked together, the two men decided to combine their skills and collaborate on obtaining a license for Justh to grow industrial hemp on his Eaton property named JD Farms. After researching and following stringent rules and regulations, Justh was granted a license to grow the state's first legal crop of certified organic industrial hemp. His was the first license to grow hemp in New York in eighty years. Because of this milestone accomplishment Justh offered Dolgin equal co-ownership of the farm, which was happily accepted. JD Farms planted and harvested its first crop of organic industrial hemp in 2016.

With hemp in the ground, it was time to build a line of products that let whole hemp seeds shine. That's when Mark and Dan called upon seasoned brand and marketing leader Bryan D'Alessandro. Bryan spent more than fifteen years working in the brand and marketing world with CPG companies such as Unilever, J&J, PepsiCo and then launched a values-driven branding agency, The Humans. With a focus on responsible brands largely in the food and wellness space, and an avid fitness junkie and certified yoga instructor, Bryan was the perfect man for the job. Bryan, Mark, and Dan set out to build Eaton Hemp as cofounders.

Dan and Mark's farm consists of 2,500 acres of organic land nestled in the tranquil hills of Eaton, New York. Named after the area in which it is located, Eaton Hemp "operates on the principles of reverence, stewardship, and transparency." This philosophy guides its owners in their treatment of both the land and the company's employees. The team is driven by a mission to restore hemp to its rightful place in the American agricultural scene.

The farm's original plan was to grow the hemp as an organic ground cover, but nature had other plans. They quickly fell in love with the plant's nutty, buttery flavor and quickly learned that hemp is a delicious source of protein, fiber, omega fatty acids, and other heart-healthy fatty acids. To satisfy consumers' concerns, the owners of Eaton Hemp want folks to know that "hemp is legally defined as having less than 0.3 percent THC, which means that ingesting the plant in any form will *not* get you high."

One very popular product of Eaton Hemp is their organic hemp seed super snacks. With Bryan at the healm as CEO, the team worked hard to get the right products formulated and ready to market. The super snacks are made of whole hemp seeds that are free of added sugars and preservatives.

In January 2020, the company announced the launch of their USDA organic CBD line, complete with two full-spectrum, unfiltered CBD oils and a topical CBD salve. Their CBD products are made from 100 percent organic hemp which is grown, processed, and packaged in upstate New York. They infuse their CBD directly into their own 100 percent organic hemp seed oil and salve. The company has set the gold standard by releasing one of the first full-spectrum, unfiltered USDA organic CBD products on the market. The owners of Eaton Hemp believe that USDA organic certification is the best way to know the product's legitimacy. For them, "If it isn't certified, it isn't verified." To ensure optimal quality and efficacy, they leave their oil unfiltered, which maintains the full benefits of naturally occurring cannabinoids and terpenes, the way that nature intended.

Eaton Hemp's cofounders, Mark Justh, Dan Dolgin, and Bryan D'Alessandro, consider the farm's organic certification to be one of its most valued assets. The folks at the farm know that growing products organically can be more challenging but, as stewards of the land, are willing to do so rather than add chemicals as a shortcut. For them, the resulting damage to the land and the health of the folks who live there are too much of a sacrifice. Today, the farm grows a portion of the hemp used by the Eaton Hemp brand with the remaining production coming from a network of organic farmers across the United States.

VEGETARIAN STUFFED SWEET POTATOES

by EATON HEMP   **MAKES** 8 servings as an appetizer or 4 servings as a main dish

> **EATON HEMP:** Stuffed sweet potatoes with a crunch. Loaded with toasted hemp seeds, chickpeas, and red bell peppers, these are sure to hit your comfort food cravings. Be warned, these stuffed sweet potatoes are borderline addicting. But hey, who's complaining when you're getting nature's perfect omega 3 to 6 ratio, tons of fiber, and a protein punch that will keep your body feeling strong.

SWEET POTATOES

4 medium sweet potatoes, scrubbed and patted dry

Extra-virgin olive oil, as needed

Salt and freshly ground black pepper

CHICKPEA FILLING

1 (15.5-ounce) can cooked chickpeas, drained, rinsed, and patted dry

1.34-ounce package of Eaton Hemp Ancho Chili BBQ Toasted Hemp Seeds

2 scallions, chopped

1 medium red bell pepper, seeded and coarsely chopped

2 tablespoons extra-virgin olive oil

1 teaspoon garlic salt

1 teaspoon onion powder

1 teaspoon turmeric powder or smoked paprika

½ teaspoon chili flakes, optional

¼ teaspoon ground cumin

Salt and freshly ground black pepper

GARNISHES

¼ cup vegan sour cream

3 tablespoons fresh chopped cilantro, or to taste

1. To bake the sweet potatoes: Preheat the oven to 425°F. Line a baking sheet with foil. Set aside. Rub the potatoes with the oil. Place the potatoes on the prepared baking sheet. Season with salt and pepper to taste. Using the tines of a fork, pierce the potatoes 6 to 8 times. Bake until the potatoes are fork-tender, about 1 hour, depending on the size of the potatoes.

2. To make the chickpea filling: Thirty minutes before the sweet potatoes are done, roast the chickpeas on another oven rack with the potatoes. Line a quarter-size rimmed baking sheet with parchment paper or foil. Set aside. In a medium bowl, combine the chickpeas, hemp seeds, scallions, red bell pepper, olive oil, garlic salt, onion powder, turmeric, chili flakes, and cumin. Adjust seasonings with salt and pepper to taste. Spread the chickpeas on the prepared baking sheet in a single layer. Roast, and using a spatula, gently toss the chickpeas on the baking sheet every 10 minutes, until slightly crispy on the outside and still soft on the inside, about 30 minutes.

3. To assemble: Once the potatoes are cool enough to handle, slice the potatoes down the middle. Fluff the flesh with a fork. Top with the chickpea mixture. Adjust seasoning with salt and pepper to taste. Garnish with a dollop of sour cream and sprinkles of cilantro. Serve at once.

Many of us strive to eat healthy, or at least make an attempt to demonstrate this desire, by serving certain foods to our families and guests that are known for their nutritional benefits. Enter the sweet potato, a colorful addition to any dinner table with its white, cream, yellow, orange, or deep purple flesh. Although the sweet potato can be found in most markets year-round, it is in season during the months of November and December.

This vegetable is a dicotyledonous plant that belongs to the bindweed or morning glory family. Scientists have researched the sweet potato and believe that it was domesticated in Central America thousands of years ago, making it one of the oldest vegetables in cultivation. It is said that Christopher Columbus brought sweet potatoes back to Europe after his first trip to the Americas. Because of its hardiness and adaptability, the sweet potato is now grown in more developing countries than any other root vegetable.

There are roughly four hundred varieties of this root vegetable. Some of them are shaped like white potatoes, and others are long and tapered. The best-known sweet potatoes are the orange- or red-skinned with orangey flesh. The intensity of this orange flesh corresponds to its beta-carotene content. Our bodies produce vitamin A, a strong antioxidant, from this beta-carotene. Sweet potatoes with white, cream, or orange skin are most commonly found in grocery stores. The purple-skinned variety, with its antioxidant and anti-inflammatory properties and purple flesh, is a rare find. It is interesting to note that you cannot always tell a sweet potato's flesh color by its outer skin.

Buying certified organically grown sweet potatoes reduces the possibility of their having been exposed to pesticides and heavy metals. To find organically grown products in supermarkets, look for the USDA logo. You can eat the entire potato, including the skin, of those that are organically grown. Remove the skin of the nonorganic variety, as it may have been treated with dye or wax.

There are two groups of sweet potatoes as determined by texture when cooked. The first type is firm, dry, and mealy while the second is soft and moist. Over one million tons of sweet potatoes are grown in the United States each year. Half of these come from the southern states, especially North Carolina.

Sweet potatoes are often mistaken for yams, but they are not the same. Yams come from the yam plant and have white flesh that is dry and starchy. They are usually larger than sweet potatoes. Commercial production of yams in the United States is rare; even though the sign in the grocery store may say "Yams," you are probably buying sweet potatoes. When shopping for yams, it is best to go to a specialty store that carries foods from tropical countries.

Sweet potatoes are a good source of vitamins A and C, manganese, copper, pantothenic acid, and vitamin B6. They also supply potassium, dietary fiber, niacin, and vitamins B1 and B2, as well as phosphorous. When trying to decide between a sweet potato that has more fiber and vitamin A, or the traditional white potato that is higher in essential minerals, it really all boils down to personal preference. Both have the same number of carbs per serving. Choose sweet potatoes that are firm, free of cracks, bruises, and soft spots. Avoid those that are displayed in the refrigerated section of your produce aisle, because cold temperatures tend to alter their unique flavor.

There are a number of ways to prepare sweet potatoes, from simply baking and adding cinnamon and nutmeg to boiling and mashing with a bit of butter. Cutting the potato into ½-inch slices and quickly steaming for 7 minutes is the perfect way to bring out its flavor and maximize nutritional value. Toss a few cubed and chilled potatoes into your salad to add a distinctive touch. Try them in casseroles, pot pies, and soups in lieu of the traditional version.

The potato's sweetness lends itself to the creation of heavenly desserts, sweet potato pie being a mouthwatering favorite. Feeling adventurous? Make that a sweet potato meringue pie, or tantalizing sweet potato tart decorated with a sea salt caramel drizzle. Ending the meal with this sort of scrumptious flourish might even get folks to help with the dishes, especially if you offer them a sweet potato doughnut as a reward!

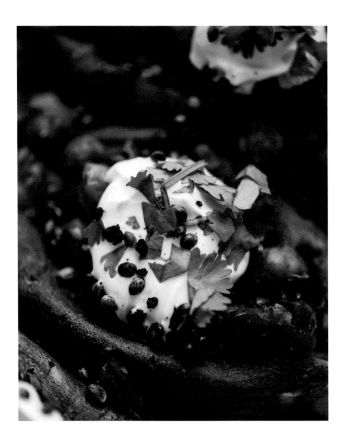

SPICY MAPLE CAULIFLOWER "WINGS"

with a Toasted Hemp Seed Coating

by EATON HEMP

MAKES 4 to 6 serving as an appetizer

EATON HEMP: There's a new Buffalo dish in town for our vegan friends! Get ready to indulge in this classic American dish without the need for deep-frying or unhealthy oils. The crust is made with our maple-flavored toasted hemp seeds, creating a unique flavor profile and the perfect crunch. You'll be asking your local wing spot to start making these bad boys.

BATTER

1½ cups all-purpose flour

1½ teaspoons garlic powder

1½ teaspoons paprika

1½ teaspoons onion powder

1 teaspoon freshly ground black pepper

1 teaspoon fine sea salt

1⅛ cups unsweetened soy milk

⅔ cup water

CAULIFLOWER

1 large (about 2 pounds 4 ounces) cauliflower head, cut into medium florets (about 8 cups)

SPICY MAPLE SAUCE

Makes about 1⅛ cups

1 tablespoon cornstarch

1 tablespoon water

3 tablespoons unsalted vegan butter

¼ cup maple syrup, dark

4 tablespoons hot sauce, such as sriracha

2 tablespoons soy sauce

1. Preheat the oven to 400°F. Line 3 baking sheets with parchment paper. Set aside.
2. To make the batter: In a large bowl, stir together all the dry ingredients. Slowly add the soy milk and water, whisking until completely smooth.
3. Add all of the cauliflower florets into the batter at once, tossing to coat evenly, shaking off the excess batter. Using tongs, transfer the florets to a cooling rack over one of the prepared baking sheets to drain off the remaining excess batter, about 5 minutes.
4. Evenly divide the florets on the remaining 2 prepared baking sheets. Bake in the oven for 25 minutes, flipping the florets over, using tongs, halfway through.
5. While the florets are baking, start making the spicy maple sauce 10 minutes before the cauliflower florets are done. Place the cornstarch and water in a small bowl. Using a fork, whisk together until completely smooth.
6. Melt the butter in a small saucepan over medium heat. Add the maple syrup, hot sauce, soy sauce, and apple cider vinegar, whisking until well combined. Whisking constantly, add the cornstarch and cook until the sauce thickens to a gel, about 6 minutes. Remove from the stove top and fold in the hemp seeds. Season with salt and pepper to taste. Set aside.
7. Reduce the oven temperature to 350°F.

Ingredients list continues on page 173

Recipe continues on page 173

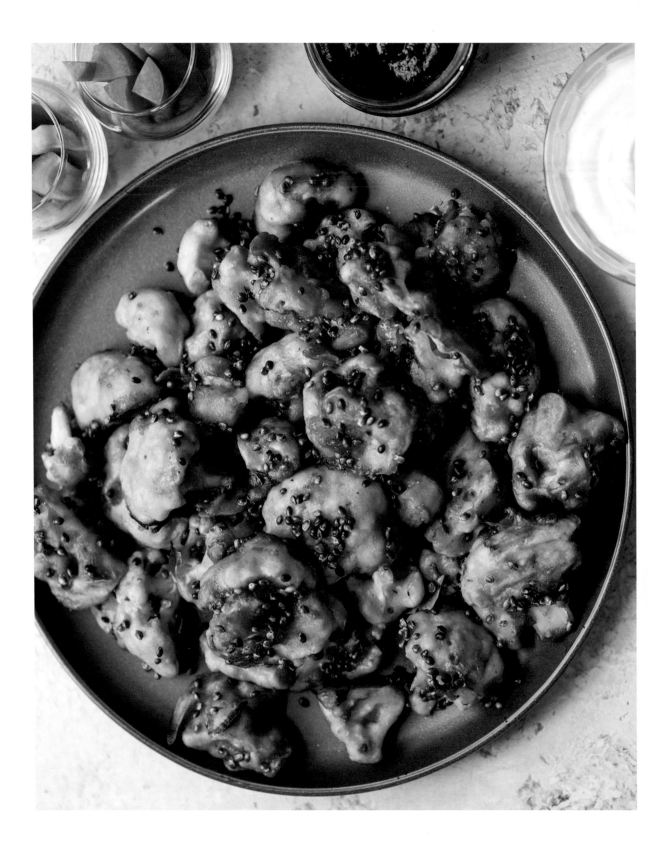

1 tablespoon apple cider vinegar

½ cup hemp seeds, preferably two 1.34-ounce packages of Eaton Hemp Himalayan Pink Salt Toasted Hemp Seeds

GARNISH

2 scallions, trimmed, thinly sliced on the bias into rings, white and green parts, for garnish

FOR SERVING

3 large carrots, peeled and cut into sticks

3 large celery stalks, trimmed and cut into sticks

Vegan sour cream

Vegan Ranch dressing

8. Using tongs, dip each floret into the spicy maple sauce and return to the baking sheets. Using a pastry brush, brush the extra hemp seeds remaining in the bottom of the saucepan on the florets. Return the baking sheets to the oven and bake until the florets are golden around the edges, about 25 minutes.

9. Garnish with scallions. Serve immediately with carrot and celery sticks, sour cream, and ranch dressing alongside.

WILD RICE
with Roasted Butternut Squash
and Ancho Chili BBQ Toasted Hemp Seed Tofu

by EATON HEMP   **MAKES** about 3 quarts; seven 1½ cup-sized servings

EATON HEMP: A vegetarian's best friend. This delicious whole-grain salad is made with wild rice, roasted butternut squash, and our Ancho Chilli BBQ Toasted Hemp Seeds. The perfect combo of sweet and savory, with tons of health benefits. Get ready to add a serious protein punch to your favorite bowl!

TOFU

1 (14-ounce) container organic tofu, extra-firm

WILD RICE

Makes 3½ cups cooked rice

Note: Thirty minutes before you plan to start the wild rice, start pressing the tofu.

2 cups organic wild rice

4 cups vegetable stock

¾ teaspoon salt

ROASTED BUTTERNUT SQUASH

1 (about 1½ pounds) butternut squash

2 tablespoons extra-virgin olive oil, divided

Sea salt, extra-fine grain

ANCHO CHILI BBQ TOASTED HEMP SEED MARINADE

¼ cup soy or organic tamari sauce

2 tablespoons extra-virgin olive oil

1 teaspoon smoked paprika

½ teaspoon chipotle powder

1. Line two baking sheets with parchment paper. Set aside.
2. To prepare the tofu: Pat the tofu dry with paper towels. Slice the tofu lengthwise into **7** even slabs, about ¾ inch to 1 inch thick. Place the tofu slabs on a paper-towel-lined plate. Set a heavy frying pan on top of tofu and weigh it down with a heavy can or brick for 30 minutes. Remove the weight and discard any liquid from the tofu.
3. While the tofu is being pressed, start the wild rice. Place the wild rice in a fine-mesh strainer, then put the strainer over a bowl. Fill the bowl with cold water and let the rice soak for 5 minutes. Repeat this process 2 more times, draining off any excess water with each soak. Place the rice, vegetable stock, and salt in a large saucepan. Bring to a boil over medium-high heat. Reduce the heat to a simmer; cover and cook, checking occasionally, until tender and some of the grains have burst open, about 50 minutes.
4. Preheat the oven to 400°F.
5. While the rice is cooking, prepare the squash. Using a sharp knife, remove both ends of the squash and discard. With a sharp vegetable peeler, remove the skins and discard. Cut the squash in half lengthwise and scoop out the seeds and strings, then cut into ½-inch rings. Slice the rings into long rectangles and then into ½-inch cubes. Note: You will have about 4 cups of cubed butternut squash. Transfer the squash cubes to a prepared baking sheet and toss with 1 tablespoon olive oil. Season with salt and set aside.

½ teaspoon garlic powder

½ teaspoon onion powder

½ teaspoon finely ground sea salt

⅛ teaspoon freshly ground black pepper

⅔ cup almond flour

½ cup Ancho Chili BBQ Toasted Hemp Seeds, preferably Eaton Hemp

VEGETABLES

1 small red onion, peeled, trimmed, and thinly sliced into half-moons

½ medium leek, white and light green parts only, trimmed and rinsed thoroughly, thinly sliced into half-moons

1 medium carrot, peeled and cut into tiny cubes (brunoise cut)

HERB MIX

1½ tablespoons fresh minced parsley leaves, or to taste

1½ tablespoons fresh minced cilantro leaves, or to taste

1½ tablespoons fresh minced basil leaves, or to taste

6. To make the Ancho Chili BBQ Toasted Hemp Seed Marinade: In a medium shallow bowl, stir together the soy sauce, olive oil, smoked paprika, chipotle powder, garlic powder, onion powder, sea salt, and pepper until well combined. Set aside.

7. In a second shallow bowl, whisk together the almond flour and toasted hemp seeds. Set aside.

8. Cut the pressed tofu into 1-inch cubes. Arrange the tofu cubes in a single layer on the remaining prepared baking sheet. Add half of the tofu cubes to the first bowl of soy sauce mixture and allow to marinate for 10 minutes, turning them halfway through soaking. Using a slotted spoon transfer the marinated cubes to the second bowl with the almond flour mixture, gently tossing until well coated, shaking off any excess. Repeat with the remaining cubes. Arrange the tofu cubes in an even layer on the same baking sheet. Pour any leftover hemp seed rub in the bottom of the coating bowl over the tofu cubes.

9. Roast the butternut squash and tofu cubes at the same time but on different racks. Roast the butternut squash until fork-tender, about 25 minutes. Bake the tofu until the cubes are golden brown and slightly puffed, about 25 minutes.

10. While the squash and tofu are roasting, transfer the cooked rice to a fine-mesh strainer, to drain off any excess liquid, reserving the wild rice stock for another use. Place the rice in a bowl and fluff with a fork, adjusting the seasoning with salt.

11. To prepare the vegetables: Start sautéing the vegetables 10 minutes before the squash and tofu are done baking. Heat the remaining 1 tablespoon of olive oil in a skillet over medium heat. Add the onions, leeks, and carrots and sauté, stirring frequently, until onions and leeks are soft and translucent, about 7 minutes. Season with salt to taste.

12. To assemble: Transfer the squash, onions, leeks, and carrots to the bowl with the wild rice, tossing until well combined. Fold in the herbs until well combined. Adjust seasonings with salt to taste. Gently scatter the tofu cubes on top. Serve at once.

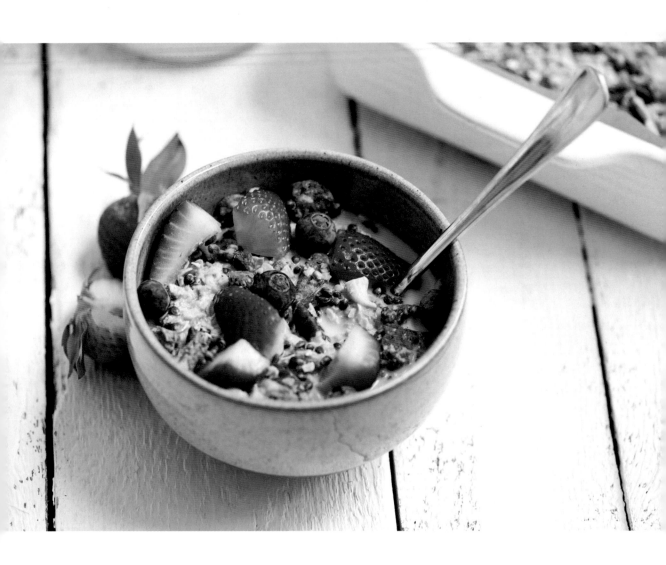

APPLE WALNUT CINNAMON BAKED GRANOLA

by EATON HEMP

MAKES approximately 10 cups, depending on the size of the granola pieces

EATON HEMP: Craving sweets without the guilt? This Apple Walnut Cinnamon Baked Granola recipe will leave your taste buds in awe while keeping your body at peak performance.

2 cups old-fashioned rolled oats

2 (4-ounce) packages Eaton Hemp Walnut Super Squares, broken into ¼-inch pieces

½ cup toasted hemp seeds, preferably Eaton Hemp Maple Cinnamon

1 cup mixed coarsely chopped raw nuts, such as pecans or walnuts

⅓ cup pepitas

⅓ cup sweet shredded coconut

½ teaspoon fine-grain sea salt

½ cup pure maple syrup

⅓ cup melted refined coconut oil

1. Arrange a rack in the middle of the oven. Preheat the oven to 350°F. Line a half-sheet rimmed baking sheet with parchment paper. Set aside.

2. In a medium mixing bowl, combine the oats, square pieces, hemp seeds, nuts, pepitas, shredded coconut, and salt, mixing until well combined.

3. Pour in the maple syrup and coconut oil, tossing until evenly coated.

4. Pour the granola onto the prepared baking sheet and spread the granola out into an even layer. Using a spatula, press the granola down into the pan or place the bottom of a second baking sheet on top of the granola and press the two sheets together to compress the granola. Note: It is important to have the granola tightly packed to help it stick together.

5. Bake until lightly golden, about 15 minutes, stirring and recompressing only once halfway through cooking.

6. Remove from the oven and let cool completely on the baking sheet for about 1 hour, then break the granola into desired-size pieces. Note: If you enjoy large clumps of granola, press it down once more before it cools to help it clump together.

7. The granola can be stored in an airtight container, in a cool dark place, for up to one week. Remember to label the container with the date and contents.

8. To serve: Enjoy the granola with milk and fresh blueberries and strawberries, or scattered over yogurt, or use as an ice cream topping.

BEN BANKS-DOBSON, MELANY DOBSON & FREYA DOBSON

Founders, Hudson Hemp

Hudson Hemp is a company that cultivates and produces hemp-based products for medicinal and culinary use. It is located on a 2,700-acre organic, regenerative farm in New York's Hudson Valley. Regenerative farming focuses on topsoil regeneration and revitalization, with attention to water management and fertilizer use. In 2013 Hudson Hemp's farms, Old Mud Creek and Stone House Grain, began transitioning to certified organic and non-GMO practices. Stone House Grain grows a variety of certified organic and non-GMO grains for milling, animal feeds, cover crops, malting, medicinal, and culinary use, while Old Mud Creek is used primarily for hemp production. The folks at Hudson Hemp know that healthy soil produces clean food (minimally processed) which improves health benefits and the betterment of our planet, people, and society.

Ben Banks-Dobson cofounded Hudson Hemp in 2017 with Abby Rockefeller. Dobson's sisters, Melany and Freya, soon were asked to became part of this venture. The company was one of the first in New York State to receive a permit to cultivate hemp. Its founders know that growing hemp, using regenerative and organic practices, improves the ability to clean the soil, sequester carbon, and prevent erosion, all of which are paramount to supporting healthy life on earth. The folks at Hudson Hemp work together to enrich the earth within the boundaries of the agricultural and industrial system.

The business has created their own in-house hemp extract (CBD) product line called Treaty. The Hudson Hemp team worked with the International Cannabis and Cannabinoids Institute (ICCI) to research and verify Treaty's formulations. These formulas were developed according to nature's prescription to help users stay calm, find focus, recover better, and maintain balance.

Treaty products are inspired by the Hudson Valley landscape, using a selection of bioregional plants that thrive together in nature and on a molecular basis in the body. The tinctures are made with Hudson Hemp's broad-spectrum hemp extract (CBD) and a blend of the highest quality botanicals ingredients. The bioregional ingredient palette is designed to regenerate local supply chains. The manufacturing of Treaty involves a monthlong extraction that utilizes both certified organic grain alcohol and oil infusion (maceration). The extraction process distills different chemical compounds from the plant, preserving its ingredients, integrity, and potency.

The end product is designed to be taken sublingually, by using a dropper to dispense the recommended dosage into the mouth, allowing the product to melt beneath the tongue before being swallowed. All of Hudson Hemp's products are tested by a third-party lab at various stages (from cultivation to processing, to manufacturing, to sales) to comply with state and federal guidelines.

With the passage of the 2018 Farm Bill, hemp is now a legal category of cannabis. It contains below 0.3 percent THC and cannot get you high, whereas marijuana refers to plants that contain higher amounts of THC. Hemp has been grown for over 60,000 years. When it comes to food, fiber, textiles, and medicine, hemp offers a healthy alternative to traditional practices.

The team at Hudson Hemp strongly believe that farmers are the caregivers of the land and producers of food. Chefs have the ability to bring that food into culture and elevate conversations around the source of that food. Farmers and chefs can break the stigma around cannabis. Many people still only think of cannabis as a drug, in isolation from society, and not as an agriculture crop. Eating is an incredible opportunity to open folks' minds to all cannabis can do. It is essential to engage with the plant in ways that bring people together and stimulate conversations. Farmers and chefs need to be at the forefront of this movement; one cannot exist without the other, and they play equally important parts.

HUDSON HEMP

There is a distinction between infusing food with CBD and cooking with the raw hemp plant. CBDa is one of the compounds present in the leaves and flowers of the hemp plant. CBDa turns into CBD only after the leaves and flowers have been decarboxylated by a heating process. Research and testing have shown that raw cannabinoids have excellent medicinal effects. Raw hemp contains cannabinoid acids, antioxidants, magnesium, potassium, calcium, iron, zinc, phosphorus, and fiber. It is rich in polyphenols, omega-3 and omega-6 fatty acids, and digestible globular proteins.

All mammals have an endocannabinoid system. Endocannabinoids bind to different receptors in the body and help regulate the immune and nervous systems and bone function. Consuming raw cannabinoids can bring your endocannabinoid system back to optimal function and improve conditions associated with the other systems.

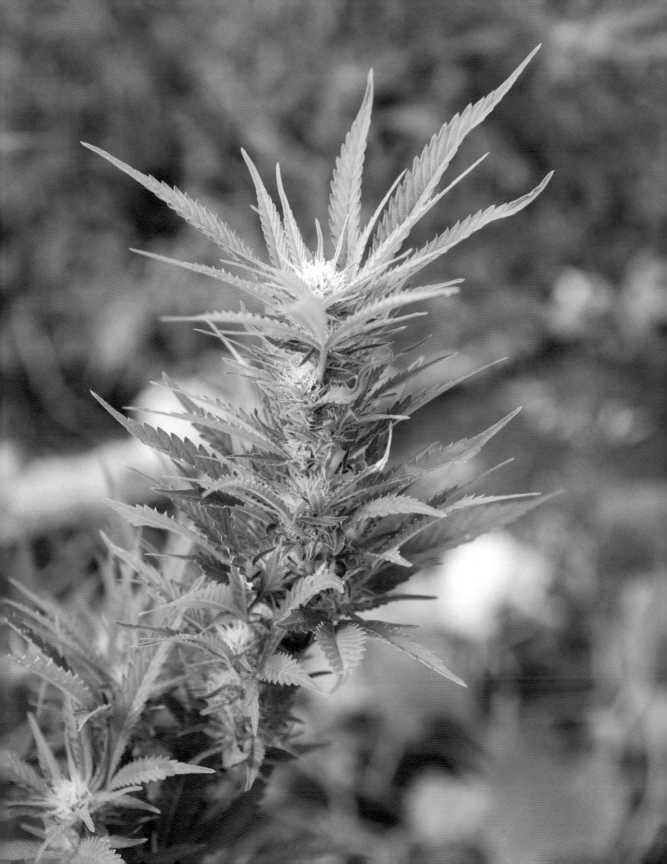

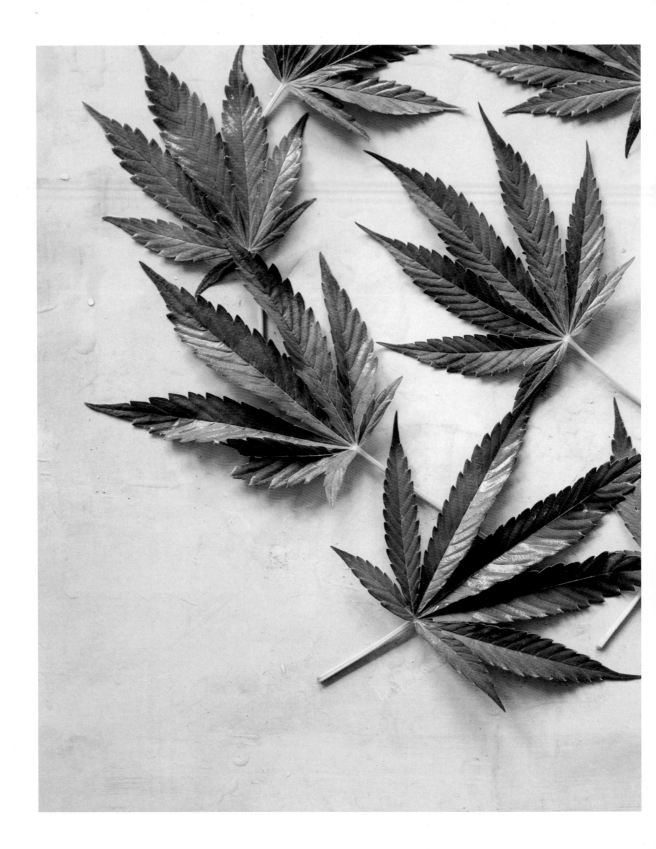

FRESH PRESSED HEMP JUICE

by HUDSON HEMP

MAKES approximately 4 cups

> **FREYA DOBSON:** The hemp recipes are inspired by summer days on the farm. The acres of hemp filling the landscape with lush greens, the aromatics filling the air. Many days I would find myself walking the fields and giving attention to the plants by pruning them, allowing each one to reach its full potential. A deep connection was made by doing this work: no part of the plant should go to waste. Soon I began experimenting with the leaves in some of my favorite recipes. The pesto and fresh pressed juice worked out beautifully because of the bounty of fruits and vegetables on the farm. My goal through sharing these recipes is to inspire people to think about food as medicine and to begin healing themselves through cooking and eating.

4 medium organic cucumbers, ends removed and discarded, cut into large chunks

2 cups organic hemp leaves, lightly packed

4 organic celery ribs, trimmed

1 large organic apple, cored and quartered

1 organic lemon or lime, peeled, ends removed, and cut into chunks

1-inch piece of fresh ginger, peeled and chopped

Honey, optional

GARNISH
Cucumber wheels, optional

1. Run the produce, one at a time, through a cold press juicer. Pour into glasses, adjust sweetness with honey if desired, and garnish with a cucumber wheel. Serve at once.

NOTES

For a sweeter juice, purchase Red Delicious, Gala, or Golden Delicious apples. For those desiring a tarter juice, use Granny Smith or Pink Lady apples.

A cold-press juicer (a.k.a. masticating juicer) is recommended for this juice because it doesn't generate as much heat as a centrifugal juicer, which may convert the CBDa to CBD. The juice is best enjoyed right away; however, leftovers can be refrigerated for up to 3 days or frozen into ice cubes and stored in the freezer for several months. If refrigerating, store in mason jars with tight-sealing lids and shake well before drinking.

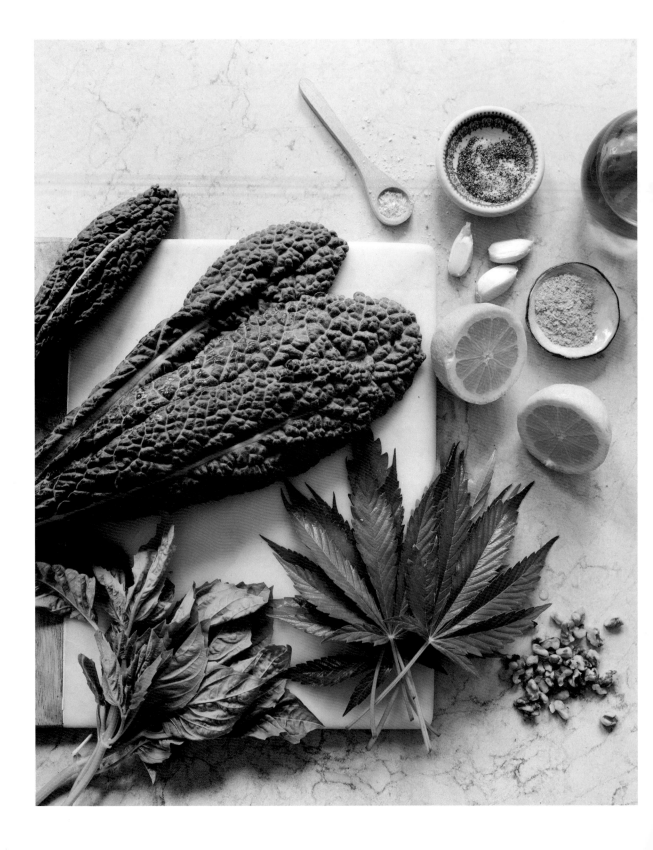

RAW HEMP LEAF PESTO

by HUDSON HEMP

MAKES approximately 1 cup

> **FREYA DOBSON:** For those wishing to add CBD oil to the pesto, I recommend adding 10 milligrams of Treaty Balance per serving. Treaty's parent company is Hudson Hemp. The Balance formula includes only the farm's proprietary organic hemp, grown and processed at our regenerative farm. It's the simplest formula for experiencing the benefits of broad-spectrum hemp extract in isolation.

3 or 4 medium cloves garlic, peeled and coarsely chopped

3 tablespoons organic raw pine nuts, walnuts, or cashews

1 cup fresh organic hemp leaves, woody stems removed, lightly packed

1 cup fresh organic basil leaves, lightly packed

½ cup coarsely chopped organic kale leaves, stems and inner ribs removed and discarded, lightly packed

Juice of 1 lemon, or to taste

½ cup extra-virgin olive oil or hemp seed oil

3 tablespoons nutritional yeast, or to taste

Pink Himalayan sea salt, fine-grain

Freshly ground black pepper

1. Process the garlic and pine nuts in a food processor until minced. Add the hemp, basil, kale, and 2 tablespoons of the lemon juice, and process until well combined. While the food processor is running, slowly add the oil in a steady stream until well blended, scraping down the sides of the bowl as needed.

2. Spoon the pesto into a decorative bowl and fold in the nutritional yeast. Adjust seasonings with additional lemon juice and nutritional yeast, if desired. Season with salt and pepper to taste. To serve, spread on toasted bread rounds topped with sliced cherry tomatoes or lightly drizzle pesto over and around your favorite eggs. Note: See fried egg recipe (page 186).

NOTES

The pesto can be stored in the refrigerator, covered with a thin layer of olive oil, for up to 2 days.

Raw hemp leaves are rich in cannabidiolic acid (CBDa). It is a nonintoxicating, inactive cannabinoid. When CBDa is heated (activated) through a process known as decarboxylation, it converts to CBD. Since this recipe uses raw hemp leaves that have not gone through a decarboxylation or extraction process, CBD is not present.

FRIED EGGS
with Raw Hemp Leaf Pesto

4 tablespoons unsalted butter

4 extra-large eggs

4 toasted baguette slices, about ¼ inch thick

Raw Hemp Leaf Pesto

1. Melt the butter in a nonstick skillet over medium heat. Fry the eggs, cooking two at a time, until the yolks are runny, or until desired doneness is achieved. Serve over toasted bread. Top with Raw Hemp Leaf Pesto (page 185).

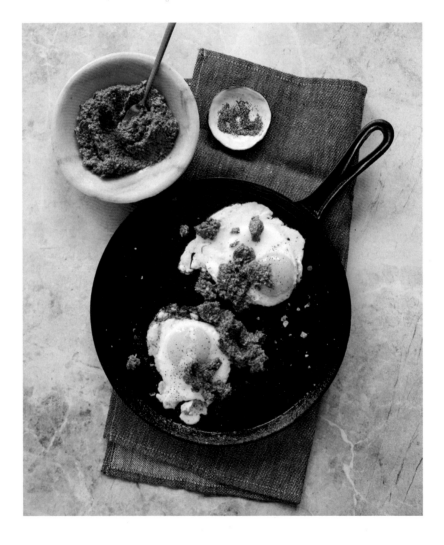

HEMP SEED CRUNCH

JOSEPHINE PROUL, LOCAL 111 RESTAURANT   **MAKES** approximately 1½ quarts

This makes more hemp seed crunch than you will need for the Sunflower Seed and Tahini Goat Milk Yogurt (page 189). Save the extra and sprinkle it over your favorite salad, ice cream, or oatmeal. The crunch can be stored in an airtight container, in a cool dark place, for up to one month.

½ cup unsalted butter, softened

¼ cup brown sugar, firmly packed

¾ cup organic dark rye flour

1 cup hemp seeds

¼ cup sunflower seeds, hulled

⅛ cup old-fashioned rolled oats

½ heaping teaspoon of chopped thyme leaves, about 2 thyme sprigs

½ teaspoon ground caraway seeds

¼ teaspoon kosher salt, or to taste

⅛ teaspoon freshly ground black pepper, or to taste

1. Arrange a rack in the middle of the oven. Preheat the oven to 325°F. Line a rimmed baking sheet with parchment paper.

2. To make the dough: In the bowl of a stand mixer, cream together the butter and sugar on medium speed until light and fluffy, about 3 minutes. Add the flour and mix on medium-low speed until just combined.

3. In a separate bowl, combine the hemp seeds, sunflower seeds, oats, thyme, and caraway seeds, salt, and pepper. Add the hemp seed mixture to the dough and mix on medium-low speed until combined, about 3 minutes. Note: If you do not own a stand mixer, you may also mix with a sturdy spoon.

4. Using your hands, gently press the dough out to the edges of the prepared baking sheet, then flatten it out into an even layer with the back of the spatula.

5. Bake until lightly golden brown, about 15 to 20 minutes.

6. Remove from the oven and let cool completely on the baking sheet, about 20 minutes. Once cooled, break into desired piece sizes.

7. To serve: Scatter the hemp seed crunch over the Sunflower Seed and Tahini Goat Milk Yogurt (page 189).

TIP

The bottom of the crunch gets browner much faster than the top. To avoid overcooking, when it's almost done, break off a small corner and peek underneath to check for doneness. Once cooled, the crunch will be broken up into pieces, so this will not harm the final product.

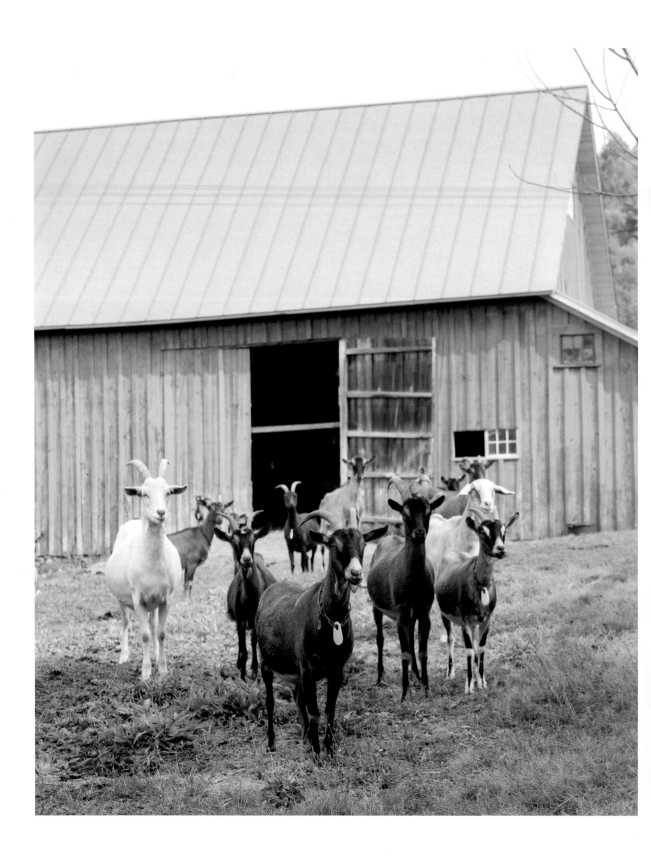

SUNFLOWER SEED AND TAHINI GOAT MILK YOGURT

with Hemp Seed Crunch

by JOSEPHINE PROUL, LOCAL 111 RESTAURANT

MAKES 6 servings

This savory yogurt is all about textures and depth of flavor. Each component adds a different texture and flavor, from the creamy, tangy goat milk yogurt to the nuttiness from the Hemp Seed Crunch (page 187) to the tender texture of the sunflower seeds.

SUNFLOWER-TAHINI PURÉE

1 cup sunflower seeds, hulled

½ cup tahini

3 tablespoons THC-infused olive oil, homemade or store-bought

¼ teaspoon kosher salt, or to taste

⅛ teaspoon freshly ground black pepper, or to taste

YOGURT

1 quart grass-fed goat milk yogurt

Hemp seed crunch (page 187)

GARNISHES

Fresh mint leaves, thinly sliced

Pomegranate seeds

1. To make the sunflower-tahini purée: In a blender, combine the sunflower seeds, tahini, olive oil, salt, and pepper until smooth.
2. Place the yogurt in a mixing bowl and fold in the sunflower-tahini purée. Adjust seasonings with salt and pepper to taste. Top with Hemp Seed Crunch (page 187). Garnish with mint and pomegranate seeds.

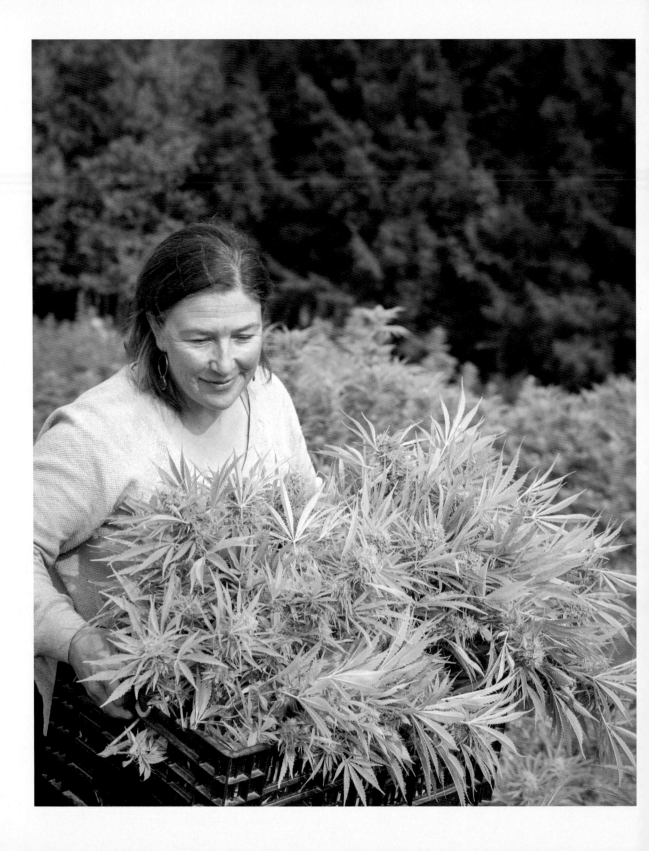

JOE & REBECCA PIMENTEL

Founders, Luce Farm Wellness

When Joe and Rebecca Pimentel visited Luce Farm Wellness, nestled on the rolling hills of rural Stockbridge, Vermont, it was love at first sight. The two organic vegetable farmers had always dreamed of owning an antique hill farm. They were delighted to learn that the 1820s farmhouse, with its cluster of barns and accompanying 206 acres, was for sale. Drawn to the beauty of the land, the couple frequently returned to this peaceful place. It was during one of their visits that they met and became friends with Leah, the farm's caretaker. As time passed, they shared with her their dream of one day owning the picturesque farm. It came as a complete surprise when their realtor told them that Luce Farm's owner knew of their interest in the property. Soon after, they were amazed to learn that their new friend, Leah, was the farm's owner. With her approval, the sale was a done deal and the Pimentels' dream had become a reality.

The Pimentel family moved into their new home on Thanksgiving Day, 2015. As they organized a business plan, the couple soon realized that organic vegetable farming, with its low profit level, was no longer going to work for them. It didn't take long before they changed direction and decided hemp was the new way to go. Joe was familiar with the cannabis debate in Montpelier, Vermont, which had piqued his interest in CBD. During the ensuing eight months, he made it his mission to learn as much as possible about all aspects of the hemp industry.

In 2016, the couple, partnering with a group of hemp entrepreneurs, planted an experimental 100-plant patch of the product in the farm's greenhouse. The goal was to learn how to grow, process, and market hemp. By the winter of 2017, Rebecca and Joe were experimenting with the beautiful crop they had grown, working with the hemp flowers and developing recipes. They shared the products that they produced with friends and family and were delighted with the positive feedback.

Rebecca and Joe grow organic sustainable hemp on a diverse farm, allowing them to rotationally graze their livestock and interchange pastures with cover crops and hemp fields. Their hemp is *Cannabis sativa* that has been bred to produce high concentrations of CBD and low concentrations of THC, therefore classifying it as hemp. All the hemp plants are raised from seed and then transplanted into fertile fields enriched with manure from the farm's flocks of poultry and herds of goats. The seeds are started under grow lights in April and planted in late June, with harvesting, drying, and trimming of flowers from mid-September through October. Each plant is individually hand-pruned during the growing season to increase and concentrate its terpene and cannabinoid content.

During harvest, the flowers are removed and carefully dried. Joe takes the dried flower buds to a CO_2 extraction facility in Northern Vermont that processes the full-spectrum oil. An environmentally friendly supercritical CO_2 method is then used to extract the terpenes, cannabinoids, and other nutritional compounds. The result is a terpene- and cannabinoid-rich CBD oil that is then analyzed and assayed for THC (less than 0.3%) as well as CBD content. Legal hemp products must have less than 0.3 percent THC. The oil is then sent to an independent lab in Massachusetts for third-party testing. That CBD oil goes into the products that the team manufactures in their state-inspected commercial kitchen in downtown Bethel, Vermont.

It is Rebecca's job to create new products and handle e-commerce while Joe focuses on supply management, research, and development. Luce Farm Wellness currently makes nine CBD & hemp–infused products that include original and peppermint-flavored organic full-spectrum hemp extract and CBD oil, hemp-infused honey, hemp-infused CBD coconut oil, and topical hemp-infused balms blended with farm-grown botanicals. Their product line is based on wellness, requiring only the best-quality organic hemp.

The farm is now growing more than double the number of hemp plants than in past years; still, they are unable to keep up with the requests for their hemp-infused products. To meet the growing demand, the Pimentels have formed Luce Farm Collective. This is a group of eight selected growers who share the farm's values and commitment to sustainability. These growers are supplied with seeds, or plants, which must be grown to Luce's standards. They are encouraged to start with a small number of plants, enabling them to provide the best care possible. Their goal is to grow the healthiest and highest quality hemp without using shortcuts or gimmicks.

Luce Farm Wellness is a values-based botanical wellness business. They use glass and metal packaging, not plastic. Their farm team and production crew employ thirty people, a mix of full and part-time help. Its owners are proud to state that 75 percent of their employees are women.

Joe and Rebecca Pimentel are excited about hemp's potential to revive American farming. They are convinced that this plant can be a winner for local farmers across the United States. Every decision that the owners of Luce Farm Wellness make revolves around family, farm, employees, wellness, and community. The hemp and medicinal herbs that they grow are an extension of this belief.

Luce Farm Wellness

In this rapidly growing world of hemp, being an educated consumer is important. Here are some questions to ask yourself as you shop for hemp-infused products:

Where and how was the hemp in this product grown (organically, outdoors, etc.)?

How were the cannabinoids (CBD, CBG, CBN, etc.) extracted from the hemp plant (CO2 extraction, ethanol extraction, etc.)?

How many milligrams of CBD are you getting per serving? (In other words, what is the concentration of CBD in the product?)

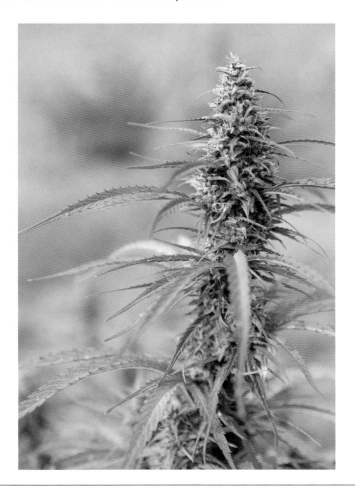

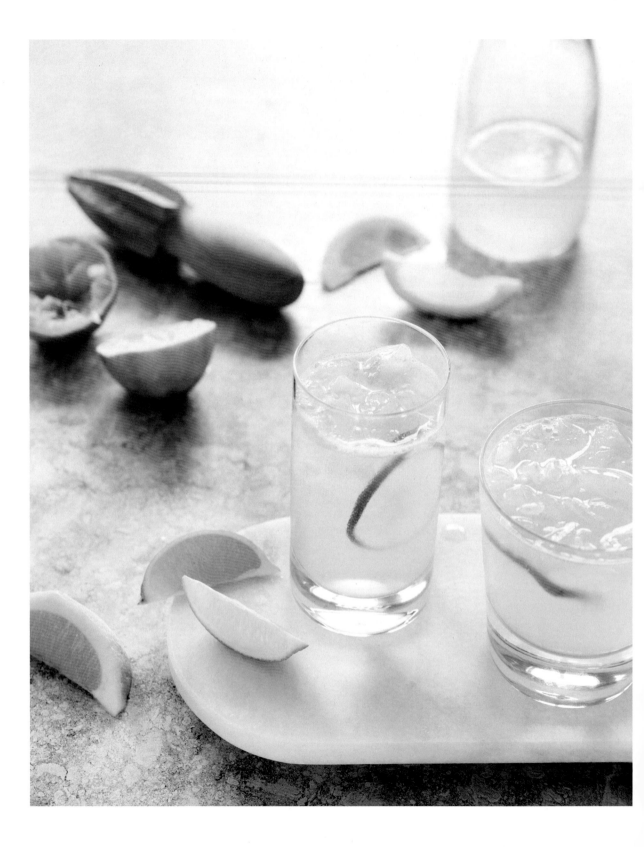

HEMP-INFUSED HONEY CITRUS TONIC

by LUCE FARM WELLNESS

MAKES 2 servings

REBECCA PIMENTEL: Tonic recipes shouldn't be limited to cold season. This wonderful elixir is commonplace at the farmhouse, loved by all ages, and a great alternative to sugary juices. Add some peeled ginger and pour into a fancy glass for an elevated "mocktail" recipe.

2 cups coconut water

Juice of 2 limes

Juice of 1 lemon

1 tablespoon hemp-infused honey, preferably Luce Farm Wellness

⅛ teaspoon salt

1. Place all the ingredients in a blender and process until well combined. Pour over ice and serve.

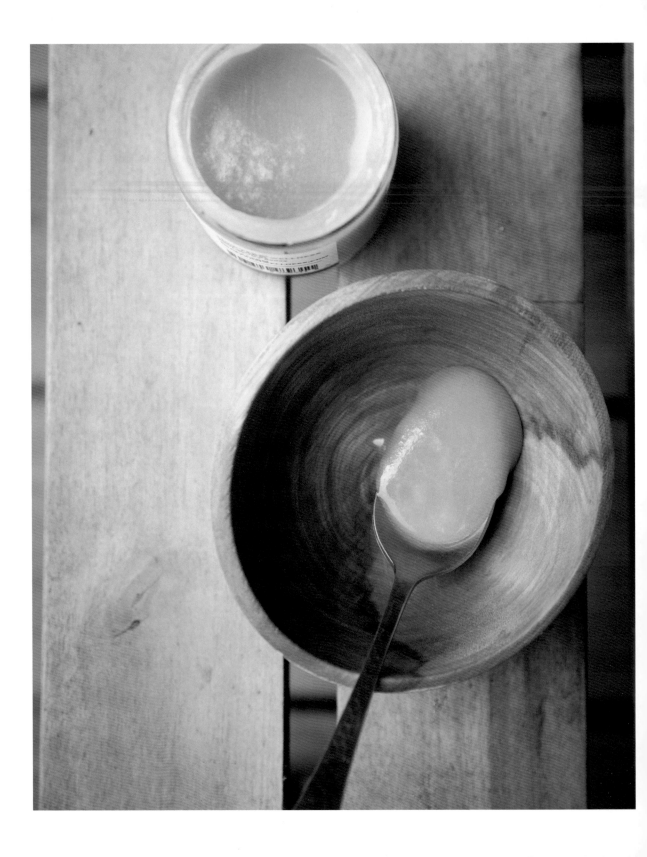

HEMP-INFUSED CHOCOLATE COCONUT BARS

by LUCE FARM WELLNESS

MAKES 12 large bars; 12.5 milligrams CBD per bar
or 24 smaller bars; 6.25 milligrams CBD per bar

REBECCA PIMENTEL: Make this recipe for your next dinner party. These sweet and simple bars are a delicious addition to your wellness routine.

COCONUT BARS

1 cup organic sweetened condensed milk

5 tablespoons melted hemp-infused oil, preferably Luce Farm Wellness

5 cups unsweetened finely shredded coconut

1 teaspoon kosher salt

CHOCOLATE BASE

2 cups best quality semisweet chocolate chips

2 teaspoons melted organic extra-virgin coconut oil

2 teaspoons honey

1. Line a rimmed baking sheet with parchment paper. Set aside.

2. In a small bowl, combine the condensed milk and oil until well combined.

3. Place the condensed milk-oil mixture, shredded coconut, and salt in the bowl of a food processor and process, scraping down the sides of the bowl as needed, until the dough is fully combined.

4. Place two pieces of parchment paper slightly larger than 9×13 inches on a clean work surface. Turn the dough out onto one piece of the parchment paper. Top with the second sheet of parchment paper and flatten with your hands, then roll the dough out to a 9×13-inch rectangle. Carefully place the dough, along with the parchment paper, onto a 9×13-inch baking dish. Remove the top piece of parchment paper, leaving the bottom piece under the dough. Transfer to the freezer and freeze until firm, about 30 minutes.

5. Remove from the freezer, then cut into 12 even rectangles (larger bars) or 24 even rectangles (smaller bars), then return to the freezer while tempering the chocolate.

6. To make the chocolate base: Place the chocolate chips, coconut oil, and honey into the top pan of a double boiler. Set aside.

7. Pour about 1 inch of water into the bottom pan and bring to a simmer. Place the top pan with the chocolate on top, making sure the bowl does not touch the simmering water. When half of the chocolate chips have melted, gently stir the mixture until the chocolate has fully melted.

Recipe continues on next page

8. Remove the bars from the freezer and dip the bottom side of each bar about ⅛ inch into the chocolate, shaking off any excess. Place the bars chocolate-side down on the prepared baking sheet. Repeat with the remaining bars.

9. Dip the tines of a fork into the remaining chocolate mixture and drizzle over the top of each bar. Place in the refrigerator until the chocolate has set and hardens, about 20 minutes. Serve chilled. The bars can be stored in an airtight container in the refrigerator for up to one week.

NOTE

You can increase the milligrams of CBD in this recipe by using Luce Farm Wellness hemp-infused honey.

STEVE GONZALEZ & SCOTT KETCHUM

Chef/Co-owner and Co-owner, Sfoglini Pasta Shop

When Steve Gonzalez and Scott Ketchum met in 2010, their mutual love of the culinary arts created a connection that destined them to become lasting friends. Steve was a chef who had a degree in culinary arts from the Art Institute of Colorado. He was introduced to the technique of handmade pasta at the elegant Vetri Cucina in Philadelphia, and has worked at renowned restaurants in Spain and Italy during his career. Returning to America, he opened his own restaurant in Philadelphia, eventually selling his share and moving on to New York to work in some of that city's upscale dining establishments.

Scott Ketchum received a degree in graphic design from Iowa State University. For eighteen years, he worked as a creative director and graphic designer in San Francisco and New York, where he observed an interesting connection between design and the culinary arts. This correlation inspired him to travel to Italy, France, and Belgium and assimilate the food and beverage cultures of those countries.

After Ketchum returned home, he was quick to note the lack of artisanal pasta in the New York City area. He reached out to his friend Chef Gonzalez, and the two discussed the idea of creating a superior locally produced pasta that could be specifically branded as a product of New York. Their mission was to bring classic Italian-style pasta back to New York City by sourcing top-quality American organic grains. While producing their first batches during the research and development stages, the two men discovered that the grains grown in America stood out in both taste and quality. This was especially true of the organic wheats, which made them decide early on that organic was the way to go.

The company's name, Sfoglini, was inspired by the pasta makers of Bologna, Italy, who were called "Le Sfogline." These people have made pasta by hand for generations using traditional techniques passed down from generation to generation. This is exactly what Ketchum and Gonzalez hoped to do with their new company: inspire and teach folks in the United States to follow the Sfoglines' example. In July 2012, the business opened its doors in a 750-square-foot pasta shop in Brooklyn, New York. The two men decided to make dried pasta, keeping in mind that in Italy it is as well thought of as the fresh version. They brought the Italian technique to their product, also creating a fresh variety to sell to local restaurants.

When the Sfoglini brand was first introduced, most pasta found on restaurant menus and local market shelves consisted of shapes like rigatoni, fusilli, and penne. Because the business at first serviced restaurants, Chef Gonzalez and Ketchum wanted to focus on shapes that would complement each eatery's pasta offerings. When it became available on retail shelves in local markets and grocery stores, the product's unique shapes helped to distinguish the Sfoglini brand. Chef Gonzalez created recipes to accompany and emphasize the distinctive characteristics of each shape, making it easier for consumers to choose a sauce or other ingredient that would partner well with their selection.

What sets Sfoglini Pasta apart from other brands is the quality of the product's ingredients. The company uses a process that heightens flavor and nutrition. They work with local flour mills in upstate New York to source whole-grain flours, including local grains like "emmer." A partnership with Bronx Brewery & Empanology has enabled Chef Gonzalez to create a pasta that uses "spent" grain, which is a by-product of brewing. In comparison, most store-bought pasta is made from commodity flour, manufactured using completely automated production lines.

In June 2018, the company expanded to a 40,000-square-foot facility in Coxsackie, New York, nearly ten times bigger than their Brooklyn complex. The move increased distribution nationwide and allowed the facility to be closer to the farms and mills they work with. The company has purchased new equipment from Italy; once producing 1,000 pounds of pasta a day, they are now making 1,200 pounds per hour! Their new pasta machine, called a pasta extruder, is very much like a huge Play-Doh machine. A bronze die on the machine has a tool insert that creates the unique pasta shapes. The shape of the pasta can make the sauce cling better, keeping it from slipping to the bottom of the bowl. Sfoglini has brought back shapes that other pasta makers no longer use, such as zucca and reginetti. When the pasta making process is completed, the finished product is slow dried at low temperatures to preserve nutrition and lock in flavor.

The company's enduring relationships with local farmers began by meeting them at farmers' markets in New York City, using small amounts of their grains and ingredients, and then coming back for more and more. As time went on, strong bonds developed. When production amounts increased, the business began to promote these partnerships on their packaging to help each other grow. Sfoglini Pasta is committed to producing quality products and supporting the large network of farms and mills that provide their essential ingredients.

Sfoglini makes twenty-six different pastas each year, including their limited seasonal offerings. Chef Gonzalez's cooking philosophy is based on seasonal cooking options, "Use what is available and fresh each month of the year." Their seasonal pasta uses local ingredients and is only made when these become available. There are ramps and nettles in the spring, followed by mint, basil, and chiles during the summer, all of which are purchased directly from local farms.

A friend introduced Chef Gonzalez and Ketchum to JD Farms in Eaton, New York. The men were excited to hear that the farm was the first to be licensed to grow organic hemp in New York State. They asked for samples and made test batches that had a wonderfully unique taste that they thought their customers would love. The hemp added a nuttiness that enhanced the pasta's flavor.

The company makes three distinct hemp pasta shapes: radiators, rigatoni, and zucca. Since their shapes soak up and trap sauces, the radiators and rigatoni work well with pasta dishes that have thicker sauces and cheeses. Zucca is good with dishes that have chopped ingredients, as they tend to get trapped in the clamshell opening of this pasta. Hemp rigatoni is one of the company's top five best-selling pastas.

Sfoglini Pasta is for sale at retail locations in thirty states and on the company's website. Chef Gonzalez heads the pasta production and Ketchum manages the business end. Both men believe that the key to the company's success is the fresh locally produced ingredients that they buy from New York State farms. They work with GrowNYC Grains to support local farms across the Northeast, helping to build a market for local grains. The ties to regional farmers have strongly anchored Sfoglini Pasta in the local food movement.

ORGANIC HEMP

Sfoglini Pasta Shop

Organic hemp is heart-healthy; it is high in fiber and protein and contains fatty acids, essential amino acids, and minerals. Rich in antioxidants, hemp helps to maintain low cholesterol levels. Chef Gonzalez has found that the hemp pasta's nutrient-dense quality and nutty flavor enhance the character of his recipes.

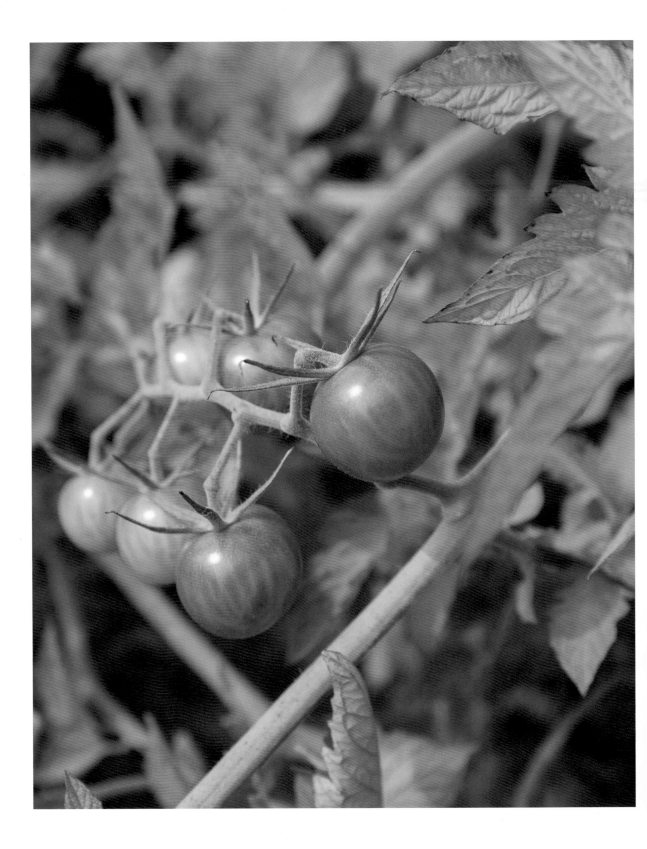

SFOGLINI HEMP RIGATONI

with Shrimp, Corn, and Cherry Tomatoes

by ELIZABETH BOSSIN

MAKES 5 to 6 servings

SCOTT KETCHUM: Pairing hemp foods can be difficult for early adopters of hemp. One great combination we discovered early on was hemp with seafood, and this dish is one of our favorites.

1 (16-ounce) box Sfoglini Hemp Rigatoni

3 tablespoons olive oil, divided, plus more for drizzling

1 pound large shrimp, peeled and deveined

½ teaspoon kosher salt, divided

½ teaspoon freshly ground black pepper, divided

2 cups fresh corn kernels (cut from 2 to 3 ears of corn)

1 medium shallot, peeled and minced (about ⅓ cup)

2 tablespoons minced garlic (3 medium cloves)

1 cup dry white wine

3 cups assorted colored cherry tomatoes, halved

¼ teaspoon crushed red pepper flakes, or to taste

½ cup thinly sliced fresh basil, plus more for garnish

1. Bring a large pot of salted water to a boil over medium-high heat. Add the pasta and cook according to the package directions. Drain, reserving ½ cup of the pasta water. Set aside.

2. While waiting for the pasta water to boil, start cooking the shrimp. Heat 2 tablespoons of oil in a large heavy-bottomed saucepan or Dutch oven over medium heat. Add the shrimp and season with ¼ teaspoon of salt and ¼ teaspoon of pepper. Sauté the shrimp until it starts to turn pink and is just cooked through, about 2½ minutes per side. Using a slotted spoon, transfer the shrimp to a plate and tent with foil. Set aside.

3. Add the corn, the remaining ¼ teaspoon of salt, and the remaining ¼ teaspoon of pepper, stirring often, until golden brown around the edges, about 7 minutes.

4. Add the remaining 1 tablespoon of oil, shallot, and garlic and cook, stirring often, for 1 minute.

5. Add the wine and bring to a simmer, stirring occasionally, until the liquid is reduced by half, about 4 minutes. Add the tomatoes and cook until softened, about 5 minutes.

6. Stir in the red pepper flakes and ¼ cup of the reserved pasta water until well incorporated.

7. Add the shrimp and pasta and toss until evenly coated, adding more pasta water to taste, if desired.

8. Stir in the basil, tossing until well combined. Season with salt and pepper to taste. Transfer to individual pasta bowls. Garnish with basil and drizzles of olive oil. Serve at once.

SFOGLINI HEMP RADIATORS

with Ricotta, Peas, and Lemon

by TRACEY MEDEIROS

MAKES 4 servings

> **TRACEY MEDEIROS:** This satisfying one-dish meal is always a hit at home and can be prepared quickly after a busy day! The milky, sweet flavor of the ricotta cheese is the perfect complement to the texture of the plump peas and the bright citrus notes from the lemon zest.

PASTA

1 (16-ounce) box Sfoglini Hemp Radiators

RICOTTA, PEAS, AND LEMON SAUCE

1 cup high-quality, whole-milk ricotta

1 cup fresh or frozen green peas, cooked

2 tablespoons extra-virgin olive oil, plus extra for drizzling

2 tablespoons lemon juice, or to taste

1 tablespoon lemon zest

2 medium cloves garlic, grated

1 teaspoon kosher salt

½ teaspoon freshly ground black pepper

½ cup freshly grated Parmigiano-Reggiano cheese

¼ cup thinly sliced fresh basil

1. Bring a large pot of salted water to a boil over medium-high heat. Add the pasta and cook according to the package directions. Drain, reserving ¼ cup of the pasta water. Set aside.

2. In the same pot used to cook the pasta, make the ricotta, peas, and lemon sauce. Remove the pot from the stove top and mix together the ricotta, peas, olive oil, lemon juice, lemon zest, garlic, salt, and pepper until well combined. The sauce will have a thick texture similar to loose mashed potatoes or cream of wheat. Note: For a thinner consistency, add some of the reserved pasta water, 1 tablespoon at a time, stirring until desired texture is achieved.

3. Fold in the pasta, tossing until well coated. Adjust seasonings with salt, pepper, and additional lemon juice, if desired.

4. To serve: Divide the pasta between four bowls. Drizzle with olive oil and sprinkles of cheese over the top. Garnish with basil. Serve at once.

SFOGLINI HEMP ZUCCA

with Roasted Butternut Squash and Kale

by ELIZABETH BOSSIN

MAKES 4 servings

> **SCOTT KETCHUM:** Fall vegetables like zucchini, pumpkin, and squash create fantastic sauces when prepared with our hemp pastas. This recipe featuring caramelized butternut squash has turned out to be a Sfoglini fan favorite.

1 medium (about 2 to 2½ pounds) butternut squash

2 tablespoons extra-virgin olive oil

1 teaspoon kosher salt, divided, or to taste

½ teaspoon freshly ground black pepper, divided, or to taste

1 (16-ounce) box Sfoglini Sfoglini Hemp Zucca

2 tablespoons unsalted butter

4 tablespoons minced shallots

1 medium bunch Tuscan kale, center ribs removed, cut into thin strips

2 tablespoons fresh minced sage leaves

¼ cup freshly grated Parmigiano-Reggiano cheese, plus extra for serving

½ tablespoon lemon zest, or to taste

1. Preheat the oven to 400°F. Line a baking sheet with parchment paper or foil and set aside.

2. To prepare the squash: Using a sharp knife, remove both ends of the squash and discard. With a sharp vegetable peeler, remove the skins, and discard. Cut the squash in half lengthwise and scoop out the seeds and strings, then cut into ½-inch half-moons. Slice the half-moons into long rectangles and then into ½-inch to 1-inch pieces. Note: You should have about 5 cups of cubed butternut squash, depending on the size of the pieces. Transfer the squash pieces to the prepared baking sheet and toss with the oil until evenly coated. Spread the squash out into an even layer and season with ½ teaspoon of salt and ¼ teaspoon of pepper. Roast, stirring occasionally, until fork-tender, about 30 minutes. Set aside.

3. Meanwhile, bring a large pot of salted water to a boil over medium-high heat. Add the pasta and cook according to the package directions. Drain, reserving 1½ cups of the pasta water. Set aside.

4. Melt the butter in a large skillet over medium-high heat. Add the shallots and sauté until soft and translucent, about 2 minutes. Add the kale and sage and cook, stirring often, until the kale is softened but not wilted, about 3 minutes.

5. Reduce the heat to low. Add the butternut squash, 1 cup of the reserved pasta water, the remaining ½ teaspoon of salt, and the remaining ¼ teaspoon of pepper and cook, stirring often, until the sauce becomes creamy, about

Recipe continues on next page

5 minutes. **Note:** You may need to add additional pasta water to loosen the sauce, if desired.

6. Fold in the pasta until evenly coated. Adjust seasonings with salt and pepper to taste. Divide among pasta bowls. Garnish with cheese and lemon zest. Serve at once with additional cheese along with some crusty bread, if desired.

WEST

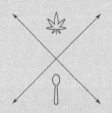

DAVID DOTLICH & DOUG ELWOOD

Cofounders, OrcaSong Farm

O rcaSong Farm is located on Orcas Island in the San Juan archipelago north of Seattle, Washington, in the Salish Sea. The farm's name is a tribute to the resident orca whales who call the Salish Sea home. Using ecologically regenerative practices, the folks at the farm are working hard to restore the land that they steward.

David Dotlich and Doug Elwood are the cofounders and owners of OrcaSong Farm. They purchased the property in 2013 with the idea of building a community-based botanical farm that would work to regenerate the land, sustain local farming, and serve as a community destination for visitors and locals. Both men live on the island year-round. It is their goal to provide

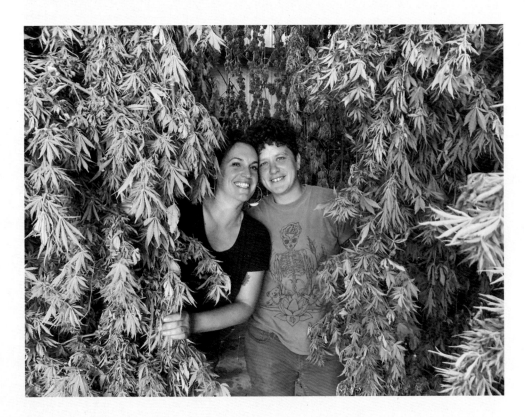

plant medicine and wholesome food and offer educational programs inspired by nature. The two men want their farm to foster an enjoyment of healthy eating, herbal medicine, and practical farming by connecting with others. To remind folks of this desire, the farm has adopted the tagline, "Our mission is to inspire change, heal the world and its inhabitants, and connect people to the food and medicine that they live by."

Framed by picturesque Turtleback Mountain, OrcaSong Farm consists of 120 acres of sunny pastures, lush forests, and beautiful gardens. There are eleven acres of mixed lavender consisting primarily of Grosso and Provence varietals. Grosso is a lavender oil producer, while Provence offers fragrances of honey and light-smelling flowers. Lavender, a medicinal and sustainable plant, has many uses and benefits. The farm's second-most-popular crop is hemp (*Cannabis sativa*), which can be used for medicine, fiber, and food. It is also a strong soil remediator. At OrcaSong Farm, harmful and hazardous chemicals are never used.

The farm grows many of the plants that are featured in their botanical line on their organic botanical and hemp farm. The goal is to celebrate nature by curating blends of high-quality botanical ingredients, infusing them with cannabinoids, while adding rapid-delivery technology to increase their efficacy. Hemp CBD products are crafted with the highest-quality hemp using steam distillation and CO_2 extraction methods. OrcaSong Botanicals strives to create organic and natural products that work better than anything else that may be found on the market. Their botanicals are packaged in compostable, recyclable, and reusable containers.

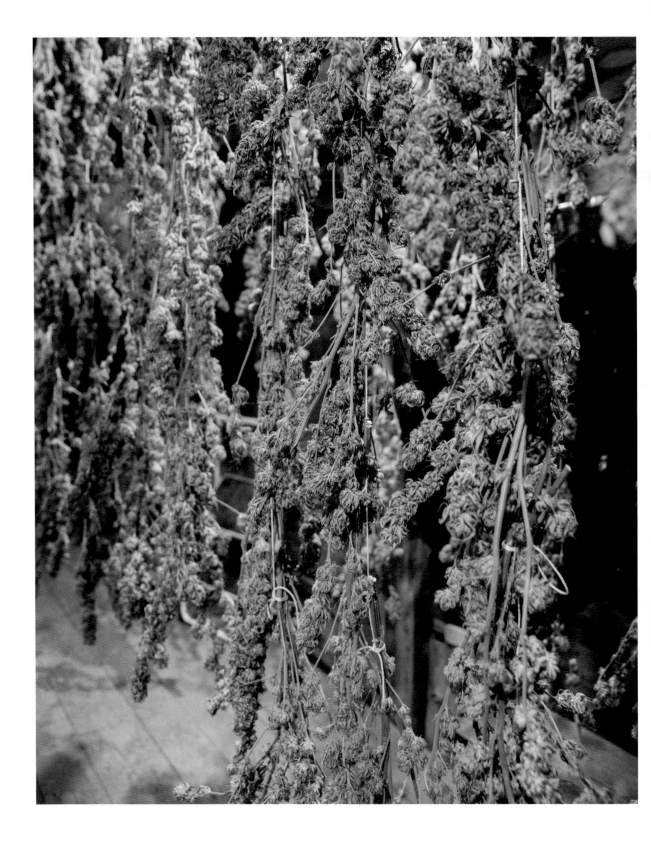

ORCASONG DREAMER'S TEA BLEND

ARIANA TERRENCE, ORCASONG FARM

ARIANA TERRENCE (FARM MANAGER): This caffeine-free herbal blend was created to evoke powerful and colorful dreams. It is especially blended for the dreamer, stimulating vivid and easily recalled dreams. A cup of Dreamer's Tea is enjoyable after a rich or large dinner or as a perfect nightcap after a long day. A blend of organic hemp, mugwort, lavender, chamomile, hops, and calendula instantly calms, raises consciousness, and eases your entry into the colorful world of dreams. Working with your lucid dream life is a vast and fascinating new way to learn more about yourself and your deepest desires.

½ teaspoon dried organic hemp

½ teaspoon dried organic mugwort

½ teaspoon dried organic lavender

½ teaspoon dried organic chamomile

⅛ teaspoon dried organic hops

⅛ teaspoon dried calendula petals

8 ounces cold filtered water

Honey, optional

1. Place all the herbs into a stainless-steel mesh tea ball or tea strainer with handle. Set aside.
2. Bring 8 ounces of cold filtered water to a boil. While the water is coming to a boil, warm the teacup by adding hot water halfway up the cup, and carefully swirl a few times. Once the teacup is warm, discard the water.
3. Place the tea ball into the teacup. Pour the boiling water over the loose herbs and steep for 4 minutes. Carefully remove the tea ball and discard the tea solids. Adjust sweetness with honey, if desired. Serve at once.

NOTE

If using fresh herbs, triple the quantities.

OrcaSong Farm

Hemp—All the benefits of the cannabis plant without the THC.

Mugwort—This smokable herb leads to a euphoric and dreamlike feeling. Smoking mugwort at night arouses lucid and colorful dreaming.

Lavender—It assists in reducing restlessness and sleeplessness as well as alleviating headaches, muscular pain, and flatulence.

Chamomile—May be used for relaxation and improving sleep for those suffering from anxiety and tension.

Hops—Has a long and proven history of use medicinally, being employed mainly for its soothing, sedative, tonic, and calming effect on the body and the mind.

Calendula—Known to bring better dreams while you sleep. Bear, the originator of the blend, believes that calendula flowers also help you remember dreams more clearly.

SARAHLEE LAWRENCE

Co-owner, Rainshadow Organics

People return home for many reasons after graduating from college and experiencing a bit of what life has to offer. For Sarahlee Lawrence, the catalyst was an article that she had read, written by one of her favorite authors, Michael Pollan, who writes about where nature and culture intersect. After reading the piece, she experienced an epiphany, feeling that she owed it to herself, family, and community to try her hand at stewarding her family's land and becoming part of the next generation of farmers. At this juncture in her life, Sarahlee had received an undergraduate degree in sociology and a master's degree in environmental science. She had traveled the world and seen many of its wonders and in 2010 was ready to return to the family's farm in Terrebonne, Oregon, the place where she had grown up.

The family-owned-and-operated farm has been in the Lawrence family since the early 1970s, and now Sarahlee and her husband, Ashanti Samuels, were taking over its two hundred sprawling acres. Sarahlee, a third-generation farmer, knew that she could make a difference. The farm has twenty-seven of its acres under rotational cultivation, seven additional acres are pig pastures, sixty are used for cows, and two utilized for chickens. The rest of the land is native habitat where plants attractive to pollinators are cultivated. The farm is nestled in the "rainshadow" of the Cascade Mountains, a geographical term for its low rainfall. Because of its location and organic certification, it seemed only natural to rename the new venture Rainshadow Organics.

Rainshadow is a certified organic, full-diet farm, which means that it supplies food to the community all year long through its CSA. It produces dozens of varieties of organic vegetables, herbs, berries, flowers, pork, chicken, eggs, turkeys, beef, honey, and grains. They use only sustainable practices with no pesticides, fertilizers, or herbicides. Most of the vegetable farming is done by hand with some equipment used for the long beds in the larger fields. The two-acre garden is almost all done by hand, biodynamically.

A farm store was opened in 2017 with a commercial kitchen that serves farm-to-table lunches, dinners, and delicious wood-fired pizzas on Saturdays. Full-time chef Travis Taylor only cooks with what the farm produces, demonstrating to folks what food security and independence look like. The award-winning chef hosts farm-to-table dinners and pizza gatherings while also serving visitors and the crew who work on the property. The farm offers an intensive seven-month curriculum through Rogue Farm Corps. Interns live on the farm learning how to raise its many crops while gaining an understanding of the business of farming. The owners of Rainshadow Organics believe that the United States needs more farmers and are doing their part to help.

Everything that is grown at Rainshadow Organic Farm is distributed within a fifty-mile radius of the property through CSA programs, local restaurants, grocery stores, and farmers' markets. By doing business in this way, the farm's owners do not have to worry about shelf life or preserving their foods' appearance because everything is freshly picked. Consumers should know that this type of produce offers more nutrients, a big difference from the products sold by commercial produce companies that sometimes take days to get their vegetables to market.

When cannabis became legalized in Oregon, it prompted Sarahlee to think that the plant would be a wonderful addition to the farm's crop rotation. The farm's hemp crop is unique, raised biodynamically and organically, surrounded by rows of vegetables, cover crops, and grains. The hemp lives among a community of other plants which support its growth and

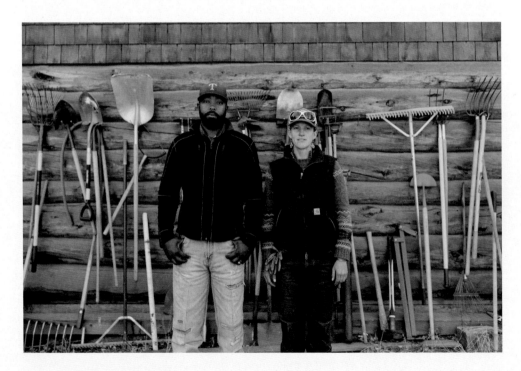

health. When the time is right, it will be distilled into oil. The distillers use a method of cryo-genic extraction, with organic food-grade ethanol, to create full-spectrum hemp extracts that Rainshadow Organics infuses into its products. The owners work closely with the processor.

Rainshadow Organics' new brand, Desert Green Hemp, was launched in September 2019. The brand was created to stand for wellness and pure and natural healing. The extraction method preserves the essential compounds of the plant, including the terpenes and flavonoids that are lost in other processes. Internal well-being is supported by Desert Green's natural and nutrient-dense products. Oils are blended with herbs and native medicinal plants that are foraged on the farm. Products are designed based on what the land can provide. The lavender, chamomile, yarrow, and mint that are used in the tinctures and salves are all supported by Central Oregon's climate and have been cultivated on the farm for years. The region's volcanic mountain soil, dry climate, and directly sourced mountain spring waters are what produce uniquely pure and powerful CBD products.

Sarahlee likes to test new products and challenge herself as a farmer. Knowing that hemp is a bio-accumulator, she stresses that you simply must know your farmer. It is with pride that the folks at Rainshadow Organic Farm contribute to the regeneration of the social, economic, and environmental health of our planet.

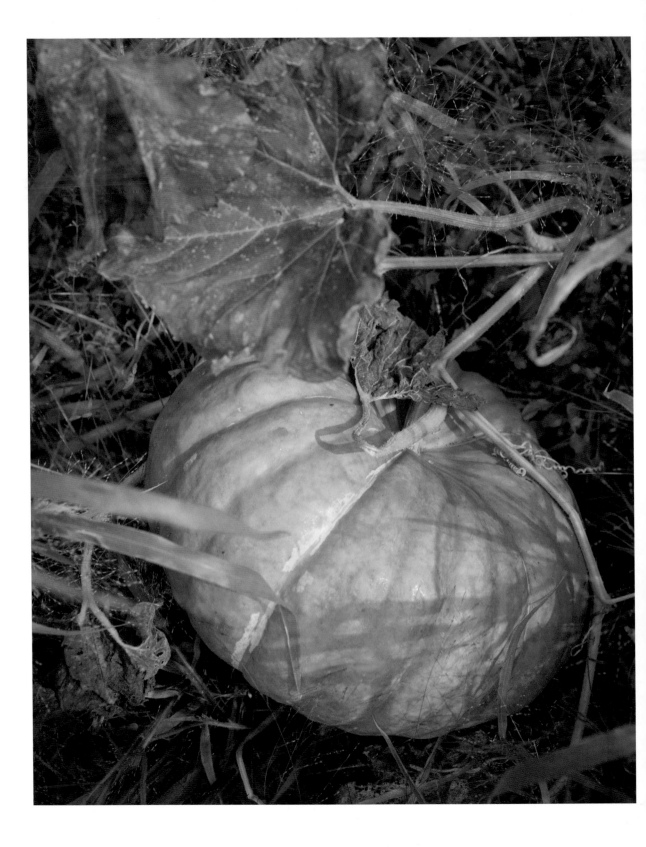

ADAPTOGENIC HEMP ELIXIR–INFUSED PUMPKIN CHOCOLATE CHIP COOKIES

by RAINSHADOW ORGANICS

MAKES about 23 large cookies;
16 milligrams of CBD per cookie

These simple-to-make cookies have a cake-like texture with hints of earthiness from the Adaptogenic Hemp Elixir. The pumpkin purée is a nice complement to the elixir, plus, it adds an extra boost of fiber, antioxidants, vitamin A, and vitamin C. When using canned pumpkin purée, be sure not to use pie filling (it's totally different), which is spiced and sweetened.

2½ cups organic hard white wheat flour, preferably Rainshadow Organics

2 tablespoons organic unsweetened cocoa powder

1½ teaspoons aluminum-free baking powder

1¼ teaspoons baking soda

½ teaspoon pink Himalayan salt, extra-fine grain

½ cup organic unsalted butter, softened

3 tablespoons organic shortening, softened

1¼ cups organic sugar

¼ cup light brown sugar, packed

2 large organic eggs, room temperature

⅔ cup canned organic pumpkin purée

1 (3-fluid-ounce) bottle Adaptogenic Hemp Elixir, 365 milligram Full-spectrum CBD, preferably Desert Green Hemp

1 teaspoon pure vanilla extract

1½ cups (10-ounce bag) high-quality organic milk chocolate chips

1. Preheat the oven to 325°F. Line three baking sheets with parchment paper or silicone baking mats. Set aside.

2. In a medium bowl, mix together the flour, cocoa powder, baking powder, baking soda, and salt until well combined.

3. In the bowl of a stand mixer with the paddle attachment, on medium speed, cream together the butter, shortening, and sugars, scraping down the sides of the bowl as needed, until smooth. Add the eggs, one at a time, and beat on medium speed, scraping down the sides of the bowl as needed, until just smooth. Add the pumpkin purée, Adaptogenic Hemp Elixir, and vanilla and mix to combine. Turn the mixer to low speed, then add the dry ingredients and mix until smooth. Add the chocolate chips, then increase the speed to medium, and mix until well combined.

4. Using a ¼ cup measuring scoop (2-ounce cookie scoop) and a spatula, drop the cookie dough onto the prepared baking sheets, about 3 inches apart.

5. Bake the cookies in batches, rotating the sheets halfway through, until the cookies are just slightly soft to the touch in the middle, the edges are set, and the bottoms are lightly golden brown, about 25 minutes. Allow the cookies to cool on the baking sheets for 5 minutes, then transfer to cooling racks and allow to sit at room temperature, uncovered, for 2 hours to firm up.

SOUTH

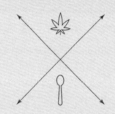

FRANNY TACY

First Female Hemp Farmer in North Carolina, Owner, Franny's Farm

Born Frances Tacy, but known to all as Franny, she holds the distinct honor of being the first woman to farm hemp in North Carolina. Before arriving at that point in her life, she had tried her hand at many different professions. Franny went to agricultural school, transferred into forestry, received a degree in biology, and was Idaho's first female firefighter. She then returned to college to earn a master's degree in education and taught for six years before entering the field of pharmaceuticals. This career enabled her to become financially secure enough to purchase what is now known as Franny's Farm.

In 2012, Tacy, realizing a lifelong dream, purchased Franny's Farm, which practices regenerative agriculture. Her plan was to use a conservation and rehabilitation approach to food and farming systems. Growing up on her father's cattle farm, she always knew that agronomics would at some point be her life's work. Located in Leicester, North Carolina, the picturesque thirty-eight-acre farm is home to heritage chickens, turkeys, sheep, and goats. The farm grows organic vegetables, herbs, and flowers and has pollinator and bee gardens. Visitors to the farm store will find seasonal fresh produce, poultry, and a variety of other tempting items for sale. For those folks who wish to stay for a while longer, lodging may be found in cozy cabins, campsites, or a custom Barn House. Beautiful views make the location the perfect venue for private and public events, as well as the very popular Goat Yoga. Goat Yoga is an interactive yoga class where you meditate and bend alongside adorable baby goats. In the summer there is a Farm Camp for children. Overlooking the rolling hills and valley of South Turkey Creek, Franny's Farm is conveniently located only ten miles from downtown Asheville with its hip restaurants and music scene.

Franny owned the farm for seven years before hemp even became an order of business. With the passage of the Federal Farm Bill in 2018, which decriminalized hemp agriculture, Franny's Farm became one of the first to receive a grow permit. That year, Tacy became the first recorded female farmer in North Carolina to plant industrial hemp from seed. She has always been a supporter of cannabis, from fiber to food. Always interested in plant medicine and herbs, Franny is passionate about what hemp can do for farmers and the US economy. As an advocate for the industry, she has helped with collaborations that deal with data and research.

The first Franny's Farmacy hemp dispensary opened in 2018. Currently, there are seven dispensaries with four in North Carolina and one each in Greenville, South Carolina, Westport, Connecticut, and Athens, Georgia. Their North Carolina operations are located within ten miles of each other, which contributes to the brand's vertical integration, reduces their carbon footprint, and ensures quality medicinal products. The company, called Franny's Farmacy, is involved with their product every step of the way, beginning the process with growing the hemp on Franny's Farm and other affiliate grow farms. The goal is to serve as a role model for future hemp farmers, both nationally and globally.

Franny is proud to say that her line of products is one of only a couple in our nation that are grown, processed, and brought to market locally. The company manufactures over fifty products using critical CO2 extractions as one of their main extraction methods. Hemp oil is a popular example. The majority of their products are full spectrum. Franny's brand and business divisions are setting the standard for this industry in growing, processing, manufacturing, labeling, testing, and education. They lead the way in transparency by providing QR codes on all products that link to the Certificate of Authenticity. There are topical and edible divisions, each supported by the very busy distribution center, which ships to every state in the country. The company will soon be entering the international market.

Tacy trains women hemp farmers through the "Women in Hemp" nonprofit organization that she cofounded. She is finding ways to support these women, giving them a voice, while also helping to raise funds for the female researchers at North Carolina State who are doing data collection and trials on the farms involved with the project. "Women in Hemp" finds it encouraging that the number of female farmers has grown by 27 percent in the last five years.

The busy entrepreneur works with a variety of chefs in Asheville, as well as when traveling to different areas of the United States and around the world. Hemp has become one of her favorite ingredients in cooking. She has participated in a diverse assortment of projects that have introduced chefs to hemp-infused cooking and is overjoyed to find that many local chefs have now featured hemp on their menus. Franny believes that "Farmers and chefs are the heart and soul of the movement, the influencers, the ones that will inspire and educate, share and provide the opportunities for people to experience hemp-inspired food." Her company now has a corporate chef, Frank Jordan, who specializes in "Clean" food and creative dishes that use hemp as a component.

The company's most popular hemp-based items are tinctures, salves, and pet treats followed by chocolates and gummies. Franny's Farmacy's website offers a full line of products, including those formulated for athletes, babies, seniors, and pets, providing options for everyone. As the company's mission statement proclaims, "Seed to Shelf, Hemp and Health."

VEGAN HEMP CREAM OF MUSHROOM SOUP

by FRANNY'S FARM

MAKES 4 servings

FRANCES TACY: Rich, flavorful, and "creamy," this vegan hemp-inspired cream of mushroom soup is deliciously satisfying, even to non-vegan foodies, and it works for gluten-free folks, too. This recipe is a true crowd-pleaser that makes a savory appetizer, or a main dish, accompanied by your favorite side.

2 tablespoons hemp oil

1 medium onion, minced

¼ cup minced celery

1 teaspoon dry oregano

1 teaspoon dry basil

1 bay leaf

10 ounces fresh shiitake mushrooms, cut into ¼-inch-thick slices

8 ounces fresh baby bella mushrooms, cut into ¼-inch-thick slices

2 large (about 7.5 ounces) portobello mushrooms, cut into ¼-inch-thick slices

4 ounces fresh oyster mushrooms, cut into ¼-inch-thick slices

2 medium cloves garlic, minced

1¼ cups vegetable broth, divided, or as needed

2 tablespoons soy sauce or tamari

2 cups hemp milk, unsweetened, room temperature

½ teaspoon fine-grain sea salt, or to taste

½ teaspoon freshly ground black pepper, or to taste

GARNISHES

Fresh thyme leaves

Fresh chopped parsley

1. Heat the oil in a large stockpot or Dutch oven over medium heat. Add the onions, celery, oregano, basil, and bay leaf and cook, stirring often, until the onions are soft and translucent, about 6 minutes.

2. Increase the heat to medium-high, then add the mushrooms, stirring until evenly coated. Cover and cook, stirring occasionally, for 8 minutes.

3. Uncover and continue to cook, stirring often until most of the water from the mushrooms has evaporated, about 8 minutes.

4. Stir in the garlic and cook until fragrant, about 30 seconds.

5. Stir in ¼ cup of the vegetable broth and the soy sauce, and deglaze the pot, scraping up the bits up from the bottom of the pot. Stir in the remaining 1 cup vegetable broth until well combined.

6. In a slow and steady stream, stir in the hemp milk, salt, and pepper. Reduce the heat to a simmer, and continue to simmer for 10 minutes. Remove and discard the bay leaf. Note: For a thinner soup, add additional vegetable stock, if desired. Adjust seasonings with salt and pepper to taste, if desired.

7. Ladle into soup bowls and garnish with sprinkles of thyme and parsley over the top. Serve with crusty bread and a side salad, if desired.

VEGAN FETTUCCINE ALFREDO

by FRANNY'S FARM

MAKES 6 servings

FRANCES TACY: This alfredo sauce needs a little advance prep, but it is well worth it. Especially for those who want a rich and creamy sauce, this will not disappoint. Add this flavorful, delicious, and satisfying recipe to your go-to list of comfort foods. It's freezer friendly, too, so make extra.

VEGAN ALFREDO SAUCE

Makes 3¾ cups

Note: You will need to soak the raw cashews in water for at least 2 hours on the counter, or up to 12 hours in the refrigerator, before you intend to use them.

½ cup raw cashews

1½ cups russet potatoes, peeled and cut into 1-inch pieces, and boiled until fork-tender

1 cup unsweetened hemp milk

1 cup vegetable broth

¼ cup hemp seeds

2½ tablespoons nutritional yeast, plus extra for serving

2 tablespoons fresh lemon juice

1 tablespoon flour

1½ teaspoons salt, or to taste

½ teaspoon garlic powder

2 tablespoons vegan butter

3 medium cloves garlic, minced

1. To prepare the raw cashews: Place the cashews in a medium bowl. Fill the bowl with water, making sure the cashews are completely submerged. Soak the cashews for at least 2 hours on the counter or for up to 12 hours in the refrigerator. Drain and rinse.

2. To make the vegan alfredo sauce: Place the cashews, potatoes, hemp milk, vegetable broth, hemp seeds, nutritional yeast, lemon juice, flour, salt, and garlic powder in a blender or food processor and process until smooth and creamy. Adjust seasonings with salt to taste. Set aside.

3. To make the fettuccine pasta: Bring a large pot of salted water to a boil over medium-high heat. Add the pasta and cook according to package directions, until al dente. Drain, then transfer to a large bowl and toss with 1 tablespoon oil until evenly coated.

4. To make the bell peppers: While waiting for the water to boil, heat the hemp oil in a medium skillet over medium heat. Add the peppers and salt, then sauté until just tender, about 10 minutes, or until desired texture is reached. Set aside.

5. While the pasta is cooking, finish the alfredo sauce. Heat the butter in a large skillet over medium-low heat. Add the garlic and sauté until fragrant, about 30 seconds. Increase the temperature to medium heat and slowly add the alfredo sauce. Cook, whisking often, until the sauce slightly thickens, about 3 to 4 minutes.

Ingredients list continues on page 225

Recipe continues on page 225

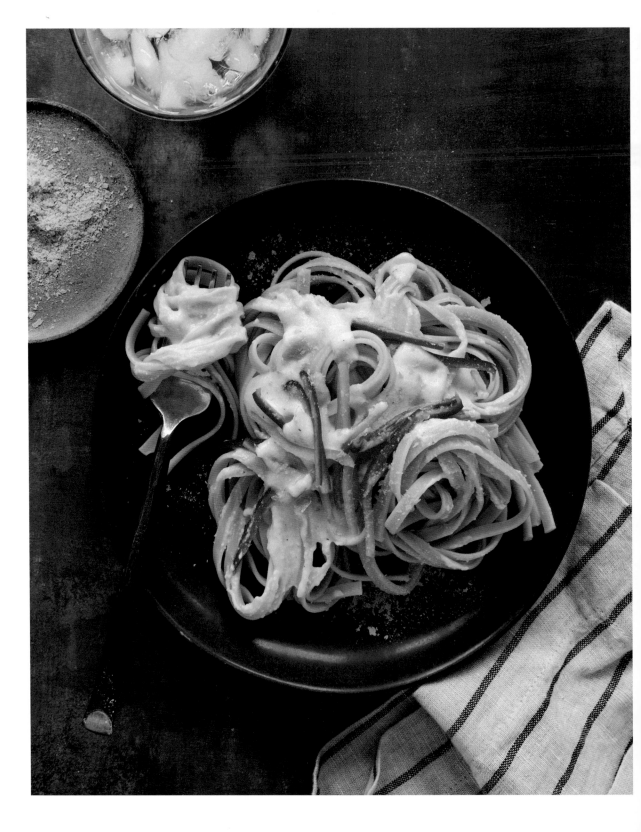

PASTA

16 ounces fettuccine, such as lentil, chickpea or whole-grain

1 tablespoon hemp oil, or as needed

BELL PEPPERS

1 tablespoon hemp oil, or as needed

2 small bell peppers, assorted colors, cut into thin strips, about 1½ cups

¼ teaspoon kosher salt, or to taste

Chopped fresh flat-leaf parsley, minced, for garnish

Adjust seasoning with salt. Reduce the temperature to low heat to keep the sauce warm, stirring occasionally, until the pasta is done cooking.

6. To assemble: Add 2 cups of the sauce to the pasta, tossing to evenly coat, adding more sauce as desired. Adjust seasonings with salt and pepper, if desired. Top each mound of pasta with peppers. Garnish with sprinkles of parsley. Serve at once with additional nutritional yeast, if desired, passing the remaining sauce at the table along with some crusty bread.

NOTE

This recipe makes more alfredo sauce than you will need for the recipe. It can be stored in an airtight container in the freezer for up to 6 months. Before using, thaw first, then run the sauce through a blender to eliminate any lumps and heat through before serving.

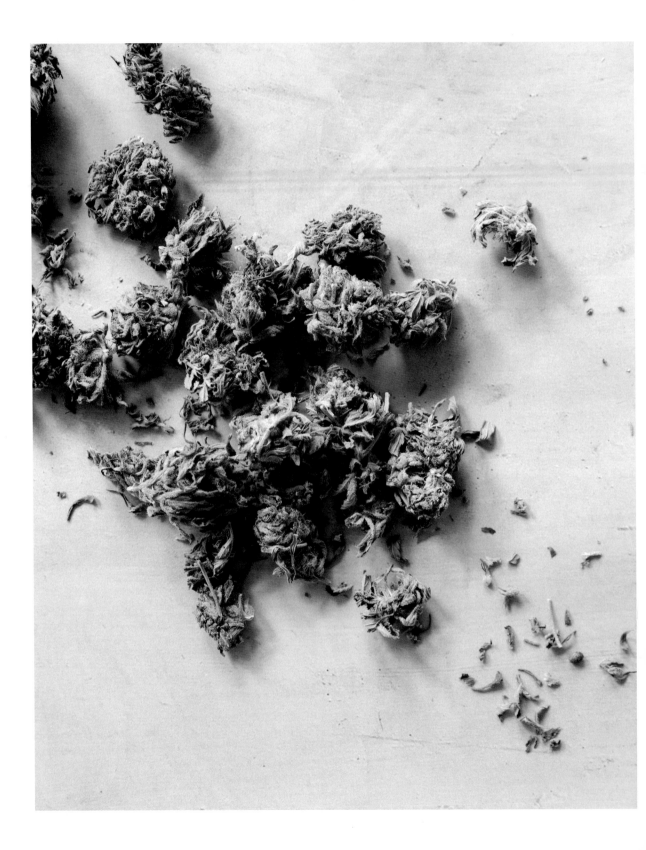

CHAPTER 3

THC—TETRAHYDROCANNABINOL

Tetrahydrocannabinol, also known as THC, is the primary psychoactive ingredient of the cannabis plant that produces a high or euphoric feeling. It is one of more than eighty-five chemical compounds found in cannabis. Some of its side effects include drowsiness, reduction of concentration, and disruption of short-term memory.

Because of its specific molecular structure, THC affects certain areas of the brain more than other active cannabinoids like CBD. THC binds to receptors in the brain that have an effect on the neurotransmitters (the chemicals that communicate between brain cells). This effect gives rise to euphoria and other psychoactive responses. THC also binds to other receptors throughout the body that produce its additional medicinal effects. Once planted in the brain, it can cause euphoria, alertness, or calmness. A THC high that is too strong can bring about dizziness, depression, anxiety, and fatigue. Each person is unique in the way that THC may affect them.

THC's medical uses include its antiemetic properties that inhibit vomiting, a factor which is useful for people on chemotherapy. Because THC increases appetite and reduces vomiting, it has started to be utilized in the treatment of anorexia and other eating disorders. It is notorious for giving folks the "munchies." THC creams are used to treat certain physical symptoms, helping to relax and soothe sore muscles and assist with other forms of pain relief. THC has also been beneficial in the care of some cases of PTSD, Tourette's syndrome, insomnia, asthma, and glaucoma.

Edibles are the easiest and strongest consumption method for introducing THC into a person's system. It is recommended that beginners consume a small quantity of edible to start, waiting at least two hours before taking another dose. A bite-size amount can take 60 to 120 minutes for effects to reach their peak, which can vary with the individual. The wisest rule is to start small, be patient, and increase slowly, especially for an inexperienced person. As should be done with any new medicine or supplement, it is always best to consult with your doctor before using cannabis.

NORTHEAST

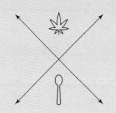

DAVID YUSEFZADEH
& SEAN CURLEY

Chef/Co-owner, Eat Sacrilicious/Ice Cream Maker and Director of Business
Development, Cloud Creamery/Co-owner, Eat Sacrilicious

During his culinary career, David Yusefzadeh has worked as a chef at Michelin-starred restaurants from Hong Kong to Chicago. He now resides in the Boston area. After spending nineteen years working in the hospitality industry, his life radically changed in 2011, when he was diagnosed with Crohn's disease. Unfortunately, the medications that were prescribed for him were of little help, and the side effects were horrific. This problem motivated Yusefzadeh to obtain a medical cannabis card, allowing him access to local dispensaries where he hoped to find edibles that would make him feel better. Disappointed that he could find few or no edibles that were made with real food and no preservatives at these dispensaries, he nonetheless decided to try a few of the products to understand their effect. The results were less than stellar, motivating the chef to begin making his own edibles at home. This whole experience opened Yusefzadeh's eyes to an opportunity that was virtually untapped in the cannabis market: infusing high-quality food with the highest-quality cannabis. The end result was the creation of Cloud Creamery and Eat Sacrilicious, exciting new culinary adventures.

Eat Sacrilicious debuted in the Boston area, as a dinner series, during the summer of 2018. Supported by his friend and business partner, Sean Curley, Yusefzadeh has created a series of high-end infused multicourse meals. Curley is also the director of business development of Cloud Creamery.

Even though the locations for the private dinner series are always changing, each setting has an intimate, elegant ambience. Yusefzadeh is the designated chef at these events, although, on occasion, a guest chef may be invited to host the affair. Tickets range in price from $100 to $225 per guest including a cannabis mocktail reception, eight-course meal, and an Eat Sacrilicious membership. After a ticket is purchased, the guest is sent a quick survey to gather data on their cannabis habits. Before the dinner begins, guests can request a low, medium, or high dose of CBD or THC. The goal is to create a menu where each course is infused differently. It is also possible for members to request a CBD- or THC-free meal that is treated as a dietary restriction. Yusefzadeh hopes to attract professionals from the business sector who are seeking a cannabis-infused culinary experience, although many people who attend these events have never used cannabis before. The staff is always checking to make sure that participants are feeling how they want to feel and are not overwhelmed, or uncomfortable. Every guest's dosage is monitored in the kitchen by a grid system that allows the relevant components in each dish to be adjusted if need be.

Chef Yusefzadeh supports area farmers and food producers, strongly believing in the importance of using sustainably sourced products. The dinner menu showcases the local ingredients supplied by these hardworking folks. The goal is to expand the offerings of premium edibles, hopefully keeping people from turning to harder pain management drugs, and celebrating cannabis.

The busy entrepreneur is also the owner of Cloud Creamery, a cannabis edible company with ice cream as its flagship product. This Framingham-based artisanal edible business is chef driven. The folks who run it are food and cannabis experts. The company makes cannabis-infused ice cream for hospitals and dispensaries. Local milk from grass-fed cows, organic cane sugar, and all-natural ingredients go into the product. Each batch of ice cream is tested and highly regulated to ensure accurate dosing. Wanting the emphasis to be on more than just cannabis, the name Cloud was chosen to signify a product that is "light, airy, and comfortable."

Cloud Creamery uses 100 percent natural sustainably sourced ingredients, working with local farmers to use their excess crops in its creations. Most of the flavors will be available year-round, along with seasonal choices such as Apple Cider Sorbet in September, and Butternut Squash in November. Two very popular summer selections are Blueberry Sweet Corn, which is mixed with sweet corn kernels, and Tomato Sorbet made from fresh local heirloom tomatoes.

The ice cream is served at private events with Cloud Creamery recently receiving permission to sell to dispensaries and hospitals. The business does not yet have a permit to sell directly to customers because their ice cream contains CBD, with some flavors also including THC. If things go well, Yusefzadeh would like to expand Cloud Creamery beyond the borders of Massachusetts to the rest of New England. It is his mission to make a difference in people's lives. He believes that "Nothing says comfort food more than ice cream!"

CANNABIS-CURED SALMON

by EAT SACRILICIOUS

MAKES approximately 10 servings

SUGGESTED DOSAGE: 5 milligrams of THC per serving; 50 milligrams THC per batch.

Take brunch to the next level with this perfect make-ahead delicious delicacy. The decarboxylated cannabis adds a subtle earthiness to the dry brine, allowing the buttery, silky texture of the salmon to really shine.

DRY BRINE

2 cups organic cane sugar

2 cups kosher salt

Zest from 2 large organic lemons

5 tablespoons minced fresh dill

3 tablespoons freshly ground black peppercorns

1 tablespoon coriander seed, toasted and ground

1 tablespoon cumin seed, toasted and ground

2 grams cannabis flower, ground fine, decarboxylated, testing at 27–28% THC

SALMON

One (2-pound) salmon belly, sushi-grade, skin and pin bones removed, cut into 4 equal pieces

Juice of 2 large organic lemons, about ½ cup juice

CROSTINI

1 large French baguette

2 tablespoons extra-virgin olive oil, or as needed

GARNISHES

1 large organic English cucumber, thinly sliced

5 organic radishes, thinly sliced

Crème fraîche

1. To make the dry brine: In a medium bowl, combine the sugar, salt, lemon zest, dill, peppercorns, coriander, cumin, and cannabis. Set aside.

2. Rinse the salmon under cold running water and pat dry with paper towels. In a glass baking dish (just big enough to hold the salmon) spread half of the dry brine onto the bottom of the dish. Place the salmon pieces over the mixture. Sprinkle the remaining brine evenly over the fish.

3. Slowly pour the lemon juice over the fish; gently smooth out the dry brine evenly over the fish with a butter knife. Place a sheet of parchment paper over the salmon and set a second baking sheet or small cutting board on top of the fish; top with several cans to weigh it down. Place in the refrigerator, turning and basting the fish with the accumulated juices every 10 to 12 hours. The fish will be ready to slice when the flesh is opaque, approximately 3 days, depending on the thickness of the fish.

4. Rinse the salmon slices under cold running water, removing all the salt mixture. Pat dry, then transfer to a paper-towel-lined plate. Place in the refrigerator, uncovered, for at least 1 hour. Transfer to a cutting board.

5. To make the crostini: Preheat the oven to 400°F. Lightly grease a baking sheet. Cut the baguette on the bias into ¼-inch slices. Arrange the bread slices in a single layer

Zest of 1 organic lemon

Salt and freshly ground black pepper

on the prepared baking sheet and brush with the olive oil. Bake until golden brown and crispy, about 5 minutes.

6. To assemble: Pat dry with paper towels once more, then slice the salmon against the grain on the bias into ¼-inch thick slices. Cover a crostini with salmon slices, a cucumber slice, radish slice, a dollop of crème fraîche, and sprinkles of lemon zest and pepper. Season with salt to taste. Repeat with the remaining ingredients. Serve at once.

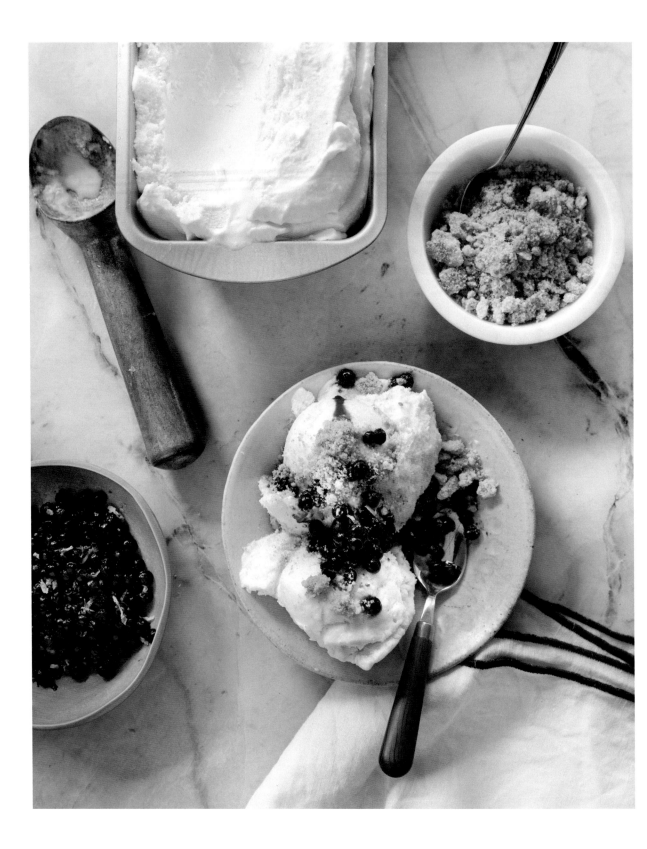

SWEET CORN ICE CREAM
with Brown Sugar Crumble and Wild Blueberries

by CLOUD CREAMERY

MAKES 5 cups; 10 half-cup sized servings

SUGGESTED DOSAGE: approximately 5 milligrams of THC per serving; approximately 50 milligrams THC per batch.

The cannabis-infused ice cream base used in this recipe pairs nicely with a strain high in pinene (or a-pinene), such as Northern Lights, to accentuate the fresh aromatic flavor of the thyme. The richness of the ice cream complements the pungently sweet, earthy, and piney flavors of this popular cannabis strain.

SWEET CORN ICE CREAM BASE

2 cups (14% milk fat) heavy cream, preferably grass-fed

2 cups whole milk, preferably organic

1 cup organic cane sugar

4 sprigs fresh thyme

1½ teaspoons kosher salt

1½ cups fresh organic corn kernels, cut from approximately 2 large ears of corn, reserving the cobs

1.75 grams (half-eighth) cannabis flower, finely ground, testing at 27–28% THC (see note below)

BROWN SUGAR CRUMBLE

Makes 2 cups

½ cup organic dark brown sugar, packed

½ cup coconut flour

¼ cup rice flour

⅓ cup cold unsalted butter, preferably grass-fed, cut into small pieces

1. To make the sweet corn ice cream base: In a heavy-bottomed saucepan, bring the cream, milk, sugar, thyme, and salt to just under boiling, whisking occasionally, over medium heat, about 20 minutes. Remove the ice cream base from the heat. Add the corn kernels, reserved cobs, and cannabis, into a large shallow pan. Carefully pour the base into the pan and allow to steep for 1 hour at room temperature. Cover with plastic wrap, gently pressing directly onto the surface of the mixture, and refrigerate overnight. Note: The wide base and shallow sides of the pan allow the ice cream base to cool more quickly.

2. Using tongs, remove the corn cobs and thyme from the base and discard. Whisk the ice cream base until well combined. Transfer half of the ice cream base to a food processor or blender and purée until smooth. Return the puréed ice cream base to the pan with the remaining mixture, stirring to combine well. Pour the ice cream base into a cold ice cream maker bowl, filling the machine no more than three-quarters of the way. Churn just until the ice cream is thick, about the consistency of soft-serve ice cream. Transfer to the freezer and freeze according to the manufacturer's directions.

3. To make the brown sugar crumble: While the ice cream is left to harden in the freezer, start the brown sugar

Ingredients list continues on next page

Recipe continues on next page

WILD BLUEBERRIES

Makes 1½ cups

1½ cups wild blueberries, washed and stems removed

1½ tablespoons organic cane sugar, or to taste

Zest and juice of 1 lemon

3 fresh mint leaves, chopped

crumble. Preheat the oven to 375°F. In the bowl of a food processor, combine the sugar and flours. Work in the butter, a few pieces at a time, and continue to pulse until the mixture is crumbly and forms pea-size lumps. Note: If working in a humid area, you may need to add a few drops of ice water to the crumble mixture. Bake on a quarter-sized baking sheet or in a medium oven-safe skillet in the oven, stirring occasionally, until golden brown, about 8 minutes. Set aside.

4. To prepare the wild blueberries: In a small bowl, gently toss the blueberries, sugar, lemon zest, lemon juice and mint until well combined. Set aside.

5. To serve: Scoop the ice cream into bowls and top each serving with brown sugar crumble and blueberries.

DAVID YUSEFZADEH'S NOTE

You do not need to decarboxylate the cannabis flower beforehand, as the heat from the cream will activate the cannabis.

DOSING

David Yusefzadeh

THC is just like anything else; it needs to be taken in moderation and in a safe environment. Alcohol can be consumed in various fashions: a glass of wine, a beer, a cocktail, or a shot of whiskey. They all have various alcohol content, vibrancy, and characteristics. They are not all equal. Cannabis is the same way. You can dose very high very quickly or you can micro-dose all day.

CARLY FISHER

Author/Journalist

Magic realism is a way of life for Carly Fisher, who believes in the transformative power of food, cannabis, and communities. Life wasn't always easy for the successful James Beard Foundation Award nominated journalist and author, who escaped a traumatic childhood oscillating between apartments, motels, and charity housing throughout the Chicagoland area before eventually putting herself through college at the University of Illinois in Champaign-Urbana, graduating with a degree in journalism and a minor in art history.

After a brief stint studying abroad at Charles University in Prague, Fisher returned to Chicago for the next several years, covering restaurants, nightlife and travel as an editor for NBC and contributing editor at Fodor's Travel, writing at large for *Food & Wine*, *Bon Appetit*, *Saveur*, and *Plate*. A transformative trip to New York City would become the first time that she felt truly at "home," and that's why in 2014, she packed her belongings and headed for Brooklyn to start a new life. She has grown to love this diverse borough for its eclectic mix of lifestyles, music, restaurants, nightlife, and culture.

Cannabis has always been a part of her life, dating back to when she was a teenager and used it to spark her creativity and manage anxiety and depression. She appreciates its many wellness components, particularly CBD, which has proven scientific benefits to help a number of chronic diseases and improve overall health. Passionate about agriculture, terroir, and cultural relationships with food, Fisher is fascinated by cannabis as a food-drug, documenting the histories of memories, perception, shared experiences, fringe cultures, and esoterica. As a result of this interest, she maintained two successful cannabis culture columns, writing for Merry Jane, a cannabis-focused digital media platform, giving strain-based astrology advice for Leafly, the largest cannabis website in the world, and routinely contributing stories to *GQ*, *High Times*, and Miss Grass. Committed to destigmatizing cannabis, Fisher believes it is the responsibility of the fast-growing cannabis industry to invest in education, research, and social equity programs to help communities impacted by the "war on drugs."

Crediting her Depression-era Jewish grandmother as the biggest culinary influence in her life, she believes in making everything from scratch and is fond of comfort foods and her family's old-world recipes. The food she serves is simple, fresh, nutritious, and delicious. For this culinarian, it is all about sharing great tasting, feel-good meals and spreading happiness with others. This busy author/journalist loves hosting and cooking for a crowd, considering leftovers a reward for her day's work.

The journalist, now turned author, has written a book entitled *Easy Weekend Getaways in the Hudson Valley & Catskills*. After two years of research, the travel guide was released in April 2020 and is geared toward curious travelers who want to explore the culture, food, nature, history and experiences of these two iconic regions. Although this book is not specifically geared toward cannabis experiences, Fisher says, with a wink and a nod, that those who are so inclined can use it as a guide to have a fun-filled weekend.

Fisher still happily lives in Brooklyn. In her down moments, she enjoys volunteering her time working with seniors and children. She also lends her talents to fundraising campaigns and partnering with public-spirited organizations for community-based outreach. Carly Fisher's journey has indeed led her home!

SH'MAC AND CHEESE

(HIGH-DOSE RECIPE—NOT FOR BEGINNERS)

by CARLY FISHER

MAKES 8 servings

SUGGESTED DOSAGE: 175 milligrams THC, each serving 21.87 milligrams THC.

CARLY FISHER: Cooking with shatter or concentrate is one of the easiest ways to infuse, and among my favorites when I am feeling too lazy to properly infuse. It's also great for entertaining, which was the case one fine summer afternoon when I made this recipe on a whim with a friend. While the wiser, older, and more respectable version of myself advises proper dosing, we both cosign this as a great way to kick back, watch some movies, and then completely zonk out. We split this recipe so that it included second helpings, which means that splitting this among ten would probably be a safer bet for those with lower tolerances, or who need to be remotely functional. Consider this a heavy-hitter-approved recipe.

¼ ounce shatter (or depending on the tolerance level)

1 pound macaroni

1 tablespoon extra-virgin olive oil

½ cup unsalted butter

½ cup all-purpose flour

2½ cups whole milk, warm

1½ cups half-and-half, warm

3 cups grated sharp white cheddar cheese

2 cups grated Gruyère cheese

1 cup mascarpone cheese

½ tablespoon salt

½ teaspoon freshly ground black pepper

¼ teaspoon paprika

¼ teaspoon powdered mustard

¼ teaspoon finely grated nutmeg

TOPPINGS

½ cup panko bread crumbs

½ cup Parmesan cheese, shredded

1. Grease a 9×13-inch baking dish with butter and set aside.
2. To decarb the cannabis: Preheat the oven to 250°F. Place the shatter in a small ovenproof glass baking dish and bake for 30 minutes. Note: This will activate the material.
3. While the oven is preheating for the shatter, start cooking the pasta. To cook the pasta: Bring a large pot of salted water to a boil over medium-high heat. Add the pasta and cook according to the package directions until just shy of al dente. Drain well.
4. Transfer the pasta to a large bowl and toss with the olive oil. Set aside.
5. Once the shatter has been decarboxylated, remove from the oven and increase the oven temperature to 375°F.
6. While the pasta is cooking, start making the roux. To make the roux: Melt the butter in a large saucepan over medium heat. Whisk in the flour and cook, whisking constantly, until fully combined and free of lumps, about 2 minutes.

Recipe continues on page 241

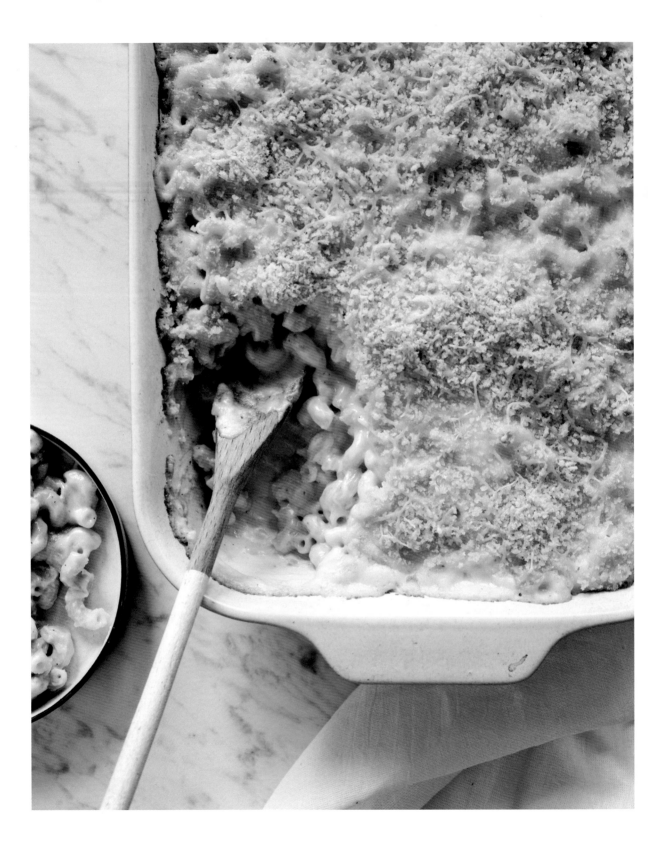

7. Slowly pour in the milk and then half-and-half, whisking constantly until smooth and thick. Add the cheddar and Gruyère cheeses in large handfuls, stirring until completely melted and smooth. Stir in the mascarpone until smooth. Whisk in the salt, pepper, paprika, mustard, and nutmeg until well combined. Using a silicone spatula, pour the melted shatter directly into the cheese mixture and stir until evenly combined. Tip: Concentrates tend to be very sticky. It is helpful to use a silicone spatula when working with concentrates to prevent sticking.

8. Add the cheese mixture to the pasta, stirring until well combined and evenly coated. Adjust seasonings with salt and pepper.

9. Pour the pasta-cheese mixture into the prepared baking dish. Evenly sprinkle the top with Parmesan cheese and bread crumbs.

10. Bake until golden brown and bubbling, about 25 minutes. Let sit for 10 minutes before serving.

WHAT IS SHATTER?

A hard form of a cannabis extract, shatter is an amber or gold, glass-like translucent concentrate. Shatter requires decarboxylation of its compounds through heat to produce the desired effects. Heating the shatter turns the extract into a runnier consistency that resembles sap, hence the commonly used nickname, "sap."

NICOLE CAMPBELL & RUPERT CAMPBELL

Co-owners, The Green Lady Dispensary

The quaint island of Nantucket became home to the Green Lady Dispensary in August 2019. This family owned company is one of only a few minority- and women-owned canna-businesses in Massachusetts. Owners Nicole and Rupert Campbell have an enduring connection to the island that they love. After working in the agricultural industry for thirty years, helping to run a family-owned fertilizer business, Nicole thought that it was time for a much-needed change. She wanted to do something new and exciting that her daughters could enjoy, the end-result being the creation of The Green Lady Dispensary.

The Green Lady Dispensary is in a facility that was formerly a dentist's office and home. The building in which it is housed looks like most of the island's residences, blending in with its surroundings and designed for discretion. Nicole calls it a "secret mystery" because from the outside the structure looks like any other building on Nantucket. Visitors can easily access the location by bike, walking, or public transportation. The company's name is a play on words; "The Green Lady" is a clever reference to Nantucket's nickname, the "Gray Lady," while "Green" refers to the cannabis at the heart of the business.

Nicole is the co-owner and chief operating officer of the company. She also serves as lab manager, as well as head of marketing, advertising, and finances. Her husband, Rupert, oversees security while their daughter, Corbet, is retail manager. Chef Eric Anderson brings his experience from working in the galleys of some of the island's best kitchens. It is his job to create Green Lady's line of handmade edibles. He is also the head farmer and manages the cultivation. The business has thirty employees and hopes to attract even more as time goes on.

The company is located on an island that is thirty miles out in the Atlantic Ocean in Federal waters. Since cannabis is federally illegal, it is not allowed to cross the territory of Nantucket Sound, or travel through airspace to reach the island. Following Federal law, it is illegal for the business to transport anything to or from the island, making it necessary for the Green

Lady Dispensary to be completely self-contained. They must produce everything that they sell in-house, with the production and sale of cannabis all done on the island.

The business is vertically integrated, which means that all products must be grown and processed by the same company that sells them. The company has a state-of-the-art cultivation facility, extraction lab with a cutting-edge supercritical CO_2 extractor, and a fully equipped commercial kitchen. They have one of the most comprehensive cannabis grow systems in the industry, completely powered by LED grow lights to reduce electric consumption. Their unique island location has allowed the Campbells to receive permission to cultivate marijuana and conduct laboratory testing on-site, instead of following the normal requirement that products must be tested at a licensed independent lab.

Clients must show a government-issued ID—driver's license, ID card, or passport. The dispensary's friendly, knowledgeable staff are expert in everything that the store has to offer. The business, which first opened as an adult use retailer, has now added medical sales to their product line. Budtenders, also known as sales agents, take time to talk with their customers, seeking to know them better. The focus is on education, helping folks who are new to the cannabis scene to learn how to use the product safely and wisely. If a visitor chooses a budtending session, they will meet with a budtender who will discuss the dispensary's different products, strains, and dosages, imparting an understanding of the items that are being purchased.

The dispensary offers a wide selection of top-quality concentrates that range from freshly pressed rosin to cold water hash. Flower, edibles, tinctures, and topicals are readily available. Customers will find everything from fan favorites to the most unusual strains, including a diverse selection of superior cannabis products. The best genetics are handpicked, alongside unique strains such as "Moby Dick," a high-THC cross between indica-dominant hybrid White Widow and sativa Haze that originated in Amsterdam. Pre-rolls are ground to the ideal size, the flower weighed and hand-packed for consistency, the joints then beautifully rolled and wrapped. The selection of topicals consist of cannabis-infused lotions, balms, and oils. THC and CBD are combined with natural plant extracts like aloe vera, lavender, and rosemary. Self-care products and cartridges are for sale as well.

Chef Eric Anderson is at the helm of the company's edible line of products. He graduated from the Culinary Institute of America in Hyde Park, New York with an associate degree in culinary arts and a bachelor's degree in management. While working as a private chef on Nantucket, he reached out to Nicole and Rupert to see if there was an opening for him on their team and came onboard soon after. Chef Anderson feels that working with cannabis is a natural evolution in his career. The chef's personal cooking philosophy is to keep things simple and fresh, believing that we truly need to eat what is local and in season.

Green Lady's small-batch bakery produces freshly baked cannabis-infused edibles that include a variety of chocolate bars, chews, ice cream cups, cookies, and brownies. Chef Anderson infuses the edibles with only the best pure THC distillate and the distillery's slow-simmered full flower cannabutter. He readily admits to having a sweet tooth, making working with chocolate and other treats an ideal way to express his creativity.

The Campbells and their Green Lady Dispensary have a mission to provide high-quality and naturally cultivated cannabis products to Nantucket's adult residents and vacationers. It is their hope that the business can be a positive example for other areas, showing that cannabis does not change the fabric of their society. They have invested in the island's future with high-paying jobs, great benefits, and an annual pledge of $10,000 to Nantucket High School's scholarship fund. The Campbells also support many Nantucket charities such as: A.S.A.P (The Alliance for Substance Abuse and Prevention), NAMI (National Alliance on Mental Illness), and NiSHA (Nantucket Island Safe Harbor for Animals). The owners of The Green Lady Dispensary are working hard to be good neighbors by giving back to their island community.

NANTUCKET PROTEIN LOGS

by CHEF ERIC ANDERSON, THE GREEN LADY DISPENSARY   **MAKES** 9 protein logs

> **CHEF ERIC ANDERSON:** Always read dosing directions on tincture packages carefully. Remember it is always better to start low and slow.
>
> **SUGGESTED DOSAGE:** 5 milligrams THC per protein log.

Scant 1 cup raw and shelled, unsalted pistachios

⅔ cup raw and unsalted cashews

Heaping ⅓ cup old-fashioned rolled oats

⅓ cup hemp hearts

1 cup dried cranberries, sweetened

2 tablespoons shredded coconut, sweetened

¼ cup plus ½ tablespoon corn syrup

Zest and juice from ½ lemon

Zest and juice from ½ lime

1 tablespoon matcha tea powder

¼ teaspoon ground ginger

Heaping ¼ teaspoon kosher salt

45 milligrams THC tincture, preferably The Green Lady Dispensary Tincture

1. Arrange a rack in the middle of the oven. Preheat the oven to 325°F. Line a baking sheet with parchment paper.
2. In a medium bowl, combine the pistachios, cashews, oats, hemp hearts, cranberries, and coconut, mixing until well combined. Pour the nut mixture onto the prepared baking sheet and spread out into an even layer. Bake until lightly golden brown, about 10 minutes, stirring occasionally. Let cool to room temperature.
3. Increase the oven temperature to 350°F.
4. Transfer the nut mixture to a bowl of a food processor and chop into medium-sized pieces. Transfer to a mixing bowl, tossing until well combined. Set aside.
5. In a separate bowl, add the corn syrup, zests and juices, tea, ginger, and salt and mix until well incorporated. Add the THC tincture and mix again.
6. While stirring continuously, slowly add the zest mixture to the dry mixture, until well incorporated.
7. Using a ¼-cup scoop, measure out the mixture into nine 2-ounce portions. Using slightly wetted hands, form each portion into 1½×2-inch logs. Place on the prepared baking sheet about 1½ inches apart.
8. Bake until soft on the inside and golden brown around the edges, about 14 minutes.
9. Remove from the oven and let the logs cool to room temperature, about 20 minutes.
10. The protein logs will keep up to 2 weeks if stored in an airtight container or up to a month in the freezer.

CLASSIC CHOCOLATE CHIP COOKIES

by CHEF ERIC ANDERSON, THE GREEN LADY DISPENSARY   **MAKES** 12 cookies

> **CHEF ERIC:** For softer, chewier cookies, decrease the bake time, and for a crunchier texture increase the bake time.
>
> **SUGGESTED DOSAGE:** 8.3 milligrams THC per cookie.

Note: You will need to make the cannabis-infused butter 1 day before you intend to use it.

¼ pound unsalted cannabis-infused butter (page 247)

⅓ cup plus 1 tablespoon brown sugar

⅓ cup white sugar

1 large egg

1½ teaspoons pure vanilla extract

1½ cups all-purpose flour

¼ teaspoon baking soda

½ teaspoon salt

¾ cup high-quality chocolate chips

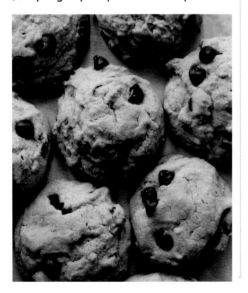

1. Preheat the oven to 325°F. Line a half-sheet-sized baking sheet with parchment paper. Set aside.

2. To make the cookies: In a bowl of a stand mixer fitted with a paddle attachment, cream together the butter and sugars on medium-high speed until light, fluffy, and creamy, scraping down the sides of the bowl as needed. While the stand mixer is running, add the egg and vanilla, scraping down the sides of the bowl, until fully incorporated.

3. In a large bowl, sift together the flour, baking soda, and salt. Working in batches, add the flour mixture to the butter mixture and mix on low speed until smooth. Do not overwork the dough. Add the chocolate chips and continue to mix on low speed until just incorporated.

4. Scoop up the dough using a ¼-cup measuring cup. Note: The cookie dough fits nicely into a ¼-cup measuring cup, but scantly, so not quite a full ¼ cup. Place on the prepared baking sheet about 2 to 3 inches apart.

5. Bake until light golden brown, about 12 to 18 minutes. Allow the cookies to cool on the baking sheet for 5 minutes, then transfer to cooling rack to cool completely.

SIMPLE CANNABIS-INFUSED BUTTER

by CHEF ERIC ANDERSON, THE GREEN LADY DISPENSARY

CHEF ERIC ANDERSON: Coarsely grind ½ gram cannabis flower, testing at 20% Delta-9-THC, with a handheld grinder. The suggested dose for the cannabis-infused butter used in the Classic Chocolate Chip Cookie recipe (page 246) will be approximately 8.3 milligrams per cookie.

½ gram cannabis flower, coarsely ground

¼ pound unsalted butter

1. Preheat the oven to 285°F. Line a baking sheet with foil. Place the cannabis on the prepared baking sheet and toast until slightly golden brown and has a nutty fragrance, about 12 minutes.

2. Melt butter in a saucepan over low heat. Add the decarbed cannabis to the melted butter and let stand in a warm place for 1 hour. Note: To prevent the butter from scorching, it is important for the temperature not to exceed 140°F. Strain the butter through a coffee filter into a clean mason jar, discarding or composting any plant matter. Let the butter cool to room temperature, then transfer to the refrigerator and allow to harden overnight. Note: If excess water forms at the bottom of the jar, you can remove the solid butter with a knife.

JOSEPHINE PROUL

Owner, Local 111 Restaurant

Visitors to Local 111 Restaurant in Philmont, New York, have described the eatery as upscale, warm and welcoming and it is that, plus so much more! Located in what was once an old service station, the space has been adapted and remodeled into a bright cheery area accented by large expanses of glass. In warm weather, the sliding glass bay doors open for outdoor dining. The restaurant itself has room enough to seat thirty-eight guests.

Owner Josephine Proul was born in California and moved to Philmont with her mother at the age of nineteen. Being of Sicilian heritage, Proul was immersed in the culture of food before she even took her first steps. As a small child, she would help her grandfather stir risottos and hand grind sausage for the family's weekly dinner gatherings. At the age of fourteen, the young girl landed her first job at a pizza parlor, an experience that offered her an early awareness of how much she loved the culinary arts.

In 2008, after graduating from the New England Culinary Institute in Montpelier, Vermont, Proul became the chef and general manager of Local 111 Restaurant in New York's Hudson Valley. Six years later, the restaurant's owners offered to pass the torch to Proul, who happily accepted. As the new owner, she believed that Philmont needed a gathering place like Local 111 to help encourage a sense of community pride.

Community involvement is the driving force behind the workings of Proul's restaurant and has become her life's mission. The dedicated chef is always striving to cultivate relationships and networks among area farmers, chefs, purveyors, and the local community. She feels that the key to accomplishing this goal is to center the selections on Local 111's menu around food that is primarily sourced from New York State. Her focus is to serve dishes that connect the restaurant's patrons to these local providers and their products, thereby creating a ripple effect of support for the future growth of farms, farmers' markets, food education, and the local food culture.

The restaurant's staff are a dedicated and close-knit group. Proul seeks out neighborhood teenagers to fill positions, striving to instill in them a sense of loyalty for the business and their community. These efforts have not gone unnoticed, as is clearly evidenced by the steady stream of customers who return to Local 111 on a regular basis, eager to sample the restaurant's latest farm-to-table creations. Because of her efforts and hard work, Proul was awarded the fourth annual Victoria A. Simons Locavore Award for her commitment to using local products and promoting community growth.

Chef Proul wears many hats—executive and pastry chef, general and front of house manager, event and catering planner, and supporter of honest food and small businesses. In her rare spare time, the busy restaurateur gardens, exercises, plays with her three dogs, and travels. Her travels offer international inspiration which she brings back to Local 111, sharing her adventures with wine, Parisian-style bread, and Spanish-inspired cuisine. Whether it may mean a menu change, or tweaking the dining room's decor, Chef Proul has a love for all that is sustainable.

The menu changes with the seasons, inspired by the bounty of local farms. The food that is served is farm fresh and sustainable, with all animals being humanely raised. Mouthwatering selections may include comfort dishes like pork porterhouse with roasted warm apples and kielbasa, li'l lamb pie, or vegetarian plates such as aged cheddar risotto. In her role as pastry chef, Proul creates delicacies such as rhubarb pavlovas, zucchini bread donuts, and cornbread shortcakes. In 2015, 2016, and 2017, Chef Proul received the best chef in Columbia County award for her delicious ingredient driven approach to cooking.

Hudson Hemp, a company that cultivates hemp-based products for medicinal and culinary use, invited the chef to create a seasonal menu which was driven, and focused, around hemp and CBD. Because they were a New York State hemp business, Hudson wanted a local chef, who had experience cooking with cannabis, to take charge of the culinary aspect of a CBD party that they were hosting. The chef readily admits that her life and food culture have always been exposed to the cannabis industry. She acknowledges the healing properties and pain management of THC and CBD and confirms the connection between the chefs and farmers who support this movement. As a like-minded member of this group, Chef Proul believes that when we take into consideration our farming, hemp, and cannabis models of agriculture, regenerative practices are supporting a future that is geared toward sustainability and biodiversity.

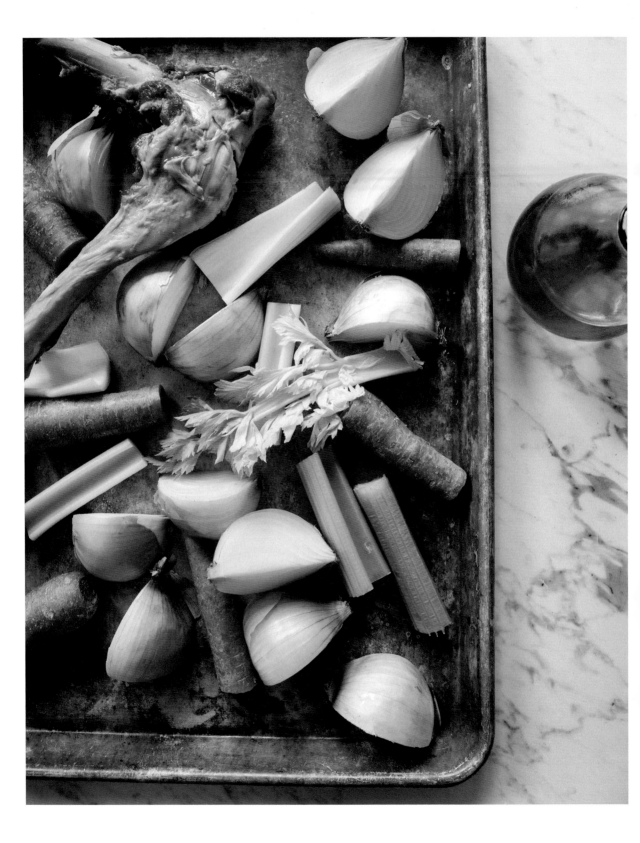

LAMB STOCK

by JOSEPHINE PROUL, LOCAL 111 RESTAURANT

MAKES approximately 14 cups

When making homemade stocks, it is important to always use high-quality bones. Roasting the bones beforehand, will enhance the color and flavor of your finished stock. Add this nourishing elixir to rice dishes, such as the Basmati Rice with Dried Fruits and Olives (page 256) for a flavor boost or as a base for the Braised Lamb with Turmeric and Lemon dish (page 253).

Olive oil, as needed

1 (about 5½ to 6½ pounds) whole leg of lamb

3 onions, unpeeled and quartered

2 carrots, unpeeled and cut into 3-inch pieces

3 celery ribs, cut into 3-inch pieces

4 quarts of water

2 cups dry red wine

½ cup tomato paste

1. To make the lamb stock: Preheat the oven to 400°F. Lightly oil a rimmed baking sheet. Set aside.

2. Trim the fat and debone the leg of lamb, reserving the bone and trimmings for the stock. Cut the meat into 1-inch cubes and refrigerate until ready to use for the Braised Lamb with Turmeric and Lemon (page 253).

3. Generously oil the lamb bone and place it along with the reserved fat and trimmings, onions, carrots, and celery on the prepared baking sheet. Roast, stirring occasionally until the bone is well browned, about 30 minutes. Using tongs, transfer the bone and vegetables to a large stockpot or Dutch oven, discarding the fat. Stir in the water, red wine, and tomato paste. Bring to a gentle boil over medium-high heat, about 20 minutes.

4. Reduce the heat to a simmer, partially covered, stirring occasionally, for 6 hours. Remove from the heat and skim off any impurities and fat from the surface. Allow the stock to cool to room temperature, about 1 hour. Using tongs, remove the large solids, and discard.

5. Strain the stock through a fine-mesh strainer into a clean, heat-resistant large bowl. Cover and place in the refrigerator overnight.

6. Using a spatula or a spoon, carefully scrape and pull off the fat that has solidified on the surface.

Recipe continues on next page

NOTES

To save on time, prepare the stock one day before you intend to use it for the Braised Lamb with Turmeric and Lemon dish. Label and date the contents, then store in an airtight container in the refrigerator.

This recipe makes more lamb stock than you will need for the recipes. Freeze the extra for a later use.

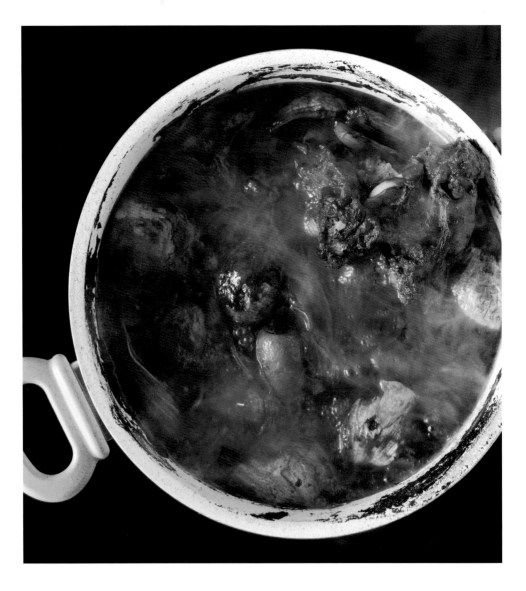

BRAISED LAMB
with Turmeric and Lemon

JOSEPHINE PROUL, LOCAL 111 RESTAURANT

MAKES 6 to 8 servings

To save on time, prepare the lamb stock (page 251) one day before you intend to use it for the Braised Lamb with Turmeric and Lemon dish.

TURMERIC SPICE MIX

Makes ½ cup

Note: This recipe makes more spice mixture than you will need for the recipe. Save the extra and sprinkle it over fish, chicken, or roasted vegetables.

4 tablespoons turmeric

2 tablespoons ground coriander

2 tablespoons sumac or grated lemon zest

1 tablespoon kosher salt

LAMB

4 tablespoons grapeseed oil, divided, or as needed

4 pounds cubed leg of lamb, trimmed of fat

4 medium onions, peeled, thinly sliced and cut into half-moons (about 4 cups)

3 tablespoons thinly sliced garlic, about 5 medium cloves

2 bay leaves

5 tablespoons turmeric spice mixture, or to taste

6 cups lamb stock, or as needed, homemade (page 251)

1. To make the turmeric spice mix: In a small bowl, combine the turmeric, coriander, sumac, and salt. Set aside.

2. In a heavy-bottomed pot or Dutch oven, heat 3 tablespoons of the grapeseed oil over medium-high heat until hot but not smoking. Pat the lamb meat dry with paper towels. Working in batches, brown the meat on all sides, adding additional oil as needed. Remove the meat from the pot and set aside. Add the remaining 1 tablespoon of oil and onions, and sauté, stirring often, until soft and translucent, about 5 minutes. Add the garlic and cook, stirring frequently, until fragrant, about 1 minute. Add the bay leaves.

3. Return the meat to the pot along with any accumulated juices. Generously coat all sides of the meat with some of the turmeric spice mix, about 5 tablespoons. Cover the meat with enough lamb stock to cover the meat completely, scraping up any brown bits on the bottom of the pot, about 6 cups. Stir in the lemon juice, then bring the mixture to a slow boil, about 15 minutes. Reduce the heat to a simmer, cover, and cook until the meat is fork-tender, about 3½ hours. Note: As the stew nears the 3-hour mark, remove the lid and check the meat to see if it is fork-tender or needs more time to cook.

4. Using a large metal spoon, skim off the fat that rises to the surface. Stir in the THC-infused olive oil, mixing until well combined.

5. Using a large slotted spoon transfer the meat and onions into a strainer over a large heatproof bowl. Carefully pour

Ingredients list continues on page 255

Recipe continues on page 255

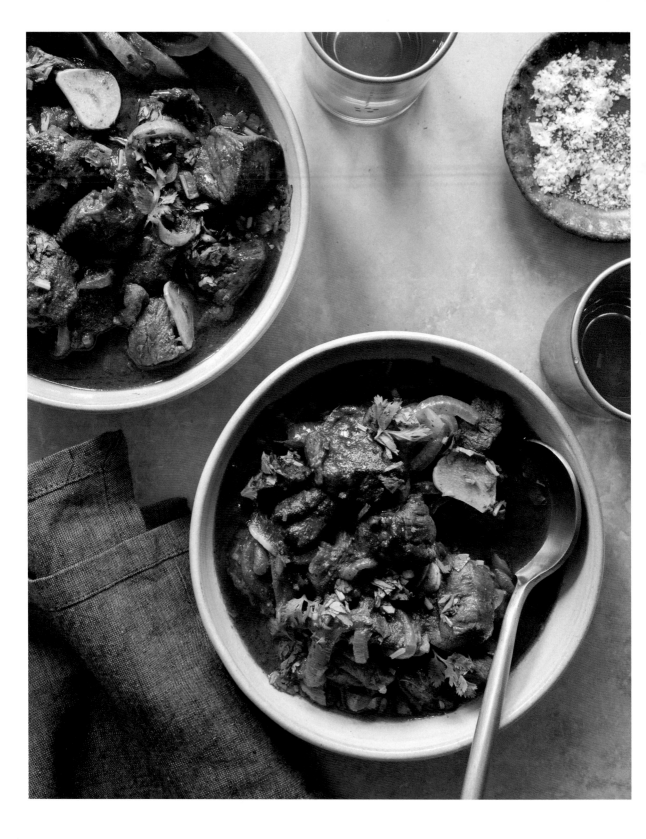

½ cup fresh lemon juice, or as needed

2 tablespoons THC-infused olive oil, store-bought or homemade

2 cups fresh minced cilantro, leaves and stems, discarding any tough stems (about 2 large bunches)

the liquid that had strained off from the meat and onions back into the pot with the reserved sauce.

6. While the meat and onions are resting in the strainer, finish making the sauce. Increase the heat to medium-high heat and cook until it is reduced by half, about 35 minutes. Return the meat to the pot. Season with salt and pepper to taste. Adjust seasonings with additional spice mixture and lemon juice, if desired. Stir in the cilantro.

7. Serve at once with Basmati Rice with Dried Fruits and Olives (page 256). Note: If you plan on serving the Basmati Rice with Dried Fruits and Olives with the lamb, it is recommended, while the sauce is reducing, start preparing the rice dish.

JOSEPHINE PROUL'S NOTE

When making the infused oil for this dish, I prefer using sativa cannabis strains.

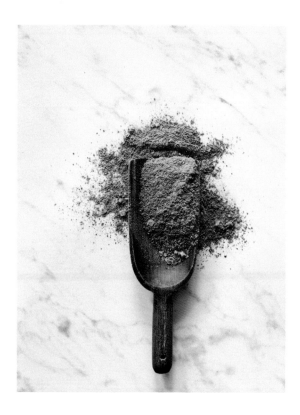

BASMATI RICE
with Dried Fruits and Olives

by JOSEPHINE PROUL, LOCAL 111 RESTAURANT

MAKES 10½ cups

Basmati rice is known for its unique, nutty aroma and fluffy texture. When selecting basmati rice, look for grains that have a slightly golden hue. Whenever possible, purchase basmati rice packaged in cloth bags labeled "extra-long grain."

2½ cups basmati rice

2½ tablespoons extra-virgin olive oil or grapeseed oil

1 large onion, peeled and finely chopped

2 carrots, cut into ¼-inch dice

3 tablespoons minced garlic

½ teaspoon kosher salt, or to taste

¼ teaspoon freshly ground black pepper, or to taste

1 teaspoon red pepper flakes

1 teaspoon ground fennel seeds

1 teaspoon ground coriander

2 thyme sprigs

2 bay leaves

¼ cup Picholine or Niçoise olives, pitted and halved

¼ cup goji berries or raisins

¼ cup chopped dried apricots

5 cups lamb stock (page 251) or vegetable stock, warm

3 tablespoons THC-infused olive oil

1. Rinse the rice in several changes of cold water, until the water runs clear. Drain well in a fine-mesh strainer. Set aside.
2. Heat the oil in a Dutch oven or in a large heavy-bottomed pot over medium heat. Add the onions and carrots, and cook, stirring often, until onions are soft and translucent, about 6 minutes. Add the garlic and cook until fragrant, about 1 minute. Season with the salt and pepper.
3. Add the red pepper flakes, fennel seeds, ground coriander, thyme, and bay leaves, and cook until fragrant, about 1 minute.
4. Add the basmati rice and stir until evenly coated. Cook the rice until the ends of the grains are almost translucent, about 5 minutes.
5. Add the olives, goji berries, and apricots, stirring until evenly coated.
6. Add the stock and stir, scraping up the bits from the bottom of the pan, and bring to a boil over medium-high heat.
7. Reduce the heat to a simmer, cover, stirring occasionally, until most of the stock is absorbed and the grains are tender, about 15 minutes.
8. Remove from the heat, and place the lid over the pot and let stand for 10 minutes. Remove and discard the thyme sprigs and bay leaves.
9. Drizzle the THC-infused olive oil over and around the top of rice and fluff with a fork. Season with salt and pepper to taste. Transfer to a decorative bowl and serve with Braised Lamb with Turmeric and Lemon (page 253).

NOTE

Approximately 50 minutes before the Braised Lamb with Turmeric and Lemon (page 253) is done, start preparing the basmati rice.

WEST

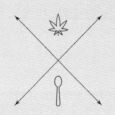

JESSICA CATALANO

Professional Culinarian/Medical Cannabis Advocate

Jessica Catalano was always drawn to the western part of the United States. She lived in Colorado for ten years, earning culinary degrees in pastry arts, culinary arts, and food service management before moving to a suburb of Seattle. While in Colorado, Catalano developed business relationships with local cannabis growers, learning how to grow the products under the tutelage of two master growers. The chef realized the importance of having trusted growers to depend on for organic flower and products, but also knew the value of being able to do the process yourself, which enables a person to be sustainable.

Chef Catalano is a medical cannabis patient, cooking for medicinal purposes with marijuana since 1997. She uses cannabis to treat her chronic migraines and to help manage the anxiety and depression associated with this problem. The chef began experimenting with strain-specific cooking and baking in 2009, launching a blog in June 2010 to share her recipes with medical marijuana patients. According to Catalano, she is the first chef in the United States to pioneer strain-specific cannabis cuisine for flavor, doing so by infusing terpenes in the preparation of her strain specific recipes. The chef has found that this method elevates the taste in the edibles that she creates.

Chef Catalano's goal is to help folks use plant medicine to create a better quality of life. She has dedicated her entire career to helping people heal with cannabis. In 2012, Jessica was offered a book deal by Green Candy Press, and *The Ganja Kitchen Revolution: The Bible of Cannabis Cuisine* was born—the very first strain-specific gourmet cannabis cookbook.

Chef Catalano is a professional culinarian and medical advocate who combines her two loves, food and cannabis, into stylishly delicious medicated dishes. She believes that the health benefits of cooking with cannabis, balanced with good nutrition, can help promote a longer and more fulfilling life. Catalano maintains that, "Plant-based medicine, when treated with respect, can be a life-changing experience. If used properly, both THC and CBD can be a healthy alternative to prescription pharmaceutical drugs. Both cannabinoids hold equal power in healing, but in different ways for different people."

CANNABIS-INFUSED COCONUT OIL

by JESSICA CATALANO

MAKES ½ cup

JESSICA CATALANO: Ideally, the best way to measure the psychoactive effect of the strain you are using is to get the bud tested in a lab, then do the math to figure out how many milligrams it is per serving of coconut oil. The reality is that this is not something everyone has access to, and you must rely on basics.

Always remember that every 1 gram of cannabis bud has 1,000 milligrams of dry weight. The average percentage of THC per gram is roughly 10 percent, with 15 percent being above average, and 20–27 percent being on the higher end. If a strain has 10 percent THC per gram lab tested, 10 percent of 1,000 milligrams would be 100 milligrams. Therefore, add the amount of cannabis for the desired dosage per tablespoon. Lastly, many factors can change the end dosage result; for that reason, keep in mind that this is an equation for approximate dosage.

½ cup raw coconut oil

3.5 grams ground decarboxylated NYC Blue or Blue Diesel (also known as Blue City Diesel)

1. Place the coconut oil into the top pan of a double boiler. Set aside

2. Pour about 1 inch of water into the bottom pan and bring to a simmer. Place the top pan with the coconut oil on top, making sure the bowl does not touch the simmering water. When the coconut oil is fully melted, add the decarboxylated cannabis and stir to make sure all the cannabis is fully saturated with the lipids. Let the oil infuse for 1 hour, maintaining enough water in the bottom part of the double boiler. While the oil is infusing, using a candy thermometer, make sure the oil temperature stays at 220–249°F. Remove from the heat and allow the oil to briefly cool.

3. Strain the infused oil through a cheesecloth-lined fine-mesh strainer into a clean heat-resistant glass jar. When cool enough to handle, gather the corners of the cheesecloth and gently squeeze out any excess oil into the jar. Discard or compost the plant matter. Label the jar with the date and contents.

Recipe continues on page 261

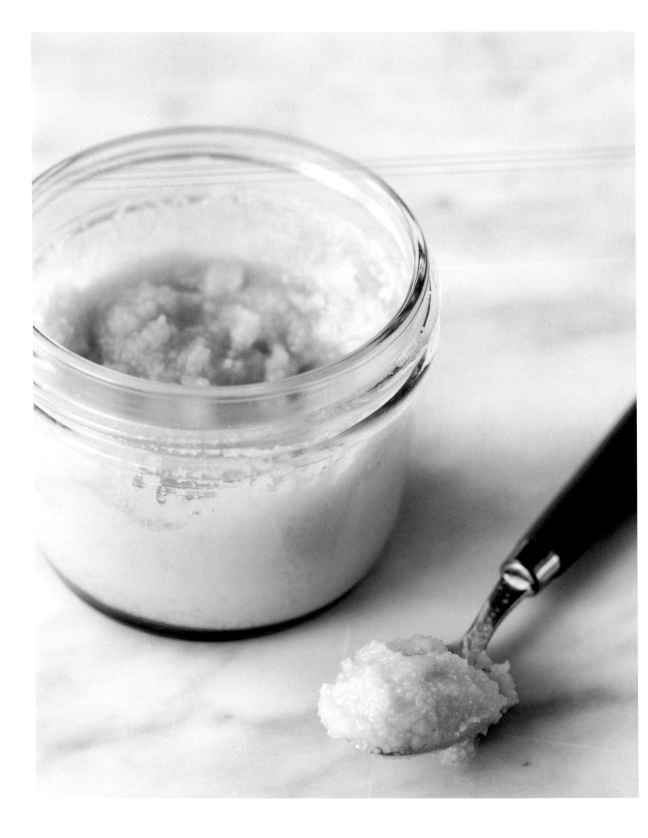

NOTE

This recipe makes more oil than you will need for the Vegan NYC Blue Fruit and Nut Chocolate Hemp Bars (page 262), so save the extra oil for another use.

JESSICA CATALANO'S NOTE

Genetically, NYC Blue is similar to the Blue Diesel (also known as Blue City Diesel) strain, but it is grown by a different breeder and has a different phenotype. I believe there are several phenotypes rolling around by different breeders. However, the Colorado one was just called NYC Blue. Blue City Diesel was originally produced by Breeder's Choice Collective.

JESSICA CATALANO'S TIP

For fats, the ideal temperature range is 220–249°F.

VEGAN NYC BLUE FRUIT
and Nut Chocolate Hemp Bars

by JESSICA CATALANO **MAKES** 24 2×2-inch bars

JESSICA CATALANO: There is a long list of fruit bars, granola bars, fruit and nut bars, and every kind of health bar that you can imagine flooding your local natural food market. Most have preservatives to keep them fresh and most unfortunately don't use the best protein sources. When I first moved to Colorado, I began experimenting with making strain-specific fruit bars, granola bars, energy bars, run recovery bars, and exercise recovery bars. I found that I could make a custom delicious health food bar without all the preservatives and with better quality protein: hemp.

When compared to soy, hemp possesses a protein profile that is more complete. This wonderful protein source contains the twenty-one most commonly known amino acids, as well as nine essential amino acids. It is rich in omega-3 and omega-6, easy to digest, less risk for an allergic reaction, and earth friendly. In my professional opinion, it is the best protein to use in these types of bars, as I have found one's body seems to benefit from it more than soy or whey. This powerful protein, combined with coconut oil, coconut flakes, dates, semisweet chocolate, cashews and flaxseed, creates a nutrient-dense health food bar without all the preservatives.

NYC Blue hails from the front range of Colorado, in historic Fort Collins, and was given to me by a good grower friend of mine, Scotty Hudson. This strain is the beautiful creation of the classic NYC Diesel (parent) and the ever-delicious Blueberry (parent). It is an indica-dominant strain (60/40) with a very sweet berry flavor mixed with diesel and floral earth undertones. This is the perfect edible for those days you just want to cruise the powder on your snowboard and relaxingly jib off a random object, in spite of the fact that your legs are sore from the other day of riding. This bar is also perfect as a nutritiously dense bar that will provide fantastic pain relief, relief from anxiety, relaxation of the body, and relaxation of the mind. The sativa spectrum of this strain will also help with energy levels. If you need the relief mentioned above but want to get things done or explore your world, this is the edible for you.

This is an extremely simple recipe that you can make in the privacy of your own home. Bring the bars with you to work, when you run errands, during a recovery exercise, or simply enjoy them in your home. Remember, if you cannot locate NYC Blue in your hometown, you can always swap it for another strain that has similar taste and smell profiles.

Note: You will need to make the infused coconut oil at least 1 hour before you intend to make the bars.

Note: You will need to soak the raw cashews in hot water for at least 15 minutes before you intend to use them.

½ cup raw unsalted cashews

1 heaping cup fresh Medjool dates, pitted (about 13 dates)

1 cup unsweetened shredded coconut

¼ cup cannabis-infused coconut oil, melted (page 259)

¼ cup semisweet chocolate chips

¼ cup organic hemp protein, chocolate

1 tablespoon ground flaxseeds

1 tablespoon almond extract

1 tablespoon vanilla extract

¹⁄₁₆ teaspoon (a pinch) fine-grain sea salt

1. To prepare the raw cashews (using the quick-soak method): Place the raw cashews in a medium bowl. Fill the bowl with very hot water (just below a boil), making sure the cashews are completely submerged. Soak the cashews for at least 15 minutes. Drain, rinse, and set aside.

2. Line a 9×13-inch baking dish with parchment paper. Set aside.

3. Pat the cashews dry with paper towels. Place the cashews in a bowl of a food processor and pulse until they are crumbly. Add the dates, shredded coconut, coconut oil, chocolate chips, hemp protein, flaxseeds, extracts, and salt and process, scraping down the sides of the bowl as needed, until the mixture is fully combined.

4. Carefully scrape the mixture out onto the prepared baking dish, then using a spatula, press it out evenly throughout the dish with a depth of about ½ inch.

5. Place in the refrigerator and chill until firm, about 1 hour. Cut into 2×2-inch bars and serve at once. *Note:* The bars will keep in an airtight container in the refrigerator for up to a week.

JESSICA CATALAN'S NOTE

Genetically, NYC Blue is similar to the Blue Diesel (also known as Blue City Diesel) strain but is grown by a different breeder and has a different phenotype. I believe there are several phenotypes rolling around by different breeders. However, the Colorado one was just called NYC Blue. Blue City Diesel was originally produced by Breeder's Choice Collective.

STEPHANY GOCOBACHI & AKHIL KHADSE

Pastry Chef/Co-owner and Chef/Co-owner, Flour Child Collectives

Stephany Gocobachi was born in the Haight-Ashbury section of San Francisco and grew up in the Bay area. From an early age she loved to cook, spending a great deal of time in her mother's kitchen lending a helping hand. By the time she was eight years old, the young chef had taken over the Thanksgiving dinner preparations in her family's San Francisco home. As Gocobachi grew older, cannabis also became one of her passions. Coming from a state that grows some of the finest cannabis to be found, she was baffled by the limited variety of edibles that were available.

While attending New York University, Gocobachi continued to nurture the dream of returning to California to start her own edibles business. During this period of her life, she also worked as a pastry chef in professional kitchens, all the while endeavoring to create recipes for her soon-to-be business venture. She met her partner, Chef Akhil Khadse, during this time. Both shared a similar dream of producing a line of edibles that would support small farms that use organic and sustainable practices.

After Gocobachi received her degree in food sustainability and social entrepreneurship from NYU in 2012, she and Khadse traveled back to California. They founded their business, Flour Child Collectives, in 2015. Flour Child is a San Francisco–based producer of sustainable cannabis edibles. Its owners work with a network of small family farms, feeling that they share the same values. Most of the company's cannabis is sourced from Bon Vivant Farms in Willits, California. The family-owned farm follows sustainable and organic cultivation practices. The two chefs want to offer consumers a more holistic edible experience, one that focuses on culinary infusion that highlights flavors, textures, and health benefits.

Flour Child makes its edibles out of whole foods that do not contain refined sugar. One of their popular products is a line of seasonal jams, each batch made by hand with fruit sourced from local organic farms. These jams are made with strain-specific, whole flower rosin that is pressed from sustainably grown cannabis. The goal is to pair each fruit and strain, enhancing, not masking, the flavor. Fans of the jam explain, "Sometimes the ingredients pair so well that it's hard to tell where the fruit ends and the cannabis begins."

Their granola product is an organic blend of oats, California olive oil, maple syrup, flax, and sesame seeds. It is finished off with Oregon salt and figs, along with Flour Child's strain-specific, house-made cannabis flower rosin. Granola was chosen because it pairs well with jam. Disappointed by what dispensaries have to offer, the chefs are determined to create gently dosed products containing quality ingredients. They believe, "When developing a cannabis cuisine, the key is distributing the effects evenly. Dosage is important. You can't just sprinkle a little weed and expect magic or consistency."

Gocobachi is proud of the fact that Flour Child's products are shelf stable, meaning that everything is packaged in reusable glass jars with metal lids to preserve freshness and be environmentally responsible. The business is working on adding a few more products to their collection, while also creating a repertoire of recipes that can be made at home.

The company offers a line of topical CBD Relief Balm for external aches and pains. It took two years of testing seventy to eighty different formulas before they found one that met their standards. The topicals use the same flower rosin that is used in their edibles. They are good for moisturizing and healing skin issues such as psoriasis, burns, and sunburns while also helping to relieve muscular and joint pain, arthritis, and sciatica.

Gocobachi hopes to one day host cannabis cooking classes where she can bring people together over their shared love of cooking, food, and cannabis. Flour Child's mission is to cultivate community through cannabis by sharing resources and providing camaraderie to like-minded entrepreneurs and consumers. Its owners are committed to "doing well by doing good."

FULL-SPECTRUM EXTRACT AND WHY IT MATTERS

Full-spectrum extract maintains the complex range of desirable compounds and properties found in the original cannabis plant without changing them through decarboxylation or oxidation. This is important, because when cannabis is used in its whole form, the synergy between each active and therapeutic compound is found to be more effective than their isolated components. This is referred to as the cannabis entourage effect or whole plant medicine, phrases coined by S. Ben-Shabat and Raphael Mechoulam in 1998. They believe that cannabinoids within the cannabis plant work together, or possess synergy, and affect the body in a mechanism similar to the body's own endocannabinoid system.

TOASTED COCONUT-TURMERIC BHANG

by FLOUR CHILD COLLECTIVE

MAKES 8 servings, 4 cups total base

SUGGESTED DOSAGE: 5 milligrams of THC & 10 milligrams of CBD per serving.

STEPHANY GOCOBACHI. This was inspired by one of the most ancient methods of consuming cannabis in India. It is there that plants grow wild in the hills, and old farmers chop down whole plants to simmer in thick milk and ghee to be used in hot drinks and psychoactive sweets. This is just the thing to have before bed or on a foggy morning. It is warming and rich with lots of medicinal spices that complement the herbal component in both flavor and function.

SPICE BLEND

3 whole green cardamom pods, seeds removed and pods discarded

3 whole cloves

3 whole allspice berries

½ teaspoon fennel seeds

1 tablespoon turmeric powder

½ teaspoon ground cinnamon

½ teaspoon ground ginger

¼ teaspoon freshly ground black pepper

⅛ teaspoon pink Himalayan or sea salt

TOASTED COCONUT

1½ cups unsweetened, shredded coconut

MILK BASE

1½ cups water, plus additional, as needed

1 cup organic full-fat coconut milk, unsweetened

½ cup rose water

1½ tablespoons honey, pure maple syrup, organic agave syrup, or organic coconut nectar, or to taste

40 milligrams THC-infused oil and 80 milligrams CBD-infused oil

1. Preheat the oven to 350°F. Line a baking sheet with parchment paper. Set aside.

2. To make the spice blend: Place the cardamom seeds, cloves, allspice berries, and fennel seeds in a mortar and grind with the pestle or in a clean coffee grinder. Add the turmeric, cinnamon, ginger, pepper, and salt and combine well.

3. To make the toasted coconut: Spread the coconut evenly on the prepared baking sheet. Toast, stirring often, until fragrant and golden brown, about 7 minutes. Set aside.

4. To make the milk base: In a 3-quart heavy-bottomed saucepan, stir together the water, coconut milk, rose water, honey, spice blend, and toasted coconut, until well combined. Bring the milk base to a simmer, stirring occasionally, for 10 minutes. Turn off the heat and let steep for about 20 minutes.

5. Using a handheld immersion blender, blend the milk base in the saucepan until smooth, or transfer to a blender and blend on medium speed until smooth. Strain the milk base through a cheesecloth-lined fine-mesh strainer, pressing on the solids with the back of a large spoon, into a clean pot or heat-resistant glass bowl to remove the solids. When cool enough to handle, gather the corners of the cheesecloth and gently squeeze out any excess liquid into the pot with the milk base, then discard the solids. Add enough water, about 1¾ cups, to make a total

GARNISHES

Chia seeds, optional

Fresh mint leaves, optional

of 4 cups, and blend together once more. Add the infused oils, and blend once more, until well combined. Adjust seasonings with salt and additional honey, if desired.

6. To serve: In a small saucepan, bring ½ cup of the milk base and ½ cup of water, for each serving, to a simmer, stirring occasionally, over medium-low heat. Using a hand milk frother, whisk the drink until it reaches the desired frothiness or pour into a blender and blend on medium speed until frothy. If serving warm, ladle into mugs and top with chia seeds and mint, if desired. If serving cold, let cool to room temperature, then stir until well combined. Fill glasses with ice and pour into the prepared glasses; garnish with chia seeds and mint. Serve at once.

NOTES

Store leftover bhang in mason jars with tight-sealing lids in the refrigerator for up to 1 week. Before storing, label the jars with date and contents.

Bhang lassi is a traditional drink from India made from cannabis flowers and leaves, milk, rosewater, spices, and sometimes yogurt. The word "Bhang," means cannabis. Stephany Gocobachi of Flour Child Collective gives this nutritious beverage a decadently delicious twist.

STEPHANY GOCOBACHI'S VARIATION

Add 1 tablespoon of ghee or grass-fed butter and 1 tablespoon of coconut oil or organic MCT oil, or extra-virgin olive oil, to the milk base, or to taste. It is also delicious blended with coffee as a milk substitute, creating a supercharged bulletproof brew that is laden with butter and oil.

STEPHANY GOCOBACHI'S NOTE

For those desiring a more traditional Bhang lassi, simply substitute infused activated cannabis flower and leaves or hashish and leave out the 40 milligrams' worth of THC-infused oil and 80 milligrams worth of CBD-infused oil. Add the cannabis flower and leaves or hashish to the milk base and allow it to simmer and steep with the other spices.

SUMMER STONE FRUIT JAM

by FLOUR CHILD COLLECTIVE

MAKES approximately 6 cups
or six 8-ounce jars

SUGGESTED DOSAGE: 2.5 milligrams of THC per tablespoon; 80 milligrams per 8 ounce jar; 480 milligrams of THC per recipe/batch

STEPHANY GOCOBACHI: This is a perfect project for a glut of summer stone fruit from the farmers' market or your excess backyard bounty. Seasonal jams were one of the first edibles we began offering at the start of Flour Child and remain a crowd favorite. There is something truly special about being able to crack open a jar of summer in the doldrums of wintertime.

We love this as an edible because it is easy to measure and stores quite well for a long time—several months in the refrigerator even if you don't water-bath this product. You can have a teaspoon, or a couple of tablespoons on toast, waffles, in yogurt, or on a cheese plate. Jams are a beautiful way to infuse more elevated desserts such as pavlova, tarts, or thumbprint cookies.

This one is much lower in sugar than traditional jams, which we love because it means far more fruit and flavor. Feel free to adjust based on your personal tastes. Fresh chopped herbs and spices are a welcome addition. Some ideas for seasonings are: vanilla beans, ginger, green cardamom, rosemary, black pepper, cinnamon, and roses . . . many flavors go well with this jam recipe, depending on what you've got on hand.

We prefer to use concentrates to infuse jams—cold water hash, rosin, or kief are ideal here. They melt right in beautifully and bind to the sugars. Decarb before beginning, and add it in once the jam has thickened up and is almost ready. You can also dissolve it into a small amount of oil or honey first, or use a purchased oil or honey infusion instead. Add it toward the end and stir very well to evenly distribute. We generally like to dose our jams at about 5 milligrams of THC per tablespoon, but you can adjust based on your personal needs. For this recipe, I lowered the per-serving dosage to give more flexibility. It can be easily doubled or scaled as necessary for the cook's personal tolerance.

4 pounds stone fruit, such as plums, pluots, peaches, nectarines, or a combination, unpeeled, pitted, and cut into 1-inch chunks

2½ cups cane sugar, or as needed

Fresh chopped herbs or spices, optional (see recipe introduction above for suggestions)*

Juice from 1 lemon

Hashish, rosin, or kief, approximately ¾ gram of 60% THC-strength concentrate, if following suggested dosage above, decarbed

1. At the beginning of cooking, place three heatproof saucers or small plates in the freezer.

2. To macerate the fruit: Toss the fruit and sugar together in a medium nonreactive bowl. Add the chopped herbs and spices, if using, to taste, and toss once more. Cover and let stand at room temperature for 1 hour, stirring occasionally, or refrigerate overnight, stirring occasionally. Note: The sugar will draw the juices out of the fruit to create a syrup.

3. Pour the fruit and syrup into a wide heavy-bottomed stainless-steel or copper pot and bring to a full boil over medium-high heat, about 12 minutes, then reduce to a simmer, stirring occasionally, with a wooden spoon or silicone spatula, to prevent scorching.

4. Continue to simmer until the fruit mixture begins to foam, about 2 minutes. Remove the pot from the stove top. Using a large, stainless steel spoon, skim any foam from the top.

5. Return the pot to the stove top and continue to cook, stirring often, to prevent scorching, until the fruit has broken down and the mixture thickens, about 1 hour, depending on the ripeness and density of the fruit. Note: You may need to reduce the heat to prevent the mixture from scorching.

6. As you approach the end of cooking, add the lemon juice and cannabis of choice, stirring until well combined. Return to a boil, stirring often, for about 2 minutes. Remove the pot from the stove top. While the fruit mixture is resting, test the doneness of the jam.

7. To test the doneness of the jam: Take one plate out of the freezer and place 1 tablespoon of the mixture into the middle of the plate. Place the plate back into the freezer and let sit for 3 minutes. Remove from the freezer. If the jam is ready, the mixture will form a skin on top that wrinkles a bit when you gently push it with the tip of your finger or spoon. If the mixture is thin and runs down the plate easily, it is not done. Cook the jam down a bit longer to reach the setting point before testing again.

Recipe continues on next page

8. Carefully ladle the jam into hot clean heat-resistant glass jars, then tightly seal the lids, and label the jars with the date and contents. Store in the refrigerator for several months or process using safe canning procedures to keep for up to 1 year.

VARIATION

This jam is delicious with other kinds of cannabis-based products such as a store-bought oil, tincture, or infused honey. Stephany recommends the brand Juna, a California-based company, for their CBD and THC oils. For a premium hemp-infused raw honey, she suggests Potli. The suggested dosage for this recipe is about 2 tablespoons (or less), however, it's always best to follow the recommended amounts on the label.

STEPHANY GOCOBACHI'S NOTE

You will lose a few ounces to the pits. If you have a scale, I suggest weighing the prepared fruit (four pounds usually yields about 3¾ pounds of cut fruit for us, however, it can vary widely with fruit). We usually start off by adding 30 percent sugar, by weight, adding more as needed, to taste. This is a rustic jam, not an exact science, so follow your heart and palate.

The term "stone fruit" conjures up all manner of imaginary offerings, none of which are likely to cause a person to salivate in hungry anticipation. Be of good cheer, readers, this sidebar is not about rocklike, tooth-chipping fruit, but rather drupe, the term used for fruit with a large stone inside. A drupe is an indehiscent fruit, which means it does not open to release seeds when ripe. Its outer fleshy part surrounds a hardened single shell which has a seed inside. Peaches, nectarines, plums, mangoes, cherries, apricots, and certain hybrids are some well-known examples of stone fruit.

The term stone fruit is used to describe the hard covering that surrounds a single large seed at the fruit's center. As the fruit hangs by its stem from the tree branch, it is supported by this stone, which provides a means for nutrients to pass from the tree to the growing fruit. Stone fruits are a species of Prunus and are members of the rose family.

Stone fruits are highly perishable because of their high levels of antioxidants and do not store well. They are high in vitamins A and C, fiber, and potassium. This is particularly true of peaches, apricots, and nectarines, which are low in fat, calories, and sugar. Their sweet flavor helps to satisfy a desire for less-healthy snacks and, because of this, helps with weight management.

There are two types of peaches, clingstone and freestone. Clingstone fruit doesn't fall off its pit, making it good for eating but hard to slice. The freestone variety is easy to separate from its pit. You cannot tell the difference between the two by their looks, but clingstones are usually the first to arrive at farmers' markets. Nectarines have smooth skin, and peaches are fuzzy. Like that of peaches, the nectarine's flesh may be yellow or white. The advantage of nectarines is that they have no skin to peel. In actuality, they are smooth-skinned peaches.

Peaches, nectarines, plums, and their hybrids are best when ripened at room temperature, stem-end down. It is best not to refrigerate this fruit before it is ripe as it may cause the skin to wrinkle and become mealy. To speed up the ripening process, put peaches and plums in a paper bag on the counter for twenty-four hours. Ripe fruit may be stored in the refrigerator for a few days.

Cherries must be picked when ripe and can be eaten as soon as purchased. They will keep in the refrigerator for up to three days if loosely covered. Sweet cherries include Bing, Rainier, and Sweetheart varieties and are sold fresh. Most cherries grown are of the sour variety, which are canned, frozen, or dried. Both

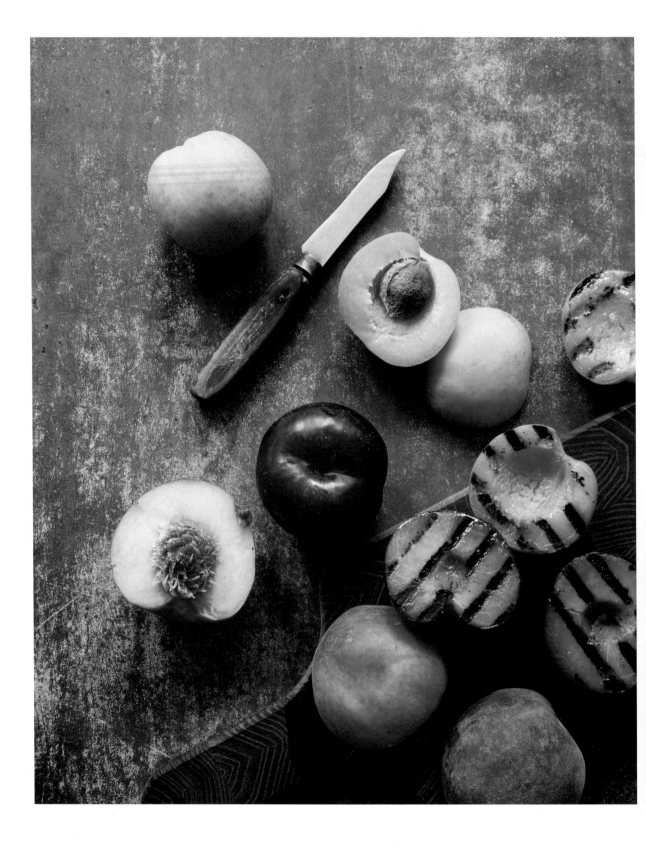

sweet and sour cherries are good sources of vitamin C and potassium and contain antioxidants. Cherry juice has been shown to fight inflammation and treat muscle pain.

Apricots are rich in pectin. Their fruit is creamy in texture when eaten ripe, and meaty when dried. They are delicious either canned or dried. Priums are a plum hybrid which is more like an apricot than a plum. They look, smell, and taste more like apricots than plums but are juicer and firmer.

There are two varieties of plums, Asian and European. Asian are larger and rounder, and the European version is smaller and oval shaped. Asian plums are always eaten fresh, while the European variety is usually dried or made into preserves. Some plums are firmer fleshed than others and have yellow, white, green, or red flesh. Fresh plums are a good source of vitamin C, and the dried variety, also known as prunes, provide fiber and vitamin A. Dried plums may be puréed and substituted for fat in cakes, quick breads, and muffins.

Mangoes can vary in size, color, and shape. They are generally sweet and when ripe can be eaten raw and used in curries and all manner of other yummy creations. This fruit is delicious when made into juices, ice cream, or smoothies or when sliced for dessert. It is a good source of fiber, folic acid, and vitamins A and C.

Breeders are coming up with a variety of interesting hybrid combinations. For example, an aprium is ⅔ apricot and ⅓ plum and has fuzzy skin much like an apricot. Hybrid pluots are similar to the aprium, but are more plum than apricot. The good news is, they do not have the plum's bitter skin. Plumcots are a 50/50 mix of plum and apricot. Today's shoppers may not know that the fruit they are buying could actually be a combination of another. For example, a nectarine may have some plum, apricot, or peach combined with it. The differences are so subtle that it can be hard to tell. Hybrids have a high sugar content, causing them to be noticeably sweeter, which makes them a wonderful addition to salads and dishes that call for stone fruit.

The season for stone fruit runs from June until September. Folks wait all year long to buy this mouthwatering fresh fruit from farm stands, farmers' markets, CSAs, and grocery stores. Creative cooks look forward to roasting, poaching, and sautéing their stone fruit while others bake pies and crumbles and make jams, sauces, and toppings. Whatever your culinary creation may be, stone fruit is sure to please the palate and make your mouth water in anticipation.

CANNABIS-INFUSED ITALIAN SALSA VERDE

by FLOUR CHILD COLLECTIVE

MAKES approximately 1¼ cups salsa verde,
enough for six 2-tablespoon servings

SUGGESTED DOSAGE: 2.5 milligrams per tablespoon; 50 milligrams per batch

STEPHANY GOCOBACHI: When serving cannabis-infused foods to a crowd, we generally like to choose one or two elements to infuse. Adding cannabis to every dish can be a slippery slope (and a long-term commitment for the whole dinner party). Dosage tolerances vary widely from person to person; therefore, we generally like to have the infused portion available on the side to allow folks to add as they please. Choose your own adventure—one tablespoon or two, or less. Condiments like dressings, relishes, jams, and chutneys are perfect vehicles for this.

Salsa verde is one of our favorite condiments to make all year round. Somewhere between a relish and sauce, it is rustic, herby, and punchy all at once. It pairs well with nearly any vegetables, eggs, or meat you have on hand. Roast chicken or grilled steaks really make it sing. Grilled and raw vegetables in the summer, roasted in the winter. You can chop it by hand, pound it in a mortar and pestle, or buzz it in a food processor or blender. Each will yield a slightly different texture. We like creating a slightly coarse and textured sauce by using a combination of hand-chopping and a mortar and pestle.

Use any combination of herbs you have on hand—parsley and marjoram (or oregano) are the most traditional flavor backbones of it, but it truly is endlessly adaptable. Add some mint if you're having it with eggplant or lamb. Sage with pork chops in the fall. Tarragon with roast chicken or potatoes. The only thing to keep in mind with your herb combos is the strength of each particular herb. Softer herbs like basil, cilantro, dill, tarragon, fennel fronds, or chervil can be used in larger quantities to partially or fully replace the parsley. Denser and more pungent herbs like rosemary, sage, oregano, thyme, and the like should be used in smaller amounts so they don't overpower the sauce as a whole.

If you are lucky enough to have a garden with a few cannabis plants, salsa verde is also a perfect outlet for your excess fan leaves. Cannabis and hemp leaves have a mild, grassy and slightly peppery flavor to them, and are highly nutritious (though they won't get you high). We love to add a handful and chop them up along with the parsley. If you have a lot of them, they will store well between damp paper towels in a container or plastic bag.

To infuse this salsa verde, we have a few options. The olive oil is the perfect carrier for either THC or CBD. Cannabis flower tends to have a more herbaceous flavor, which is often undesirable, but actually works beautifully here with the other herbs and savory notes. The terpenes already present in the sauce are the perfect foil for cannabis.

First, decarboxylate (or activate) the cannabis flower by gently heating it either in the oven or with something like the Ardent Nova Decarboxylator (a worthy investment if you make edibles often). Then the flower should go into a small amount of fat (the olive oil) and be gently heated to bind the cannabinoids to the fats. Usually, you would strain it out and then proceed, but in this recipe, we actually love the whole flower left in. Finely chopped like the rest of the herbs, it blends in really well.

You can also use raw cannabis flower and finely chop it in for a nonpsychoactive THC-A version of the sauce. Hash, kief, or rosin would also work wonderfully, as would replacing some of the olive oil with your favorite store-bought CBD or THC oil. Figure out what you want your dosage to be and work from there. For this sauce, we generally aim for a dosage of 5 mg per tablespoon. It's enough to have a spoonful to enjoy or two for those with a higher tolerance. Using flower of around 15 percent THC, a half gram is just about perfect for this. If you're using a concentrate, check the dosage if it's available to you, only about one-eighth of a gram will be necessary.

CANNABIS-INFUSED OLIVE OIL

½ cup extra-virgin olive oil, divided

Cannabis flower, finely chopped and activated, approximately ½ gram of 15-17% THC strength flower, if following suggested dosage (or if not, see notes above)

SALSA VERDE

2 medium cloves garlic, peeled

½ teaspoon sea salt flakes, such as Maldon Salt Company or Jacobsen Salt Company

1. To make the cannabis-infused olive oil: In a small skillet, heat 2 tablespoons of the olive oil and the cannabis flower, over medium-low heat until aromatic. Note: Be careful not to fry the cannabis flower. Remove from the heat and strain, if desired, or leave the cannabis flower in the oil. Allow to cool to room temperature. Transfer to a clean container with a pour spout, then add the remaining 6 tablespoons of olive oil. Set aside.

2. Place the garlic and salt in a mortar and pound into a paste with the pestle. Add the anchovies, lemon zest, red chili flakes, and pepper to taste, then pound until the paste is smooth.

3. In a medium bowl, mix together the herbs, garlic paste, capers, and lemon juice, stirring until well combined. Stir in the reserved olive oil in a slow and steady stream,

Ingredients list continues on page 277

Recipe continues on page 277

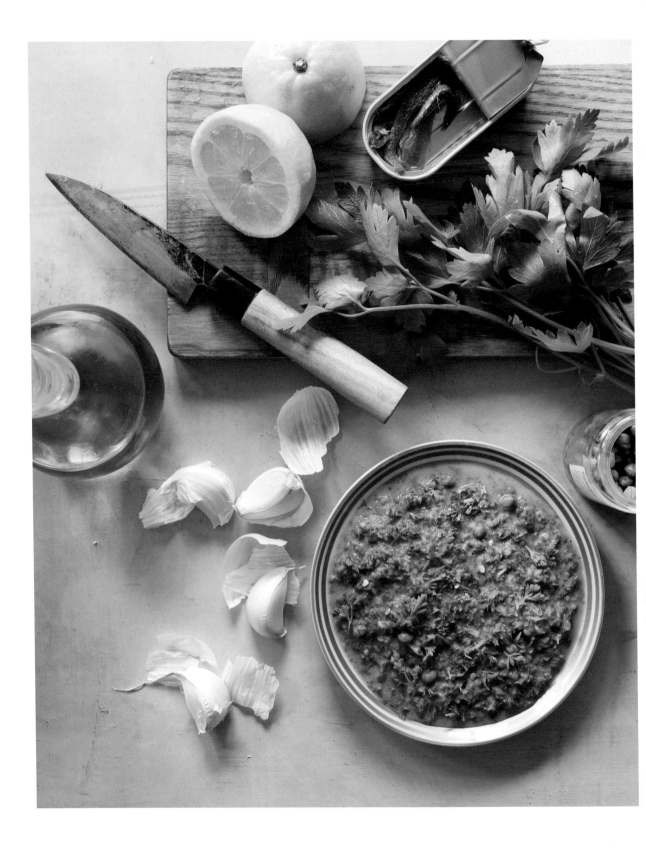

3 anchovy fillets, rinsed if packed in salt, minced

1 teaspoon organic lemon or Meyer lemon zest, or to taste

⅛ teaspoon dried red chili flakes, or to taste

Freshly ground black pepper, to taste

2 cups mixed soft fresh herbs, such as flat-leaf parsley, cilantro, mint, tarragon, and basil, leaves and thin stems only, trimmed, or fennel fronds, lightly packed, ¾ cup minced

2 tablespoons marjoram or oregano leaves, minced

1 tablespoon brined capers, drained and chopped (if using salt-cured capers, rinse, soak briefly in warm water, and drain)

Juice of 1 organic lemon or Meyer lemon, or as needed

until the salsa is loose but still coarse and textured. Adjust seasonings with additional lemon juice and zest, salt, and pepper, if desired.

4. Set aside at room temperature for 1 to 2 hours. Note: The salsa verde will need to be stirred well, right before serving to ensure even distribution of the cannabinoids in the oil. The salsa verde can be stored in the refrigerator for up to 1 day; just make sure to bring it to room temperature; stirring well, before serving.

NOTES

You will need to make the salsa at least 1 hour before you intend to use it.

If you don't own a mortar and pestle, simply place the garlic on a cutting board. Using the broad side of your knife, flatten, mash, and scrape the garlic back and forth into a paste.

ERIN GORE & KARLI WARNER

Founders, Garden Society

Garden Society, located in Sonoma County, California, is a cannabis-focused company that was started by Erin Gore in 2016. Having used cannabis in the past, Erin had again turned to the plant to help with her pain management after years of being a collegiate athlete. Seeking to deal with her pain issues and a very demanding career, she used cannabis to create what she called "High Holiday Baking Parties" with the assistance of her girlfriends. While her chef helpers created cookies, cakes, and candies, Gore applied her chemical engineering background to dose these edibles. The woman-friendly cannabis parties were a huge success and continued to be a safe place where Erin and her friends could reduce stress and find a balance in their daily existence.

These popular parties paved the way for what would soon be known as Garden Society, a company that is focused on bringing joy to women's everyday lives through the use of delicious, high-quality cannabis-infused chocolates and pre-rolls. Prior to starting Garden Society, Gore met Karli Warner through a former job connection, and the two had quickly bonded over their love of cannabis. When Gore decided to launch her business venture a few years later, she thought of Warner and their mutual interest and reached out to her. The two women formed a partnership built on Gore's chemical engineering background and her connections in the cannabis community that were strongly supported by Warner's public relations and marketing skills.

The cannabis-focused benefit corporation serves women who are looking to control the stress of their everyday lives and find peace and joy. The business creates artisanal edibles and pre-rolls that are produced by using responsible farming methods, sustainable ingredients and strain-specific cannabis. Products are handcrafted, with each cannabis strain containing a unique combination of cannabinoids that result in a specific effect or experience. The low-dose organic confections are aimed at functional relief.

The product line includes "Blissful Rest," handmade milk chocolates infused with calming indica strain of cannabis containing 10 milligrams of THC per piece. There are also "Brighter Day," rich dark chocolate with cinnamon and chili, infused with a strain of sativa hybrid available in low-dose 5 mg or 10 mg THC per serving, as well as High CBD "Calm and Focus" milk chocolate with chai. Garden Society's full-flower pre-rolls, called "Rosettes," are meant for individual enjoyment.

Made from responsibly sourced ingredients, every product is lab tested throughout the process. All are produced from full-spectrum, sun-grown cannabis. Garden Society works with local wine country chocolate makers to craft recipes that focus on flavor, texture, and specific cannabis effects. The company engages with women-owned-and-operated farms to further their commitment to support and empower women. Products are sold in dispensaries throughout California and in certain areas are available through the company's own home delivery program.

Gore and Warner are pioneers in search of ways to enrich women's lives or, as they like to say, "To turn down the daily chaos and turn up the joy." This is not your average cannabis company: Its owners are determined to break the stigma of the plant and redefine its image, making cannabis use a simple, vital part of a woman's daily routine. *Forbes* listed Erin as one of the fifteen most powerful and innovative women in cannabis right now. For the folks at Garden Society, it is about cannabis with a new woman-friendly perspective, supported by a strong belief in the power of the plant.

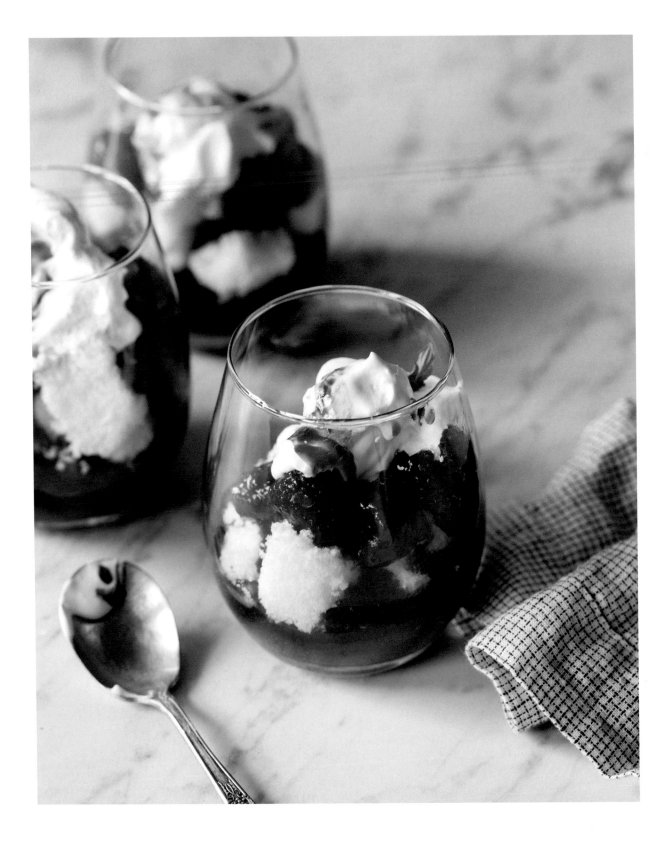

CANNABIS-INFUSED DARK CHOCOLATE SPICED PARFAIT

GARDEN SOCIETY

MAKES 8 servings

This is the perfect no-bake dessert with irresistible layers of raspberries, cannabis-infused chocolate, and store-bought angel food cake.

PARFAIT FILLING

½ cup seedless raspberry jam

¼ cup fresh orange juice

¼ cup water

2 cups heavy cream, divided

⅔ cup plus 2 tablespoons whole milk, divided

3 tablespoons sugar, divided

1 package (8 pieces) Garden Society Spiced Dark Chocolates, coarsely chopped

2 teaspoons unflavored gelatin (1 envelope Knox brand gelatin)

12 ounces (about 2 cups) fresh raspberries

8 fresh mint leaves

CAKE

Half (6-inch diameter) angel food cake, homemade or store-bought

1. To make the jam juice: In a small saucepan, whisk together the raspberry jam, orange juice, and water and bring to a boil, whisking occasionally, over medium heat, about 8 minutes. Remove from the heat and transfer to a heat-resistant bowl or measuring cup. Place in the refrigerator to chill, about 1 hour and 15 minutes.

2. Once the jam juice is chilled, in a separate small saucepan add 1 cup of the heavy cream, ⅔ cup of milk, and 2 tablespoons of the sugar and bring to a boil over medium heat, about 10 minutes. Remove from stove top.

3. Add the chocolate pieces to the hot cream mixture, and let sit for 2 minutes, then whisk to combine. While the chocolate is resting, bloom the gelatin. In a small bowl, sprinkle the gelatin over the remaining 2 tablespoons of milk. Add the bloomed gelatin to the chocolate mixture and whisk until completely smooth.

4. Pour ¼ cup of the chocolate mixture into the bottom of eight 8-ounce mason jars or wineglasses. Distribute any leftover chocolate mixture among the jars. Place the jars in the refrigerator and chill until the chocolate sets, about 1 hour.

5. While the chocolate mixture is setting in the refrigerator, start to macerate the raspberries. Combine the fresh raspberries with the chilled raspberry jam mixture in a medium bowl. Let stand at room temperature, stirring occasionally, until the juices are released, about 45 minutes.

6. At least 25 minutes before you plan to make the whipped cream, place a metal mixing bowl and metal whisk attachment from a stand mixer into the freezer.

Recipe continues on next page

7. To cut the angel food cake: Using a serrated knife, cut into ½-inch to 1-inch cubes, making sure not to press down too hard on the cake. Note: You should have about 4 cups of cake.

8. Just before serving, make the whipped cream. Remove the metal mixing bowl and whisk attachment from the freezer. Place the remaining 1 cup of the heavy cream and the remaining 1 tablespoon of the sugar into the chilled bowl and whisk in the stand mixer, scraping down the sides of the bowl as needed, until soft peaks form.

9. To assemble: Place the cake cubes evenly into each jar or glass, carefully resting them on top of the chocolate. Using a slotted spoon, evenly distribute the macerated berries on top of the cake and drizzle with about 1 tablespoon of the berry juice on top and around the cake cubes, or to taste. Top with a dollop of whipped cream. Garnish with a mint leaf. Serve at once.

CANNABIS POPCORN BALLS

GARDEN SOCIETY

MAKES 16 popcorn balls; about ½ cup size each

These simple-to-make popcorn balls combine heirloom popcorn, English toffee, and cannabis-infused chocolate to create the ultimate snack!

HEIRLOOM POPCORN

Makes approximately 9½ to 10 cups

⅓ cup heirloom popcorn kernels, such as White Cat Corn

POPCORN MIXTURE

9½ to 10 cups popcorn (see popcorn recipe above)

4 tablespoons unsalted melted butter, or to taste

¼ teaspoon sea salt, or to taste
1 cup broken pretzel sticks (½-inch pieces)

½ cup dry-roasted, lightly salted peanuts

½ cup milk chocolate English toffee bits, such as Heath

POPCORN BALLS

2 tablespoons plus 1½ teaspoons unsalted butter, divided

3 cups mini marshmallows

1 (2.7-ounce package; 8 squares) Garden Society Milk or Spicy Dark Chocolates

1. To make the popcorn: Pop the popcorn kernels on the stove top, in the microwave, or with the air-popper method, following the popcorn package and/or manufacturer's directions.

2. To make the popcorn mixture: Transfer the popcorn to a large deep bowl, and while tossing the popcorn continuously, add the butter and salt in a slow and steady stream. Add the pretzels, peanuts, and toffee bits, tossing until well combined. Adjust seasonings with additional salt and butter, if desired.

3. To make the popcorn balls: Melt 2 tablespoons of the butter in a big kettle over medium heat. Add the marshmallows and cook, stirring often with a silicone spatula, until just melted, about 3 minutes. Reduce the heat to low and add the chocolate, stirring continuously until fully melted and well combined, about 2 minutes.

4. Pour the popcorn over the chocolate mixture and stir with the spatula until evenly coated. Note: It is important to keep this mixture moving in the pot while it is warm or the chocolate mixture will clump up together and be hard to mix in.

5. Rub your fingers and hands with the remaining 1½ teaspoons of butter. Using a ½-cup measuring cup, scoop out the popcorn and compress together with your hands to form a ball. Repeat with the remaining ingredients. Each ball should be about 2½ inches in diameter. Enjoy warm or at room temperature.

HOW TO RESPONSIBLY CONSUME EDIBLES

1. Check with your doctor before consuming any cannabis products.
2. Dose on the conservative side and go slow. The best way to test for potency is to start with a low dose, wait two hours, then listen to your body and decide whether or not to consume more.
3. Hydrate with plenty of water or some herbal tea.
4. Never drive under the influence of cannabis.

PEGGY MOORE & HOPE FRAHM

Owner and Corporate Executive Chef, Love's Oven

Love's Oven has come a long way since 2009, when the Denver, Colorado, small-batch, gourmet cannabis bakery first received a medical license to produce its products. Its corporate executive chef, Hope Frahm, has been part of the company's amazing staff since 2013. Frahm always tells people that her culinary background began when she was a mechanic. While working underneath a vehicle, an accident caused her to ingest antifreeze and receive chemical burns over 35 percent of her body. Frahm's taste buds were damaged, resulting in the permanent loss of her sense of taste. After recovering, the former mechanic changed course career-wise, going to culinary school and receiving an associate degree from the International Culinary School at the Art Institute of Las Vegas.

Following graduation, Frahm worked in Las Vegas as a pastry chef in the kitchens of renowned chefs Wolfgang Puck and Thomas Keller. It was during this time that she received training from the best of the best, establishing a solid foundation for future culinary endeavors. Chef Frahm has never felt that the loss of her sense of taste has limited her cooking skills; instead, she asks the folks she works with for their feedback in that area. She also judges edibles by their smell, appearance, and texture.

In 2013, Chef Frahm had an opportunity to move to Denver, Colorado. After arriving, she noticed an ad on Craigslist for a baker's position in a small-batch marijuana bakery. To her delight, the business, Love's Oven, hired her soon after she went for the job interview. Each cook in the company's kitchen is a classically trained pastry chef who has worked in high-end kitchens for ten years or more. Chef Frahm felt that the new job was a wonderful opportunity for her to bring her skills in fine dining to this industry.

The CEO of Love's Oven, Peggy Moore, bought the company in 2013. Her two sons and younger sister serve as directors helping her to run the business. During their tenure, they have gone from a 1,700-square-foot kitchen to an 8,500-square-foot state-of-the-art facility staffed by a team of skilled chefs who are meticulous about what they do. The ingredients that they use are all natural or organic, sourced locally whenever possible. They do not use additives, preservatives, or artificial or processed flavors. Cooking methods are also natural—no chemicals, butane or propane. The folks at Love's Oven do not believe in doing things half measure.

Pretty much everything is made from scratch. Being small batch allows Love's Oven to make sure that each product they produce is handcrafted by a team of talented chefs. This ensures that each bite is consistent in potency. Chef Frahm's personal mission is to create the most dependable and best tasting cannabis edibles on the market using quality ingredients made by quality people. The emphasis is on creating edible treats that are properly infused with the right amount of marijuana, which is locally sourced. The chef's philosophy is consistency, fully aware that retaining consumers depends on making sure that they get what they expect.

Love's Oven's products are genotype (indica, sativa, and hybrid) specific. They use all-natural heat extraction for their butter, enabling them to retain the terpenes from the cannabis plant that corresponds with the genotype. This method gives the butter and edible a slight weed taste based on the strain used to produce the cannabutter. Chef Frahm has developed formulas for cannabutter and edibles that complement each other and do not allow the weed to be overpowering. The bakery's THC extraction method ensures that customers receive consistent and effective doses of cannabutter in every bite of its gourmet baked goods. The company's extraction lab, Concentrated Love, uses the highest-grade equipment, solvents, and professional staff.

Love's Oven's selection of goods includes concentrates, brownies, caramels, a wide variety of cookies, Sinsère chocolates, rosemary cheddar crackers, and an array of other tempting snacks. There is also a line of gluten-free edibles. Each serving is infused with 10 mg of cannabis with medical edibles able to be dosed higher. CBD edibles made from hemp are used for medicinal purposes. All products are sold in child safety containers with three layers of packaging, each edible individually wrapped. A clearly visible warning label is easy to detect.

In response to customer demand and tastes, the product line is constantly evolving. The company also keeps track of trends in the non-infused market. Each month two or three new products are added to the range of goods, striving to keep offerings fresh and exciting. One of Colorado's biggest pot bakeries, Love's Oven's products can be found at dispensaries throughout the state. At this small-batch bakery, everything is done with integrity, mindful that the secret ingredient is always a dose of "love."

Chef Hope Frahm, Corporate Executive Chef for Love's Oven

Hope Frahm's Notes:

This process is for any concentrate that is fully decarboxylated that has been tested for potency. Typically, potency will be reported by milligrams per gram, but can also be reported as a percentage. To convert the percentage into milligrams, simply move the decimal point to the right.

Example: 90% potency = 900mg/g

If a concentrate is not fully decarboxylated (i.e., shatters, waxes, budder, sauce, etc.) the concentrate should be fully decarboxylated prior to dosing and THC calculated by using the following formula

[THC]+([THC-A] x 0.877) = sMax THC

However, unless testing is available, then you will not be able to accurately dose, due to the uncertainty of being either fully decarboxylated or over-decarboxylated and converting your THC-A into THC into CBN.

I highly recommend using a decarboxylated concentrate over using other concentrates that need to be decarboxylated. This will give you the most accurate dosing, but if you are not worried about consistency of potency, feel free to experiment with different concentrates and terpene profiles.

1. Calculate how many milligrams are needed each per batch by multiplying the milligrams per piece by the amount of pieces per batch.

Ex: 10 milligrams per piece x 24 pieces per batch = 240 milligrams
needed per batch (10 X 24 = 240)

2. Calculate how many grams of concentrate are needed per recipe by dividing the amount of milligrams needed by the potency of the concentrate.

Ex: 240mg ÷ 900mg = .266g needed for the recipe (240 ÷ 900 = .266)

Hope Frahm's Notes:

If you do not have a scale that can accommodate that small of an amount, typically distillates will be sold in a 1ml syringe (which the conversion is almost 1:1 ml to g). Then you can just warm your concentrate in hot water (in a baggie) and dose directly into your melted fat.

If you do have a milligram scale, warm your concentrate in hot water and dose onto silicone and place that into the freezer for a few minutes. Then, simply peel the distillate off the silicone and drop into your melted fat. Highly recommend that you wear gloves when handling the concentrate, because it can get very sticky (like honey mixed with superglue).

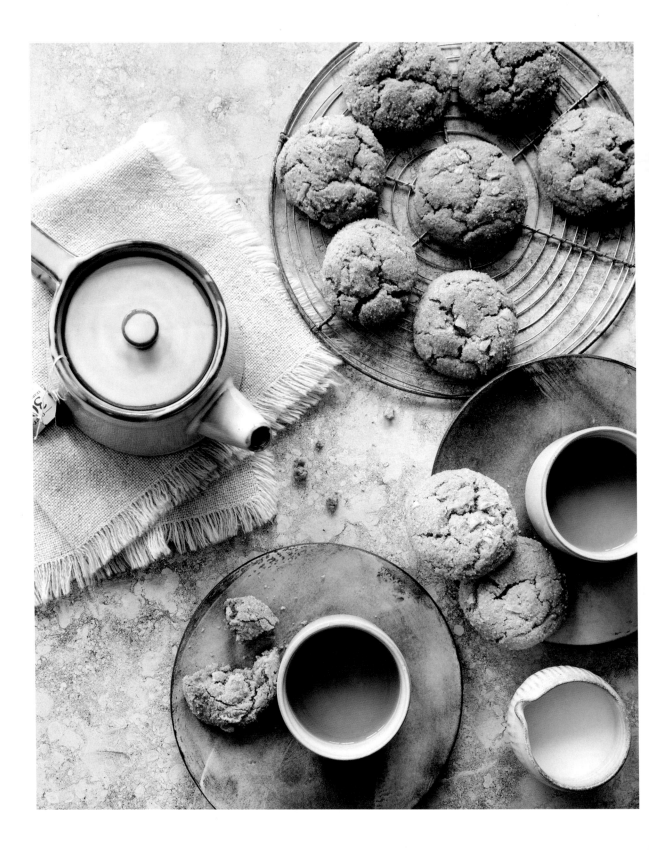

CHEWY GINGERSNAP COOKIES

HOPE FRAHM, LOVE'S OVEN

MAKES 20 cookies; 10 milligrams THC per Cookie

With a sugary exterior and slightly chewy center, these cannabis-infused cookies will become one of your must-have treats!

1½ cups all-purpose flour

½ teaspoon baking soda

¾ teaspoon ground ginger

¾ teaspoon ground cinnamon

½ teaspoon ground cloves

½ teaspoon kosher salt

5 tablespoons butter, divided

200 milligrams THC concentrate, or preferred dose

3 tablespoons molasses

⅔ cup sugar, plus ¼ cup for rolling the cookies

1 egg

⅓ cup finely chopped crystallized ginger

1. Preheat the oven to 325°F. Line two baking sheets with parchment paper or a silicone mat. Set aside.
2. In a bowl, whisk together the flour, baking soda, ground ginger, cinnamon, cloves, and salt. Set aside.
3. Melt 2½ tablespoons butter, then add the concentrate and mix until completely incorporated.
4. Soften the remaining 2½ tablespoons butter and cream together in a stand mixer with the melted infused butter, molasses, and ⅔ cup sugar on medium speed until smooth and fluffy, about 10 minutes. Note: The mixture should double in volume. You may need to beat on high speed for the last 1 to 2 minutes to achieve that volume.
5. Add the egg and continue to cream on medium speed until combined well. Add the dry ingredients in batches and continue to mix on low speed until about 50 percent incorporated. While the mixer is running, slowly add the crystallized ginger and continue to mix until all the ingredients are fully incorporated. Do not overmix.
6. Place the remaining ¼ cup of the sugar in a shallow dish. Divide the dough into 20 cookies; about 1½ tablespoons of dough weighing 1¼ ounce each. Using your hands, roll the cookies into individual balls; then gently roll each cookie around in the dish with the sugar. Place on the prepared cookie sheets about 2 inches apart.
7. Bake until the tops of the cookies start to crack, about 12–14 minutes. Repeat with the remaining cookies. Transfer to wire racks to cool.

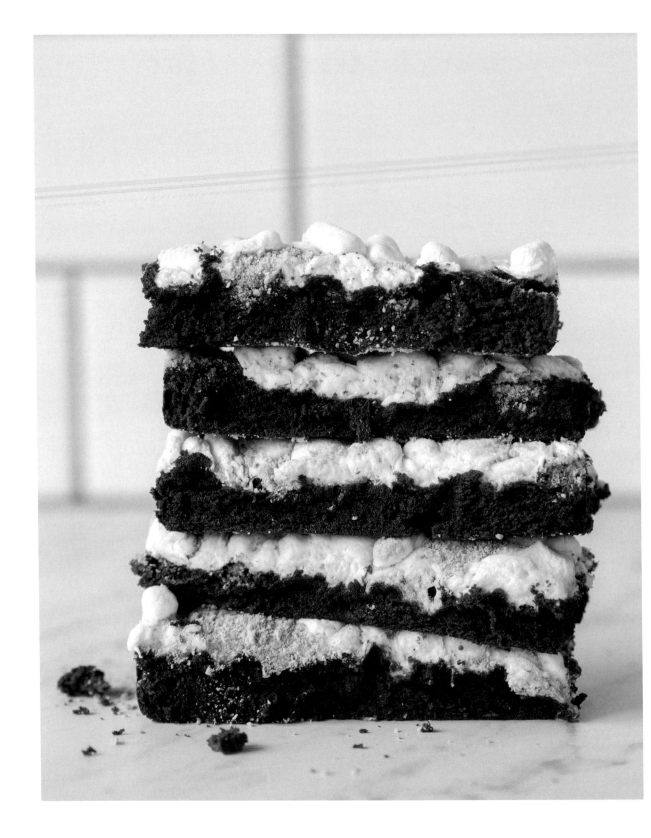

S'MORES BROWNIES

by HOPE FRAHM, LOVE'S OVEN

MAKES 20 brownies

> **HOPE FRAHM:** Chocolate chips work fine in this recipe, but higher-quality chocolates will make a richer product. Since marshmallows and graham cracker crumbs are a topping, feel free to add as many marshmallows as your heart desires. It will not affect the potency of your brownie. You can also use crushed graham crackers instead of crumbs, if desired. Also, feel free to experiment with any toppings that you wish, or none at all. This recipe is great any way you make it.
>
> **SUGGESTED DOSAGE:** 10 milligrams THC per brownie.

⅔ cup plus 3 tablespoons all-purpose flour

1 tablespoon plus 2 teaspoons dark cocoa powder

½ teaspoon baking powder

½ teaspoon kosher salt

⅔ cup unsalted butter

200 milligrams THC concentrate, or preferred dose

1¼ cups high-quality semisweet chocolate chips

1 tablespoon instant coffee powder

⅔ cup granulated sugar

3 eggs

1 teaspoon pure vanilla extract

1 cup mini marshmallows

¼ cup (2 large rectangular crackers) graham cracker crumbs

1. Preheat the oven to 325°F. Line a 9×13-inch baking pan with parchment paper on the bottom and up the sides of the pan. Set aside.

2. Whisk together the flour, cocoa powder, baking powder, and salt in a bowl. Set aside.

3. Melt the butter in a small saucepan over medium heat. Add the THC concentrate and mix thoroughly.

4. In a separate bowl, add the chocolate chips and coffee. While the butter is hot, pour over the chocolate and let sit for 3 to 5 minutes. Whisk until the chocolate is fully melted. Keep the chocolate mixture warm until ready to use. Note: You want the chocolate to be warm and slightly fluid, but not so hot as to burn the chocolate or cook the eggs when added. The chocolate temperature should be no higher than 125°F.

5. In a separate large bowl, whisk together the sugar, eggs, and vanilla until the sugar slightly dissolves. Add the reserved dry ingredients and mix until well incorporated. Add the chocolate mixture and stir until no streaks remain. Note: The batter will be thick like frosting.

6. Scoop the batter into the prepared pan, pressing it out to the edges with a spatula. Bake for 15 minutes, remove from the oven, and top with marshmallows and graham cracker crumbs, then continue to bake until the marshmallows are lightly toasted, about 15 minutes. Note: If desired, using a kitchen torch, carefully torch the marshmallows for extra toasty-ness.

7. Allow to cool completely before cutting the brownies into twenty 4½×1⅓-inch rectangles.

CHEF UNIKA NOIEL

Owner, LUVN Kitchn

Unika Noiel has become known as Seattle, Washington's premier chef of cannabis-infused soul food. Ironically, it was an edible lollipop that first introduced her to the wonders of cannabis. This experience jump-started Noiel's curiosity, motivating her to research the drug's medicinal properties, the results of which piqued her interest even more.

Noiel's grandparents were from Louisiana and introduced her to soul food and southern cooking at a very young age. With uncles who owned barbecue restaurants and a grandmother who attended culinary school, you might say that cooking was in her family's blood. Carrying on the tradition, Noiel opted to enroll in culinary school in 2013. She had tried her hand at other jobs, but the kitchen was where she felt most at home.

LUVN Kitchn is an expression of Chef Noiel's culinary history. Family, the foods she ate growing up, and those she still enjoys to this day are important parts of her culture. The letters that form the word LUVN are each of Noiel's initials accompanied by those that stand for the word love. The name embodies herself and her love for sharing food with other people.

The chef believes that food is history, fuel, and medicine. This is the reason why her popular fellowship dinners involve family-style cooking and dining, with Chef Noiel at the forefront sharing the stories behind each dish and its ingredients. She believes that people should know where their food comes from so that they can make the most nutritious choices possible. The introduction of cannabis serves to enrich the whole experience and highlight the medicinal benefits. By offering family-style dinners that integrate new foods, LUVN Kitchn strives to educate, feed, and bring folks together.

Private dinners are some of Chef Noiel's favorite occasions giving her an opportunity to collaborate with guests and bring their culinary vision to life. These cannabis-infused meals are held monthly, by invitation only, with menus that vary with each event. Infusions are inspired by soul food, ranging from southern fried chicken to catfish, with menu selections inspired by guest requests as well as seasonal and local availability. Because Noiel is from the Pacific Northwest, the cuisine is a delicious fusion of northwest and southern soul food.

The dedicated chef receives a great deal of pleasure from sharing these family-style dinners with her guests. Demand has been so strong that Chef Noiel happily acknowledges having difficulty keeping up with the requests. The owner of LUVN Kitchn enjoys producing high-quality dishes with and without cannabis for a varied audience, helping people to learn how to medicate with cannabis and eat their vegetables, too! It is her dream to expand these dinners to other communities in the not-too-distant future. Locations, dinner guests, and menu choices may vary, but at LUVN Kitchn, the importance of community remains constant.

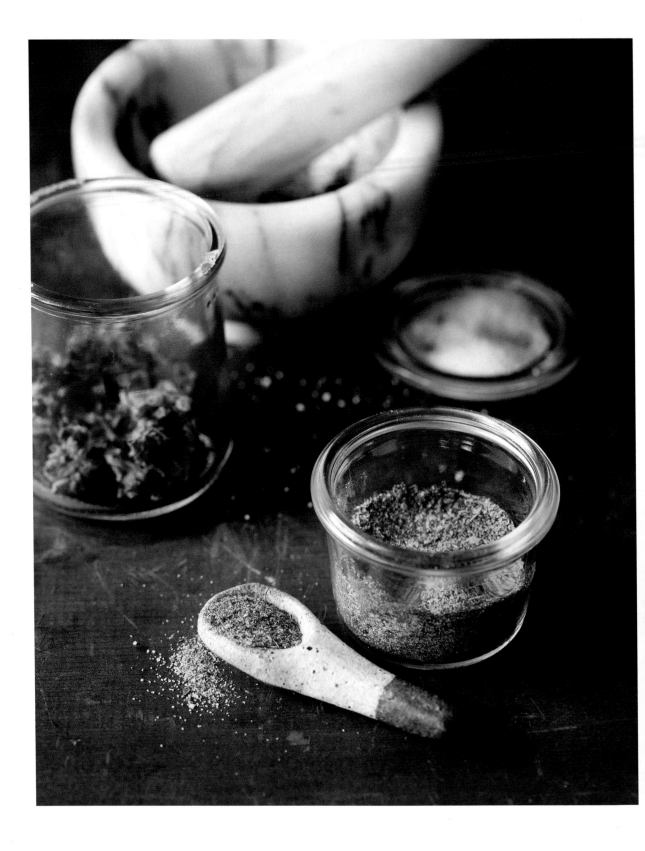

CANNABIS-INFUSED CREOLE SEASONING

by CHEF UNIKA NOIEL, LUVN KITCHN

MAKES about ½ cup

2½ tablespoons garlic powder

2 tablespoons paprika

1 tablespoon kosher salt

1 tablespoon onion powder

1 tablespoon dried thyme

1 tablespoon dried oregano

1 tablespoon cayenne pepper

½ tablespoon ground, decarbed cannabis

1. In a small bowl, stir all of the ingredients until well combined. Store in an airtight container and label with the date and contents.

NOTE

This recipe makes more creole seasoning than you will need for the jambalaya; sprinkle the extra over chicken or combine it with ground turkey for a delicious meatloaf with a twist. Remember to label and store the seasoning in an airtight container out of direct sunlight.

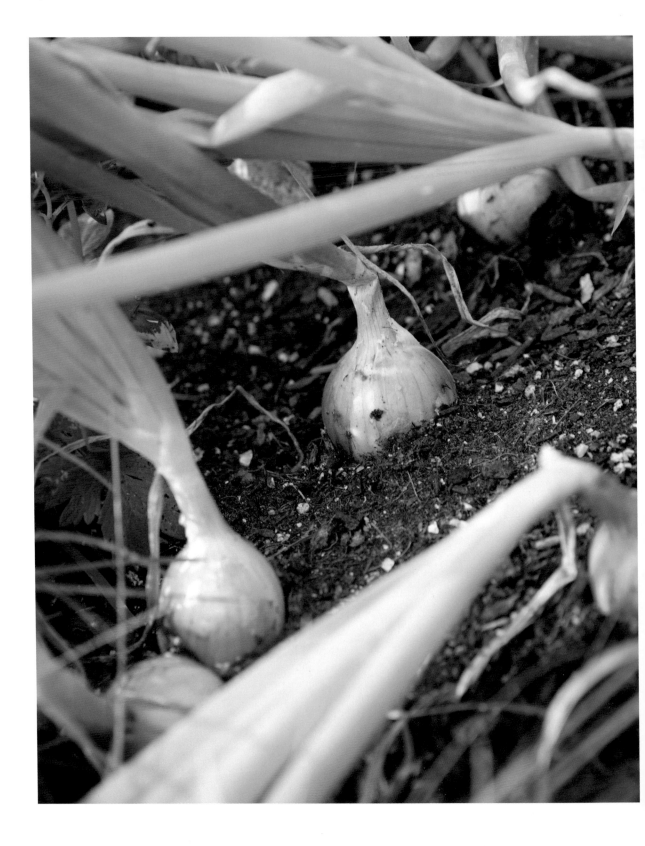

CANNABIS-INFUSED VEGETABLE STOCK

by CHEF UNIKA NOIEL, LUVN KITCHN

MAKES about 11 cups

CHEF UNIKA NOIEL: No matter what sort of savory dish you're cooking, if it calls for water, nine times out of ten it would be tastier if you used stock. Think of it this way, water can only lend a dish as much flavor as it has . . . which is *none*. So, adding fortified liquid like vegetable stock works exactly the same. If you should also happen to fortify your stock with cannabis, you will be accomplishing two objectives at the same time.

SACHET

5 to 6 fresh thyme sprigs

2 fresh parsley sprigs

½ tablespoon black peppercorns

2 fresh bay leaves

½ to 1 tablespoon coarsely ground, decarboxylated cannabis

VEGETABLE STOCK

2 medium yellow onions, peeled

4 medium carrots, washed and unpeeled

4 large celery ribs, washed

12 cups water

1. To make the sachet: Place the thyme, parsley, peppercorns, bay leaves, and cannabis in the center of a 6-inch cheesecloth square. Gather up the corners of the cheesecloth to form a bundle and tie tightly and securely with butcher's twine. Set aside.

2. To make the vegetable stock: Coarsely chop the onions, carrots, and celery and place in a large stockpot or Dutch oven.

3. Place the sachet into the pot with vegetables and cover with the 12 cups of water. Bring to just under a boil over medium-high heat.

4. Reduce the heat to a simmer, stirring occasionally, for 1 hour. Remove from the heat and allow to cool to room temperature.

5. Strain the infused broth through a cheesecloth-lined fine-mesh strainer into a clean heat-resistant large bowl.

6. Ladle the stock into an airtight storage container and label with the date and contents. Store in the refrigerator for up to 1 week or freeze for up to 2½ months.

NOTE

To save on time, prepare the stock 1 day before you intend to use it. Store in an airtight container in the refrigerator. This recipe makes more vegetable stock than you will need; freeze the extra for another use. If storing in the refrigerator or freezer, don't forget to label the storage container with the date and contents.

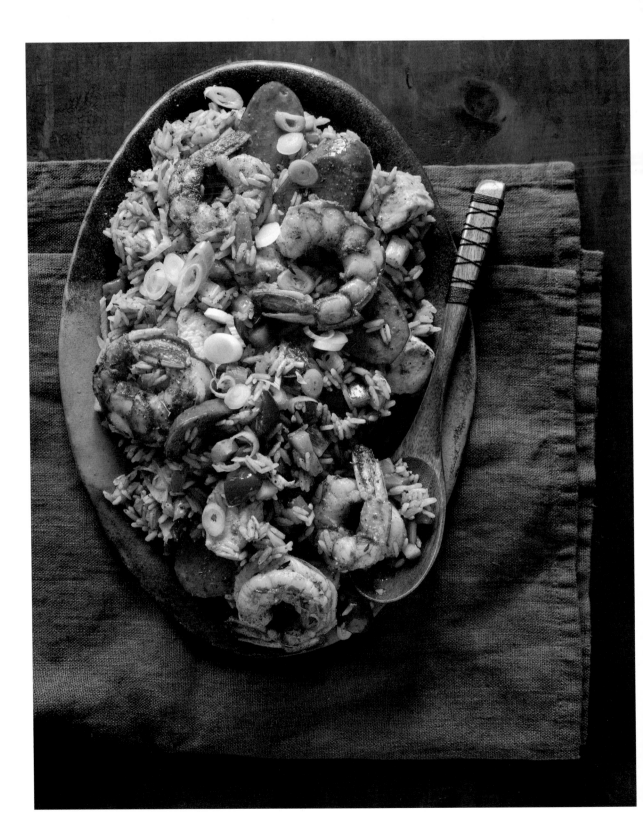

JAMBALAYA

by CHEF UNIKA NOIEL, LUVN KITCHN

MAKES 6 to 8 servings; 13 cups

CHEF UNIKA NOIEL: I've always thought of jambalaya as one of the truest culinary representations of my people; the French Pilau, or Rice Pilaf, Spanish Paella, and West African Jollof Rice come together to create this amazing Cajun/Creole dish. You'll find variations in this dish wherever you go, but take note—Creole jambalaya contains tomato, as a result of French and Italian influence. Cajun jambalaya does not. I was raised on both, but always preferred a preparation that included tomatoes. To me, the acidity they provide is necessary to help balance the richness of the rest of the dish.

DOSING: Always assume that your guests will want seconds, and dose your meals accordingly. I recommend 2–5 milligrams of THC per serving, an average of 50 milligrams per dish. If you are serving multiple infused items, stay closer to 2 milligrams. You can always consume more if you feel like you can handle it, but you can't take it back once it's in your system!

JAMBALAYA

2 tablespoons vegetable oil, divided

1 pound boneless, skinless chicken breast, cut into bite-sized pieces

1 pound andouille sausage, thinly sliced into rounds

1 cup diced white onion

1 cup diced celery

1 cup diced green bell pepper

2 tablespoons tomato paste

2 cups uncooked long-grain white rice

½ cup diced tomatoes

4½ cups cannabis-infused vegetable stock, or as needed (page 297)

2½ tablespoons cannabis-infused creole seasoning, divided (page 295)

1 bay leaf

1 pound (16/20 count per pound) raw shrimp, peeled and deveined

Salt and freshly ground black pepper, to taste

2 to 3 scallions, trimmed, thinly sliced on the bias into rings, white and green part, for garnish

Recipe continues on next page

1. To make the jambalaya: Heat 1 tablespoon of oil in a 5½ quart Dutch oven over medium-high heat. Add the chicken and sausage and cook, stirring often until the chicken is cooked through and the sausage is browned, about 7 minutes. Using a slotted spoon, transfer the chicken and sausage to a clean bowl, leaving the drippings in the pot. Set aside.

2. Add the remaining 1 tablespoon of oil to the remaining drippings in the stockpot. Add the onions, celery, and green peppers and sauté until the onions are soft and translucent, about 6 minutes. Stir in the tomato paste and continue to cook until the onions and peppers start to brown, about 3 minutes. Add the rice and stir until well combined. Add the tomatoes, stock, 2 tablespoons of the cannabis-infused creole seasoning, and bay leaf, stirring until well combined. Bring to a simmer. Cover, and reduce the heat to maintain a simmer, stirring occasionally, to make sure the rice doesn't stick to the bottom of the pot, and cook until the rice is just cooked, about 25 minutes.

3. Season the shrimp with the remaining ½ tablespoon of the cannabis-infused creole seasoning, tossing until evenly coated. Add the shrimp, chicken, and sausage to the pot with the rice mixture and cook, stirring occasionally, until the shrimp is opaque, the rice is tender, and the chicken and sausage are heated through, about 10 minutes. Remove and discard the bay leaf. Adjust seasonings with additional creole seasoning, salt, and pepper, if desired.

4. To serve: Ladle the jambalaya into bowls and garnish with scallions. Serve at once.

NOTE

After adding the shrimp, you may need to add additional stock, to help prevent the rice from sticking to the bottom of the Dutch oven.

EVERCLEAR CANNABIS TINCTURE
LUVN Kitchn

Chef Unika Noiel: This tincture is also known as "Green Dragon," and is a great way to make a concentrated dose of cannabis. Once you have made it, I recommend testing it out in ½ dropper doses until you are sure of its potency.

You can add it to a beverage or drop it straight into your mouth. You will notice its effects anywhere from 20 minutes to 1½ hours after you have consumed it. For faster action, consume on an empty stomach.

You can adjust this recipe by using the following ratio: ½ tablespoon of decarbed cannabis to 2 ounces of alcohol. I've used the amounts in the recipe provided above to ensure that you have enough tincture for the cannabis-infused sugar recipe (page 305).

When using tinctures, you should always proceed with caution, because they can be very potent!

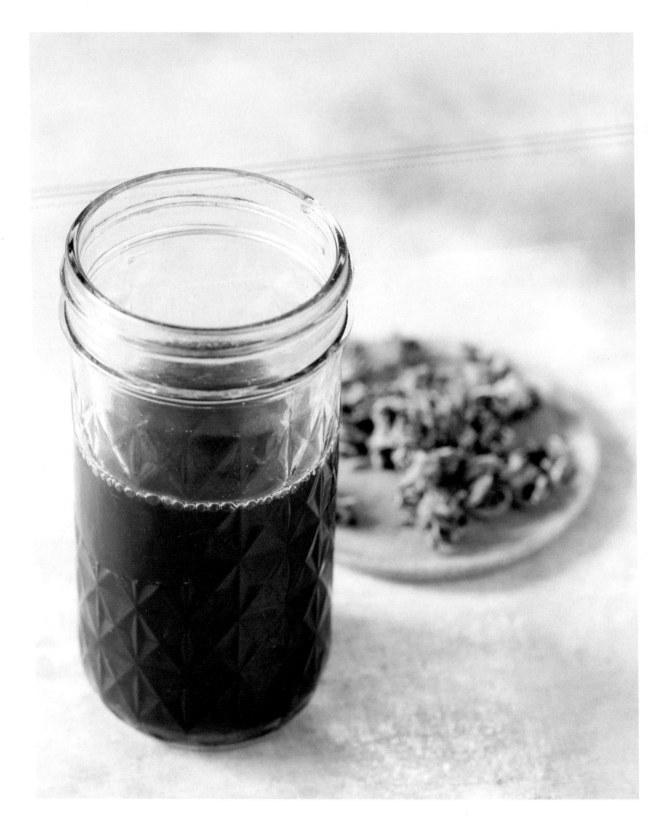

CANNABIS-INFUSED TINCTURE

MAKES 8 ounces

2 tablespoons ground, decarboxylated cannabis

8 ounces high-proof alcohol, preferably Everclear or 100 proof vodka

1. To make the cannabis tincture: Place the cannabis in a mason jar with the alcohol. Close the jar and let sit for a few weeks on the counter, out of direct sunlight, shaking it twice a day. Strain the tincture through a coffee filter or a cheesecloth-lined fine-mesh strainer into a clean container with a pour spout. Discard or compost the plant matter. Carefully pour into two 4-ounce dropper bottles. Label the bottles with the dates and contents. Store in a cool dark place.

NOTE

You will need to make the cannabis tincture a few weeks before you intend to make the cannabis-infused sugar (page 305). If you are short on time, Chef Unika offers a timesaving cannabis-infused tincture recipe on her website, LUVN Kitchn.

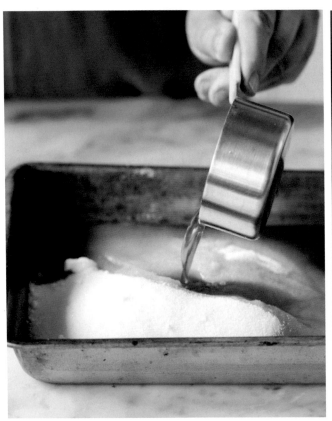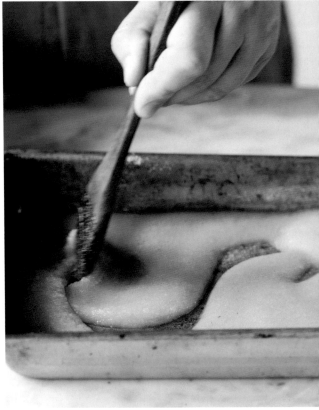

CANNABIS-INFUSED SUGAR

by CHEF UNIKA NOIEL, LUVN KITCHN

MAKES 1½ CUPS

INFUSED SUGAR

Makes 1½ cups

1 cup sugar

½ cup cannabis tincture, homemade
  (page 303)

1. To make the infused sugar: Preheat the oven to 190°F. Line a baking sheet with parchment paper and set aside.
2. In a small bowl, stir together the sugar and tincture until the sugar turns green in color and is fully hydrated. The sugar should have the texture of wet sand.
3. Evenly spread the sugar mixture out into a thin layer on the prepared baking sheet. Bake, with the oven door slightly opened (this will help evaporate the alcohol from the mixture) stirring every 10 minutes, until the alcohol has evaporated and the sugar is light golden brown and dry, about 1 hour.
4. Using the back of a spoon, press any clumped pieces of sugar through a sieve to re-granulate the sugar. Note: The sugar will look and feel very similar to regular sugar, but will have a slightly different granule shape. Cool sugar and store in an airtight container and label with the date and contents.

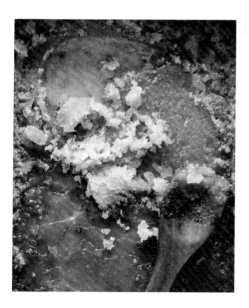

NOTES

You will need to make the cannabis tincture a few weeks before you intend to make the cannabis-infused sugar or go to LUVN Kitchn's website for a timesaving cannabis tincture recipe.

It is important to have a well-ventilated kitchen (oven fan on, open windows, etc.) when making the cannabis-infused sugar with high-proof alcohol.

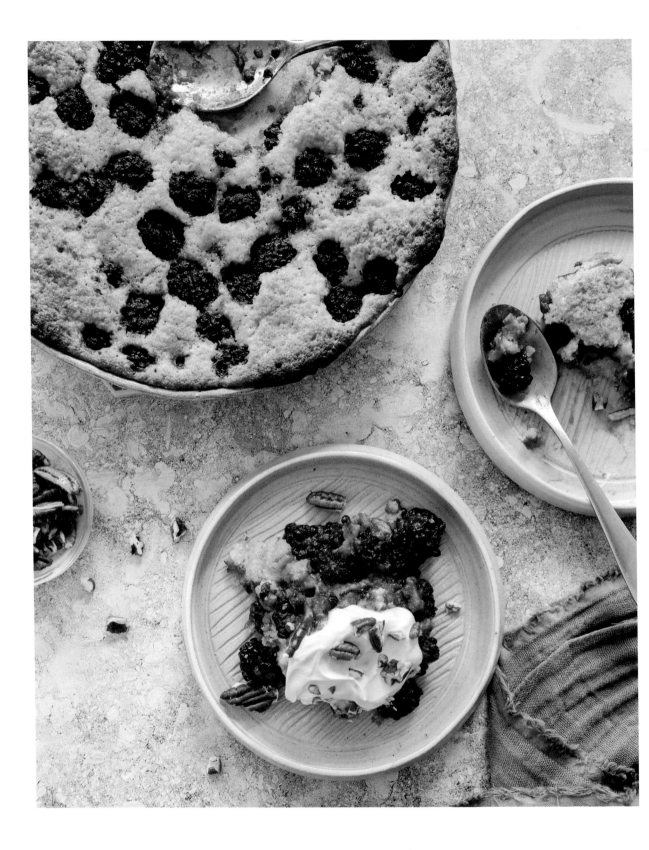

BLACKBERRY COBBLER

by CHEF UNIKA NOIEL, LUVN KITCHN

MAKES 6 to 8 servings

CHEF UNIKA NOIEL: In the Pacific Northwest, blackberries grow wild wherever nature and less-than-vigilant gardeners allow. My grandmother would send us kids outside with empty buckets and old containers, with the promise of blackberry cobbler if we returned with them full. We would spend hours looking for the biggest, juiciest berries we could find (and resist eating). As an adult, I realize it was probably a way for her to get us out of her hair, so it was definitely a win-win!

DOSING: Always assume that your guests will want seconds, and dose your meals accordingly. I recommend 2–5 milligrams of THC per serving, an average of 50 milligrams per dish. If you are serving multiple infused items, stay closer to 2 milligrams. You can always consume more if you feel like you can handle it, but you can't take it back once it's in your system!

1 cup all-purpose flour, plus extra for flouring baking dish

1¼ cups sugar, divided

1½ teaspoons baking powder

½ teaspoon salt

1 cup milk

1 teaspoon lemon zest

½ cup cannabis-infused unsalted butter, melted, plus extra for greasing baking dish

3 cups blackberries, fresh or frozen

1 teaspoon cannabis-infused sugar, homemade (page 305), optional

Whipped cream

½ cup coarsely chopped pecans

1. Preheat the oven to 350°F. Generously butter and flour a 2-quart baking dish, shaking off any excess flour. Note: The baking dish should be deep enough to allow the cobbler to rise. Set aside.

2. In a medium bowl, combine the flour, 1 cup of the sugar, baking powder, and salt. Add the milk and lemon zest and mix until well combined. Add the butter and stir until the batter is well mixed.

3. Pour the batter into the prepared baking dish. Evenly distribute the blackberries over the batter, then gently press them so the batter comes up about halfway up the berries. Sprinkle the remaining ¼ cup of sugar over the cobbler.

4. Place the baking dish in the center of the middle oven rack and bake until the top and outer edges are evenly golden and the sugar topping starts to become crisp, about 65 minutes. Sprinkle the cannabis-infused sugar over the top, if using, and continue to bake until the sugar crisps and becomes golden, about 10 minutes. Let the cobbler cool slightly before serving, about 5 minutes. Top with a dollop of whipped cream and sprinkles of pecans.

Recipe continues on next page

NOTE

If you plan on using the cannabis-infused sugar for the cobbler, this recipe takes a bit of advance planning.

CHEF UNIKA NOIEL'S NOTE

I am a fan of using purple strains when it comes to blackberries. I suggest using a strain like Presidential Kush (also called Presidential OG) by Fifty Fold for the cannabis-infused butter. Total THC: 13.17%, Total CBD: 0.11%, THCA: 14.58% (Harvest Date: 11/7/19).

KENDAL NORRIS

Founder, Mason Jar Event Group

Some individuals have a natural talent for entertaining and bringing folks together. Kendal Norris, the founder of the Mason Jar Event Group in Boulder, Colorado, is one of those people. She has always had a desire to connect friends and family around food and fun, which is the mission of her cannabis-focused event group. Norris grew up in the South where the mason jar is a cultural symbol of holidays, good times and all that bonds friends together, both old and new. These folks often exchange gifts in mason jars, a symbol of sharing and unity. With respect for these memories, Norris believes that the name she has chosen for her business perfectly represents what her company stands for, "bringing people together and creating community through shared experiences and joyous occasions."

As a passionate user, Norris has a history of hosting cannabis-themed dinners in her own home. After meeting with representatives from the cannabis industry, she decided to offer a series of celebrations to be held at private venues that would showcase that community. It was her goal to put a positive face on those who were part of the movement and try to eliminate the stigma that is so often associated with cannabis use. Norris is a strong advocate for its normalization.

Dinner themes are seasonally oriented, fashioned to suit each occasion. Norris and her stylist team work together to ensure that every detail of the evening is exceptional. Flatware, crystal, and china are handpicked for these gatherings, accented by embroidered linens and artistically designed menus. Colorful, beautifully arranged floral centerpieces reflect the celebrated season's splendor. Even the furniture has been carefully selected to set the tone for the unique gathering, which is further enhanced by the sound of live music from Mason Jar's House Bluegrass Band, "Lonesome Days."

Norris likes to use chefs who are local favorites, many of whom have never done an event such as this before. The chef and Norris will meet at the designated dispensary to learn the lineage and history behind individual strains or products and choose their favorites. Then the professional culinarian has the task of painstakingly creating a menu that will complement each of the pairings that have been selected, with desserts part of the equation. Pairings are not just limited to bud but span the many cannabis products that Colorado companies have to offer.

The first dinner was held in October 2015. Mason Jar's events are private, by invitation only. These occasions are geared toward canna-lovers and the canna-curious, with invitations much in demand and selling out quickly. To circumvent federal and state regulations, which prohibit chefs from offering cannabis-infused cuisine on a nightly basis, dinners are held at private facilities and consist of food that does not contain cannabis. These events are carefully structured to comply with Colorado's cannabis laws and meet all legal guidelines.

To facilitate matters, a shuttle service is provided to take guests to and from each event. Before the dinner, guests purchase prepared goodie bags for the occasion at a previously determined dispensary. The bags contain a variety of cannabis products that will be used as pairings for each course. Guests smoke or vaporize specific strains, free to choose how and when they would like to consume.

The busy entrepreneur likes to support local chefs who are doing interesting, innovative things with food. The chefs who host these events have carved their own niche in the culinary world, some of whom are James Beard Award winners. Guests have included Chef Hosea Rosenberg, who was the Season 5 winner of the television series "Top Chef," and is the owner of Blackberry Market in Boulder. Chef Kevin Grossi, owner of the Regional in Fort Collins, is known for his mouthwatering inventive dishes, while Chef Daniel Asher, co-owner of River and Woods Restaurant, offers community inspired recipes.

These culinary events bring top chefs, cannabis producers, and guests together for an extraordinary dining experience stylized to suit the evening's seasonal theme. Mason Jar elevates cannabis usage while educating guests to the reasoning behind each of its pairings. Norris explains that the affair is much like a wine tasting, but with cannabis instead. Highlighted by beautiful surroundings, live music and chef-driven farm-to-table cuisine, these sophisticated affairs hope to change the image of cannabis and its place in our society.

For those who want to incorporate exercise and fresh air into their routine, Norris also offers "Yoga with a View." This event consists of an hour of mindful yoga followed by a delicious farm-to-table brunch skillfully highlighted by cannabis pairings. The goal is to build bonds through both cannabis and yoga. Mason Jar Event Group is doing what it does best, bringing people together by promoting the importance of community and cannabis.

THC & CBD-INFUSED SMOKED CHEDDAR
and Green Chili Stone-Ground Grits

by CHEF KEVIN GROSSI, THE REGIONAL RESTAURANT
IN COLLABORATION WITH KENDAL NORRIS, MASON JAR EVENT GROUP

MAKES 4 servings

> **CHEF KEVIN GROSSI:** For a rich taste and creamy texture, we like to use stone-ground heirloom white corn grits.
>
> **SUGGESTED DOSAGE:** 20 milligrams THC per recipe and 3.33 milligrams THC per serving.

GRITS
Makes 6½ cups

Note: You will need to soak the stone-ground grits overnight in the refrigerator before you intend to serve them.

1 cup stone-ground heirloom white corn grits, medium cut

4 cups water

ROAST PEPPER
1 (about 6-inches long) green chile pepper, such as Anaheim or poblano

½ tablespoon extra-virgin olive oil

Kosher salt

1 cup half-and-half

¼ pound unsalted butter, divided

1 teaspoon kosher salt

2 medium cloves garlic, peeled and grated

1 cup shredded smoked cheddar cheese

4 packets Ripple Balanced 5, or two packets Ripple Pure 10

1. To presoak the grits: Place the grits and 4 cups of water in a bowl and soak overnight in the refrigerator.
2. To roast the pepper: Place the oven rack in the highest possible position in the oven. Preheat the oven broiler to high. Line a quarter-sheet-sized baking sheet with parchment paper or foil. Set aside.
3. Place the pepper on the prepared baking sheet and drizzle with oil. Season with salt.
4. Broil until the skin is charred and bubbly on all sides, turning twice with tongs, about 12 minutes.
5. Transfer to a small bowl, cover with plastic wrap, and let sit at room temperature for 20 minutes.
6. While the roasted pepper is resting, start the grits. Skim off any chaff and hulls that have floated to the top of the water. Drain and rinse the grits in a fine-mesh sieve, reserving the soaking liquid. Set aside.
7. Measure out the reserved soaking liquid, adding additional water, if needed to make 4 cups. Pour 4 cups of the reserved soaking liquid, half-and-half, 1 tablespoon of butter and salt in a 2-quart saucepan, and bring to a boil over medium-high heat, about 7 minutes. Add the grits in a slow and steady stream, then the garlic, stirring constantly with a wooden spoon.
8. Reduce the heat to just a simmer, partially cover, stirring frequently until the water is absorbed and grits are thick and tender, but still slightly runny, about 15 minutes.

Ingredients list continues on page 313

Recipe continues on page 313

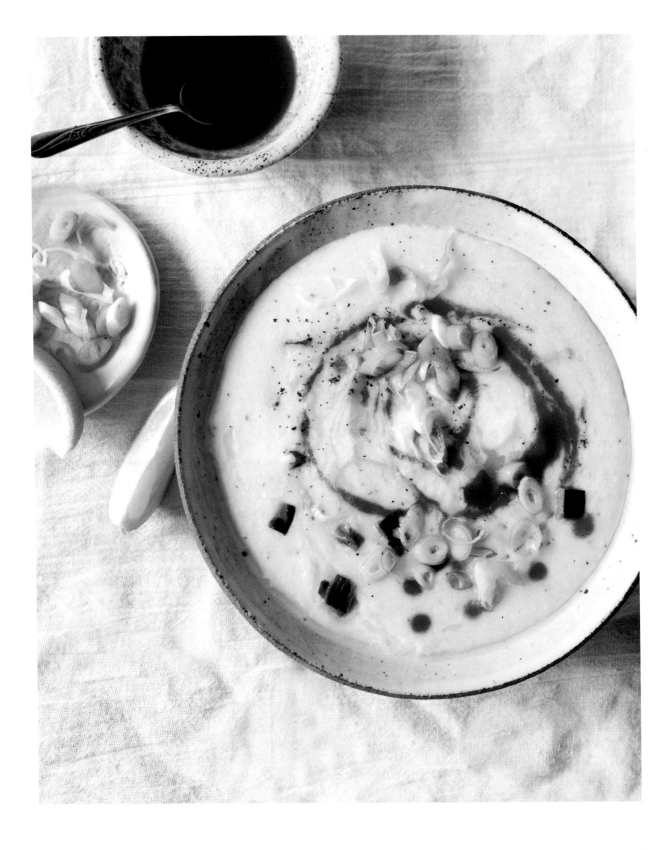

1½ tablespoons fresh lime juice, to taste

½ teaspoon freshly ground black pepper, or to taste

GARNISHES

½ cup scallion rings, thinly sliced on the bias

Hot sauce, to taste

9. While the grits are simmering, dice the pepper. Gently remove the skin and discard. Using a sharp knife, carefully cut a slit in the pepper lengthwise and discard the ribs, seeds, and stems. Cut the pepper into thin strips then dice. Set aside.

10. Remove the grits from the stove top and stir in the cheese, ⅓ cup of the roasted pepper, or to taste, the remaining 7 tablespoons of butter, Ripple, lime juice, and pepper. Adjust seasonings with additional lime juice, and salt and pepper, if desired. Garnish with a scattering of scallions over the top and a light drizzle of hot sauce, or to taste. Serve at once.

NOTE

Save the leftover roasted pepper and add to scrambled eggs, or use as a pizza topping.

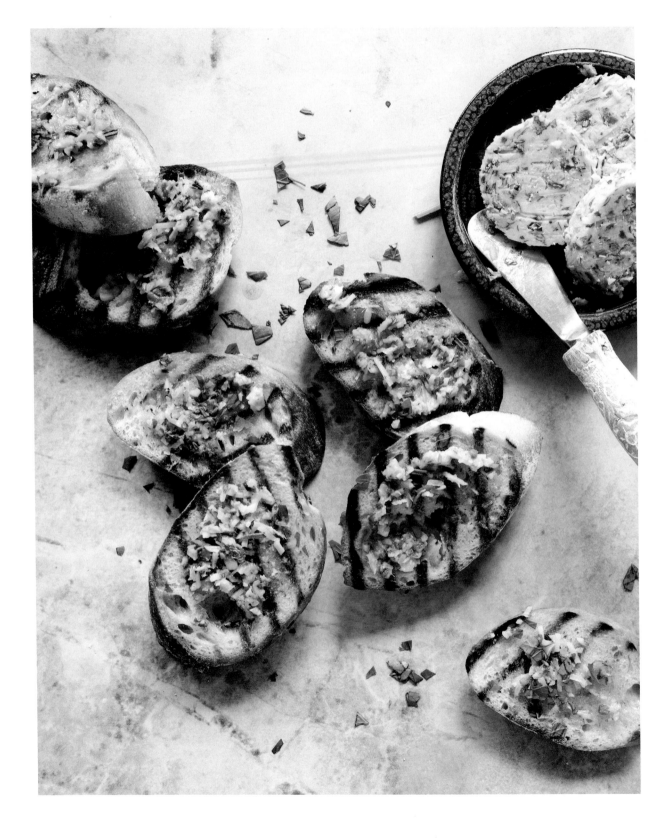

ANCHOVY BUTTER

by CHEF KEVIN GROSSI, THE REGIONAL RESTAURANT
IN COLLABORATION WITH KENDAL NORRIS,
MASON JAR EVENT GROUP

MAKES about 1⅛ cup;
approximately 1-inch
thick by 13 inches long

If you find that you have more butter than you can use, portion the leftovers and freeze. Just make sure to wrap them in plastic wrap first, then foil. Label and date the butter, then store in the freezer for up to 2 months. Be sure to allow time for the butter to thaw before using. Do not use the microwave to soften or thaw frozen butter because it could compromise the cannabinoids.

1 cup freshly grated Parmesan cheese

⅓ cup minced flat-leaf parsley

10 oil-packed anchovy fillets, drained and minced, or 1¾ tablespoons anchovy paste

4 medium cloves garlic, peeled and grated, about 1½ tablespoons

1 shallot, peeled and grated, about 1½ tablespoons

Zest of 1 lemon, about 1 tablespoon

½ tablespoon fresh minced rosemary leaves

1 stick (8 tablespoons or ½ cup) unsalted cannabutter, softened, store-bought or homemade

1. Place the cheese, parsley, anchovies, garlic, shallot, lemon zest, and rosemary in a large mixing bowl and mix until combined. Add the butter and with an electric mixer or wooden spoon, beat the butter, on medium speed until smooth and well combined, about 2 minutes, scraping down the sides of the bowl as necessary.

2. Lay out a 16×12-inch sheet of plastic wrap or waxed paper onto a clean work surface. Scrape the butter mixture onto the plastic wrap and shape into a log about 1 inch in diameter. Roll the butter up into a uniform cylinder.

3. Place in the refrigerator until firm, about 1 hour.

4. To serve: Unwrap the log and slice into coins. *Note:* It is delicious served on toasted baguette slices with garnishes of lemon zest and parsley. This butter is also excellent on steak, pork, chicken, fish, or vegetables.

NOTE

If you are making homemade cannabutter, you will need to make it 1 day before you plan to make the anchovy butter.

FLAKY PIECRUST

by CHEF KEVIN GROSSI, THE REGIONAL RESTAURANT
IN COLLABORATION WITH KENDAL NORRIS, MASON JAR EVENT GROUP

MAKES 1 dough

Part of the beauty of this recipe is that it could be used for any size pie; there might even be enough to make an upper and lower crust for a little tiny pie, or maybe a larger free-form galette sort of rustic pie thing, too!

1½ cups unbleached all-purpose flour

½ teaspoon fine-grain sea salt

¼ pound unsalted butter, cold and cut into small pieces

4 tablespoons unsalted cannabutter, cold and cut into small pieces

3–4 tablespoons ice water

1. Place the flour and salt in a bowl of a food processor, and pulse until just combined. Scatter the unsalted butter pieces over the flour mixture and cut into the flour with approximately five one-second pulses.

2. Add the cannabutter and continue cutting the butters into the flour mixture until it turns a pale yellow color and resembles coarse cornmeal, keeping some pea-sized butter pieces, about four more one-second pulses, depending on the food processor. Turn the mixture out into a large bowl.

3. Sprinkle 3 tablespoons of water over the mixture. Using a rubber spatula, fold the water into the mixture until the dough just comes together. Using your hands, press the dough together in the bottom of the bowl, adding an additional 1 tablespoon water if needed.

4. Turn the dough out onto a lightly floured surface and shape into a ball. Flatten into a 4-inch-wide disk with the heels of your hands. Wrap in plastic and refrigerate for at least 30 minutes.

5. Roll the dough out to an even thickness of ⅛ inch that will fit your pie dish. Extra piecrust may be trimmed off around the edges, then rerolled, and cut into decorative touches. Extra piecrust may also be wrapped tightly in plastic wrap and frozen for future use.

CHEF MICHAEL MAGALLANES

Owner, Opulent Chef

When it comes to the profession of cooking, Chef Michael Magallanes has redefined the meaning of the word "opulence," springboarding from traditional truffles and caviar to the use of both common and unexplored ingredients in his culinary masterpieces. Ever since he was young, Magallanes was fond of experimenting in the kitchen. This keen interest in cooking continued throughout high school and college, where he majored in philosophy and political science, not cuisine. He felt that making cooking a career, instead of a hobby, would undermine his interest and tarnish the appeal of the profession.

After graduating from college, Magallanes traveled to South America, remaining there for over a year while earning a living working in local kitchens. Upon returning to the United States, he again found himself in need of a livelihood, prompting him to return to the profession that he knew and loved. Deciding to move to San Francisco, he found employment in a select group of professional kitchens, learning how to use different types of equipment while also mastering diverse gastronomical techniques. This experience motivated him to pursue employment in upscale kitchens where he could continue to familiarize himself with the latest state-of-the-art equipment and unique ingredients.

By his late twenties, Magallanes found that he had reached an impasse job-wise. It was time for him to reevaluate his professional goals and either continue in the field of culinary arts or change his focus altogether. The decision was made simple when he was offered the rare opportunity to work his way up the line under The French Laundry chefs at San Francisco's Michelin-starred restaurant, Aziza. At Aziza he learned knife skills and distinctive cooking techniques, expanding his already growing repertoire of culinary know-how. After three years, he then moved on to open a Michelin-starred sister restaurant, Mourad, where Magallanes was essentially chef de cuisine, filling his days creating opulent innovative dishes.

Chef Magallanes left Mourad after two very productive years to start his own business, Opulent Chef, a boutique catering/private chef company located in San Francisco. The company offers exclusive dinner parties throughout the Bay Area and beyond. With help from a friend in the cannabis industry, the chef began experimenting with decarboxylation and infusing cannabis into oils, integrating the by-product into food. After educating himself on the practice of dosing, a celebratory dinner party was held for friends which was soon followed by an open-to-the-public pop-up affair.

Opulent Chef's Hightened Series is a sequence of fine-dining events, offering its guests an opportunity to enjoy gourmet food paired with various cannabis concentrates. The goal is to provide folks with an experience that is much like the one they would have at a fine restaurant where a sumptuous meal is paired with a superb wine. The chef feels that cannabis is an unexplored product in the culinary industry that has huge potential, not only as an ingredient in food but also as a replacement for wine. Through his work at Michelin-starred restaurants, Chef Magallanes has gained a hands-on understanding of what the luxury dining experience is all about. The busy chef also cooks for private clients in their own homes serving either cannabis-infused or cannabis-pairing meals. He still offers non-cannabis dinners for those who so desire.

For his cannabis dinners, the chef creates multiple courses that amount to one fully completed dish. Chef Magallanes seeks out unexplored ingredients of which guests have little or no knowledge and skillfully prepares them. His expertise with terpenes and aroma began with practice and was further enhanced through collaboration with professional hash-makers, whom he has dubbed the "wine stewards" of the cannabis world.

Events are by invitation only and require approval from the venue's owner. Chef Magallanes's favorite cannabis products are ice water hash and rosin made from ice water hash. The farmer and hash maker are invited to attend some events to talk about how they grew and made their product. They will talk about the strain and why it pairs well with a certain dish. The goal is to give guests an understanding of what concentrates are and how they are made, which offers insight into how they are paired. Each dinner contains an educational component that tries to destigmatize cannabis, presenting it as a natural element for enjoying life.

Menus change seasonally with some dishes repeated because of their popularity. Molecular gastronomy is at the forefront of every culinary experience, meaning that the chef is continually investigating the physical and chemical transformation of the ingredients that he uses in his recipes. Chef Magallanes does not like to use the cannabis flower because of its excess plant material that imparts a very strong flavor into the food, which is not to his liking. His choice is single-origin, strain-specific, outdoor-grown, clean concentrates. For this chef, ice water hash and rosin are the best expression of the plant. He avoids the use of CO_2, butane, or distillate extracts because the flavor and high aren't as good. The chef wants his guests to taste the cannabis in harmony with the food and enjoy what they are tasting.

Guests are encouraged not to drink alcohol during their meal, because it often does not mix well with cannabis. As cannabis can enhance alcohol, guests may often get too inebriated. The chef brings his intricate form of molecular gastronomy to infused cooking. He tailors the potency of each dish to suit a person's tolerance by creating unique infusions that use marijuana powders and milks.

Chef Magallanes wants his guests to become cannabis connoisseurs. To do so, he uses a modern approach to food that includes high-quality local and international ingredients. He feels that the definition of opulence in fine dining is changing, making it necessary to include cannabis as part of the equation. His artful creations and innovative techniques offer an opulent cannabis experience which is helping to erase the stigma associated with the use of the plant.

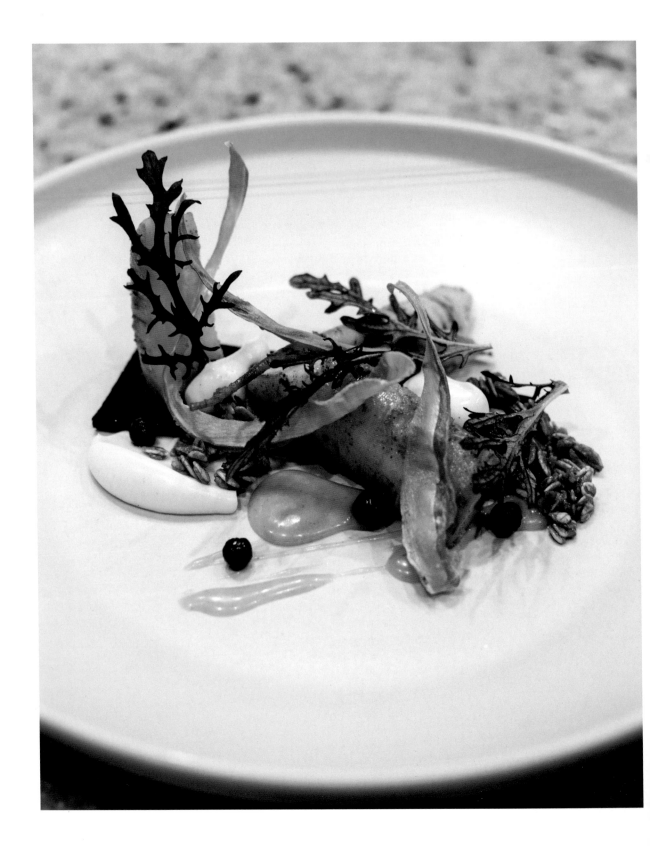

PARSLEY ROOT SALAD
with Pickled Huckleberries

CHEF MICHAEL MAGALLANES, OPULENT CHEF   **MAKES** 7 to 8 servings

CHEF MICHAEL MAGALLANES: Eating your way through this adventurous dish will ignite so many different textures and flavors, one can't help but fall in love. It's rich and savory while being bright and sweet all at the same time.

This recipe takes a bit of advance planning; it's best to approach it as several sub-recipes with multiple steps that come together as a unified whole at the end.

MICHAEL MAGALLANES'S TIPS ON MAKING THE CANNABIS-INFUSED BROWN BUTTER GASTRIQUE: First you'll make your brown butter, then you'll add your cannabis to the butter and let it infuse at 185°F for four hours, then strain it out. I recommend using the cannabis strain Astroboy, with 25 percent THCA before decarboxylation. There will be some further decarboxylation happening during the four-hour infusing time, so a full decarb isn't necessary unless you want some CBN. I think it's really whatever the person prefers. They could not decarb at all, then just infuse into the butter and get a mix of THC and THCA. I know people who prefer that method as well.

Three Days Before You Intend to Serve the Dish, Start the Pickled Huckleberries and Spice Mix.

PICKLED HUCKLEBERRIES

MAKES ½ cup pickled huckleberries

NOTE: You will need to pickle the huckleberries 3 days before you intend to serve them. If you can't find huckleberries, blueberries are a good substitute.

1 cup huckleberries, fresh or frozen

½ cup champagne vinegar

½ cup sugar

½ cup water

1. To make the pickled huckleberries: Place the huckleberries in a mason jar with a tight-sealing lid and set aside.
2. Combine the vinegar, sugar, and water in a saucepan and bring to a boil, stirring often, over medium-high heat.
3. Ladle the brine over the huckleberries. Allow the brine to cool to room temperature, about 30 minutes.
4. Tightly seal with lid and refrigerate the pickled huckleberries until you intend to serve them.

Recipe continues on next page

SPICE MIX

MAKES 1 cup

> **NOTE:** To save time, prepare the spice mix 3 days before you intend to use it. Remember to store the spice mix in an airtight container out of direct sunlight. This recipe makes more spice mix than you will need for the roasted parsley roots; serve over chicken or fish.

⅔ cup dry mint

1 tablespoon dry savory

1 tablespoon dry rose petals

1 tablespoon ground cumin

1 tablespoon ground coriander

½ tablespoon ground cinnamon

½ tablespoon ground nutmeg

½ tablespoon ground allspice

1 teaspoon ground black pepper

⅓ teaspoon ground cloves

⅓ teaspoon ground mustard seed

⅓ teaspoon ground green cardamom

1/16 teaspoon (pinch) ground fennel seed

1. To make the spice mix: Combine all ingredients in a bowl until well combined. Store in an airtight container until you are ready to use on the parsley roots.

Recipe continues on next page

CARAMEL-COATED OATS

MAKES about 1¾ cups

NOTE: To save time, prepare the oats 2 days before you intend to use them. Store the prepared oats in an airtight container out of direct sunlight. This recipe makes more caramel-coated oats than you will need; save the extra oats and serve over yogurt or add cold milk to a bowl of them for breakfast.

⅛ teaspoon coconut oil

⅛ teaspoon honey

⅛ teaspoon brown sugar

¼ teaspoon salt

1¼ cup rolled oats

1. Preheat the oven to 350°F. Line a baking sheet with parchment paper. Set aside.

2. To make the caramel: Melt the coconut oil in a small saucepan over medium heat. Stir in the honey, brown sugar, and salt and cook over medium heat until melted. Remove from the heat and add the oats, tossing until well combined.

3. To make the caramel-coated oats: Spread the oats out on the prepared baking sheet, so they are as flat of a mass as possible, and bake until golden brown, about 10 minutes. When cool enough to handle, break apart into nearly single oat flakes.

Recipe continues on next page

PARSNIP CHIPS

MAKES approximately 1¼ cups chips

NOTE: You will need to dehydrate the parsnip chips 2 days before you intend to serve them. Store the dehydrated chips in an airtight container out of direct sunlight.

1 large parsnip, about 7 ounces total

FRYING
1 cup organic safflower oil, or as needed

1. To dehydrate the parsnip chips: Using a sharp knife, slice the parsnip by hand thinly on a diagonal so that they are long oval strips. Place them in a single layer on the dehydrator trays and dry at 135°F until they are slightly pliable when done, about 2½ hours. (See note below.)

2. To fry the parsnip chips: Heat the oil in a large cast-iron skillet over medium-high heat until shimmering, but not smoking. Drop the parsnips, in batches if necessary, into the hot oil and quickly fry until golden brown, about 20 seconds. Using a slotted spoon, carefully and quickly remove and drain on paper towels.

NOTE

If you don't own a dehydrator, you can dry the parsnips in the oven. Preheat the oven to 170°F. Place a metal cooling rack on a baking sheet and arrange the parsnips in a single layer on the rack so they have air circulating around them. Dry until they are slightly pliable when done, about 4 hours.

Recipe continues on next page

One Day Before You Intend to Serve the Dish, Start the Huckleberry Base.

HUCKLEBERRY BASE

NOTE: To save time, make the huckleberry base 1 day before you intend to make the huckleberry veil. If you can't find huckleberries, blueberries are a good substitute.

NOTE: This recipe makes more huckleberry base than you will need in the veil; save the extra base and serve over ice cream, pancakes or waffles.

1 pound huckleberries

1 cup water

¼ sugar

2 tablespoons balsamic vinegar

1. To make the huckleberry base: Combine the huckleberries, water, sugar, and balsamic vinegar, in a saucepan and bring to a boil, stirring often, over medium-high heat, about 9 minutes.
2. Remove from the heat and allow to cool to room temperature, about 1 hour and 30 minutes.
3. Transfer to a blender and blend until smooth.
4. Strain the berry mixture through a fine-mesh strainer, occasionally running a spatula around the inside of the strainer to loosen up any clogged material.
5. Ladle into a mason jar, then tightly seal with a lid. Transfer to the refrigerator and allow to cool until you are ready to make the huckleberry veil.

Recipe continues on next page

Early in Day You Intend to Serve the Dish Make the Following: Huckleberry Veil, Cannabis-infused Brown Butter Gastrique, Parsnip Vanilla Creme, Roasted Parsley Roots.

HUCKLEBERRY VEIL

NOTE: You must use a pan that can hold the veil so that it is only ⅛-inch deep. Recommended pan sizes: a metal, rimmed, quarter-sized baking pan or a 9×13-inch baking dish.

NOTE: It is important to note that agar sets very quickly at room temperature.

1 cup huckleberry base (page 325)

½ tablespoon agar powder, 1.2 percent

½ cup cold water

2 teaspoons Knox gelatin powder (1 envelope) or 2 gold gelatin sheets, such as PerfectaGel

1. To make the huckleberry veil: Line a baking sheet with parchment paper. Set aside.
2. Place the huckleberry base into a small saucepan and add the agar, whisking constantly and thoroughly for 10 minutes until the agar has fully dissolved and hydrated.
3. Bring to a boil over medium heat, whisking constantly, about 8 minutes. When the base has reached a boil, turn off the heat.
4. Pour the water into a small bowl and sprinkle the gelatin over the water. Stir to combine and allow to bloom for 1 minute.
5. Strain off any excess water and add the bloomed gelatin to the hot huckleberry base. Whisk gently together until well combined.
6. Pour the base into the quarter-sized baking sheet, and tilt slightly so that the mixture runs into all of the corners. Allow the veil to cool to room temperature on an even surface.
7. Once the veil is at room temperature, use a sharp knife to cut the veil into rectangular strips that measure approximately 1½×5 inches. Using an offset spatula, gently transfer the rectangles to the prepared baking sheet until ready to use. Note: You will have approximately 12 strips.

NOTE

If using gelatin sheets instead of the gelatin powder, place the gelatin sheets in a bowl of ice water, then allow to bloom for 10 minutes.

CANNABIS-INFUSED BROWN BUTTER GASTRIQUE

NOTE: Xanthan gum has a tendency to clump when added to liquids. To avoid this, mix the xanthan gum with the sugar first before being incorporated into the liquid.

BROWN BUTTER

Makes 1¾ cups

Note: This recipe makes more brown butter than you will need in the gastrique; save the extra and serve over pasta or steamed vegetables.

1 pound of unsalted butter

GASTRIQUE

Makes 2⅓ cups

Note: This recipe makes more gastrique than you will need for the recipe, save the extra and add to your favorite tomato sauce, fish dish, or spooned over roasted vegetables.

1 scant cup sugar

1½ teaspoons xanthan gum

2½ cups plus 2 tablespoons water

Scant ½ cup sherry vinegar

Scant ½ cup champagne vinegar

1 cup plus 3 tablespoons toasted, chopped almonds

1 cup infused brown butter (see recipe above)

1. To make the brown butter: In a medium saucepan, melt the butter over medium heat. Stirring occasionally, cook until the butter turns a toasty brown color, about 15 minutes.
2. Remove from the heat and allow to cool until just warm. Strain the butter through a fine-mesh strainer or cheesecloth to remove all the solids.
3. Infuse desired amount of decarboxylated cannabis into butter at 185°F for 4 hours, depending on your individual tolerance level and strain. Set aside until ready to use in the gastrique.
4. To make the cannabis-infused brown butter gastrique: place the sugar and xanthan gum in a small bowl and mix together until well combined.
5. Place the water and vinegars in a saucepan. Whisking constantly, pour the sugar mixture in a slow and steady stream into the center of the water mixture whirlpool until the xanthan gum is hydrated.
6. Add the almonds and reduce the liquid over medium heat, whisking occasionally, until the volume is reduced by about 1⅛ cups, about 1 hour and 10 minutes. Let cool for 10 minutes.
7. Transfer to a blender. While the blender is running on low speed, add the infused brown butter in a slow and steady stream to keep the mixture emulsified.

Recipe continues on next page

PARSNIP VANILLA CRÈME

PARSNIPS

Note: Reserve the parsnip peels for another use, such as a vegetable stock.

11 ounces organic parsnips, scrubbed, ends removed, peeled and cut into chunks

½ tablespoon extra-virgin olive oil

¼ teaspoon kosher salt

⅛ teaspoon freshly ground black pepper

1. To make the parsnips: Preheat the oven to 425°F. Fill a small baking dish with enough water to cover the bottom of dish. Set aside.
2. In a small bowl, combine the parsnips and olive oil until well combined. Place the parsnips on the prepared baking dish in a single layer. Evenly sprinkle with the salt and pepper over the top. Cover with foil and bake in the oven, until fork-tender, about 25 minutes, or depending on the thickness. Reserve the parsnip meat for the crème.

GELLAN BLOCK

¼ tablespoon calcium gluconate

2¼ cups water plus ½ tablespoon, divided

1¾ tablespoons Gellan Gum, Low Acyl

1. To make the gellan block: Place a large bowl of ice water near your cooking area.
2. To make the calcium gluconate slurry: Place the calcium gluconate in a small bowl. In a slow and steady stream, whisk in the ½ tablespoon of water until the calcium gluconate is completely smooth.
3. Place the remaining 2¼ cups of water into a large saucepan. Whisking constantly and vigorously, add the gellan gum in a slow and steady stream. Bring to a boil, whisking constantly, over medium-high heat until the gellan gum is fully dissolved, about 12 minutes. Add the calcium gluconate slurry and bring the liquid back to a boil, whisking constantly, about 3 minutes. Allow to cool over the prepared bowl of ice water until thoroughly chilled and fully firm, about 40 minutes.

CRÈME

10½ ounces parsnip meat (See recipe above)

6⅓ ounces gellan block (See recipe above)

½ tablespoon vanilla paste

½ cup crème fraîche

1. To make the crème: Place the parsnip meat, gellan block, and vanilla paste into a blender and blend until very smooth, scraping down the sides as needed. Add the crème fraîche and blend until just incorporated. Pass through a mesh strainer.

Recipe continues on next page

ROASTED PARSLEY ROOT

14 small parsley roots, parsley-like tops removed, scrubbed and peeled

Olive oil, as needed

3 tablespoons spice mix (page 322)

Kosher salt

3 tablespoons unsalted butter

6 fresh thyme sprigs

1. Preheat the oven to 425°F. Fill a small roasting pan with enough water to cover the bottom of the pan. Set aside.

2. Place the parsley roots in a large bowl and drizzle with olive oil, tossing until well combined. Add the spice mix and salt, to taste, tossing until well combined.

3. Transfer to the prepared roasting pan. Place the butter and thyme around the roots. Cover with foil and bake in the oven until tender, about 25 minutes. Remove the foil and bake for another 10 minutes uncovered. When cool enough to handle, cut into the parsley roots into pieces.

GARNISHES

Red Frill mustard greens

Fleur de sel

1. To assemble: Place a swoosh of the desired amount of cannabis brown butter gastrique on a plate. Using two spoons, shape the crème into a three sided "oval" (a technique known as a quenelle) and carefully drop it on the plate. Then place 1 huckleberry veil rectangle on the crème oval. Place two to four root pieces on the plate, sprinkle 2 tablespoons of the caramel-coated oats around the root pieces and crème, followed by some of the pickled huckleberries. Garnish with parsnip chips, mustard greens, and a light sprinkle of fleur de sel, to taste. Repeat with the remaining ingredients.

VARIATION

Alternatives to Red Frill mustard greens would be Swiss chard, kale, spinach, or escarole. Thinly slice before using as a garnish.

SQUID INK RICE CRACKERS

with Poached Pickled Radishes and Avocado Purée

by CHEF MICHAEL MAGALLANES, OPULENT CHEF

MAKES about 12 servings; approximately 2 crackers each

> **CHEF MICHAEL MAGALLANES:** This canape was created as a way to easily control the amount of THC we serve our guests to commence a dinner party. We create a variety of cannabis-infused coconut oil powders at different THC strengths, making it easy to accommodate a large range of tolerance levels. This savory, creamy, bright, and crunchy bite is a fun crowd-pleaser.

POACHED PICKLED RADISHES

Note: You will need to poach and pickle the radishes 1 day before you intend to serve them.

1 bunch red radishes, trimmed and quartered (about 1⅓ cups radish quarters)

1 tablespoon extra-virgin olive oil

¾ teaspoon kosher salt

Scant ¼ teaspoon sugar

3 tablespoon fresh lemon juice

CANNABIS-INFUSED COCONUT OIL POWDER

Makes approximately 1¼ cups

Note: To save time, make the infused coconut oil 1 day before you intend to make the crackers.

Note: This makes more cannabis-infused coconut oil powder than you will need for the crackers; save the extra and sprinkle over roasted vegetables, salads, or homemade pizza. Store the leftovers in an airtight container and label with the date and contents.

1. Bring a 2-quart saucepan of water to a simmer.
2. To make the poached pickled radishes: In a medium mixing bowl, toss the radishes with the olive oil, salt, and sugar. Place the radishes along with any remaining brine into a food-grade silicone bag used for vide cooking. Roll the bag to remove any excess air before sealing the bag. Note: If you do not own a food-grade silicone bag, it is important to use a plastic bag that is made out of food-grade plastic.
3. Gently lower the bag of radishes into the water until it is completely submerged, and poach, maintaining a water temperature of 135–145°F on an instant-read thermometer, until fork-tender, about 1 hour and 15 minutes. Note: You may need to weigh down the bag to get it to fully submerge. A glass canning jar filled with a little water works well as a weight—just let it sit on top of the sealed bag.
4. Carefully remove the bag and glass jar from the water.
5. Remove the radishes and brine from the bag and transfer to a mixing bowl. While the radishes are still hot, toss with the lemon juice and allow to cool to room temperature, stirring occasionally, about 20 minutes. Cover and allow to rest in the refrigerator overnight. Note: This will allow the color of the radishes to fully brighten.
6. If you have cannabis-infused coconut oil on hand, skip this step. While the radishes are cooling, start making the cannabis-infused coconut oil. Infuse the desired amount of decarboxylated cannabis into coconut oil at 185°F for 4 hours depending on your individual tolerance level

⅛ cup cannabis-infused coconut oil, melted (page 259)

1¼ cups tapioca maltodextrin

SQUID INK RICE CRACKERS

1 cup medium-grain rice, such as arborio, Valencia, or Bomba

3¾ cups water, divided

1¼ tablespoons (16 grams) squid ink

1½ teaspoons kosher salt

FOR FRYING

2 cups rice bran oil

GRILLED SCALLION RELISH

2 bunches scallions (about 12 stalks), trimmed

3 tablespoons extra-virgin olive oil, plus extra for the grill

¼ kosher salt, or to taste

⅛ freshly ground black pepper, or to taste

AVOCADO PURÉE

Makes approximately 1⅓ cups

2 medium ripe Hass avocados, pitted and peeled

3 tablespoons fresh lime juice

Scant 1 teaspoon kosher salt

GARNISH

Edible flowers, such as pansy or radish

and strain. Allow the oil to cool completely before using (page 259).

7. To make the squid ink crackers: Preheat the oven to 185°F. Line 2 half-sheet rimmed baking sheets with parchment paper and generously grease with oil. Set aside.

8. Place the rice in a pot with the 3 cups of water and cook, covered, over low heat, stirring often until rice is mushy and all of the water has cooked off, about 30 minutes.

9. Add the rice, squid ink and salt to a blender. While the blender is running on low to medium speed (depending on the strength of the blender's motor) add the remaining ¾ cup of water in a slow and steady stream, scraping down the sides of the blender with a wet spatula as needed, until very smooth.

10. Place a small bowl of room temperature water next to your cooking area; this will be used to keep the spatula wet.

11. Pour 2 cups (400 grams) of the rice mixture onto the prepared baking sheet and spread evenly with a wet spatula. Note: Dipping the spatula into the prepared water bowl periodically will help the rice from sticking to the spatula. Repeat with the remaining 2 cups of rice mixture on the second prepared baking sheet.

12. Bake until the surface of the cracker is dry, about 1 hour and 10 minutes on one side. Note: The cracker should feel dry to the touch but still soft underneath the surface.

13. Remove the baking sheet from the oven, and carefully place another baking sheet on top of it, sandwiching the cracker between the two sheets. Holding the 2 baking sheets together with both hands at the edges, carefully flip them over so the cracker will gently land upside down on the surface of the second sheet. Carefully remove the top baking sheet and parchment paper, leaving the cracker on the new baking sheet. Repeat with the second cracker.

14. Return the baking sheets with the crackers to the oven and bake until firm and leathery, but not fully hard and dehydrated, about 1 hour and 20 minutes on the second side. Let the crackers air dry for 1 hour on the counter.

15. To fry the crackers: Break the crackers into 4-inch pieces and set aside. Pour the rice bran oil into a 10-inch cast-iron skillet and heat to 425°F. Working in batches place

Recipe continues on next page

2 pieces of the cracker at a time into the oil and fry until they puff, about 1 minute per side. Using a slotted spoon, transfer to a paper-towel-lined plate and allow to cool. Break the crackers into the desired size and shape. Repeat with remaining crackers.

16. To make the scallion relish: While the crackers are baking in the oven, preheat a gas or electric grill to medium-high heat and generously brush the cooking grate with oil. In a medium bowl, add the scallions, oil, salt, and pepper and toss until well combined. Remove the scallions from the oil and arrange in a single layer across the grill grate. Grill, covered, turning often until fully cooked and slightly charred, about 15 minutes. Transfer to a cutting board and allow to slightly cool, then finely chop. Transfer to a bowl and season with salt and pepper to taste. Set aside.

17. While the scallions are cooling, make the avocado purée: Place the avocado meat, lime juice, and salt into a blender and blend until very smooth. Transfer the purée to a plastic squeeze bottle with a tip. Set aside.

18. To finish the radishes: Slice the radish quarters into ⅛-inch-thick slices. Return the slices back to the bowl with the brine, tossing until evenly coated. Set aside.

19. To make the cannabis powder: Carefully scoop the tapioca maltodextrin into a bowl of a food processor. While the processor is running, slowly add the cannabis-infused coconut oil in a slow and steady stream until the oil is evenly distributed throughout the powder, scraping down the sides of the food processor as needed to keep the powder free-flowing. Set aside.

20. To assemble: Sprinkle the desired amount of cannabis-infused coconut oil powder onto each cracker. Place 2 small piles of the scallion relish on top. Scatter 2 to 3 pickled radish slices over the top. Place 4 to 5 dots of the avocado purée on top and around each cracker. Garnish each with a flower. Serve at once.

NOTE

Tapioca maltodextrin is designed to transform oils into powders. When transferring this very fluffy and light powder, it is helpful to use a spoon or scoop.

MICHAEL MAGALLANES'S NOTE

Garlic juice and indica cannabis strain pairs well with the cracker recipe. For the recommended dosage, I feel that it is a personal preference. One person might only need 3 milligrams, while another person might want 10 milligrams. I suggest that people figure out what their tolerance levels are and then dose accordingly.

BASIC DOSING CALCULATOR—DOSE PER SERVING

Grams used in recipe x THC per gram = Dose per recipe divide by the number of servings

CHEF DANIEL ASHER
& JOSH DINAR

Co-owners, River and Woods

At the young age of seven, Daniel Asher could frequently be found spending time in the kitchen with his mother, helping in some small way with the day's meal. His mother made everything from scratch, baking her own bread, growing her own vegetables, and curing meats. She not only taught her son technique but also instilled in him a devotion to and love of the art of cooking.

When Asher was very little, the family moved from Montreal, Canada, where he was born, to the United States. He grew up outside of Chicago, known for its culinary traditions and iconic signature dishes. Always loving anything food related, Asher started at the age of fourteen to work in professional kitchens washing dishes and peeling potatoes, slowly working his way up the culinary ladder. Asher became a sous-chef when he was in his early twenties, graduating to executive chef a few years later. A business project consultation brought him to the Boulder, Colorado, area and he has been there ever since.

Chef Asher and Josh Dinar are the co-owners of River and Woods restaurant in Boulder. Dinar is a restaurateur, cofounder of Boulder's Restaurant Week, community volunteer, and publisher of *Dining Out* magazine. The two men have known each other for many years, meeting through the magazine connection. When offered an opportunity to partner and cocreate River and Woods, the two decided to purchase a hundred-year-old homestead cottage in the heart of the city. Once a very popular dining spot, the building had been vacant for many years after its previous owner had retired. The two men saw enormous business potential and set out to revive the historic structure. Their dream was to create a community restaurant that would serve an upscale taste of Colorado comfort cuisine.

River and Woods opened for business in 2016. The restaurant's two main rooms are bright and cozy, with a seating capacity that accommodates up to sixty-five guests. A sprawling backyard offers diners a taste of the outdoors accented by rustic picnic tables, a rotisserie, and a converted Airstream trailer that serves as a unique bar. A large play area makes this the perfect place for families to enjoy a meal and commune with nature. The restaurant's name is a play on words, a whimsical reference to "Over the River and through the Woods," that illustrates the Colorado lifestyle. It's a little cottage that you happen upon in the woods, where you can walk in and warm up with delicious food and happy people.

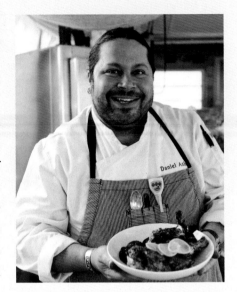

For Chef Asher, the beauty of working in a restaurant involves the connection with its guests which, over time, evolves into a true feeling of community. To encourage and further strengthen this bond, visitors are invited to submit one of their own favorite family recipes that, if chosen, will be included on the menu. The recipe could be one that they have created themselves, or a treasured heirloom that has been passed down from generation to generation. Those that are selected are interpreted by the chef in a way that reflects River and Woods' approach to natural, organic, and sustainable eating. This very novel approach is called "crowdsourced cuisine."

The restaurant's ever-changing menu lists the origin of each selection under its appropriate category: Rivers, Woodlands, High Plains, Coasts, and Farms and Fields. An item that is prefaced with @ denotes a community-inspired recipe. About a third of the menu consists of interpretations of guests' submissions. Chef Asher wants to know where the food he uses comes from. It is important for him to determine its source before he can decide if it will be a satisfactory fit for the restaurant. For him, food is a collective experience that is a collaboration of many people.

The chef works with a select group of area businesses that produce craft cannabis strains. Together they strive to offer food pairings for special occasions and events. Cannabis-infused roasted organic citrus chicken, sugar-glazed turkey, quick-pickled elephant-heart plums, maple-roasted organic garnet yams, and creamed organic kale are just a few of the culinary delights that Chef Asher has created for these affairs. All are complemented and accented by the appropriate cannabis strain. The chef believes that, "We all need to do our part to promote sustainable agriculture and healthy decisions for our planet to ensure the wellness of future generations. It's about being kind, being gentle with the earth, being thoughtful, and being a steward of the land."

CANNABIS-INFUSED MISO-SRIRACHA DEVILED EGGS

by CHEF DANIEL ASHER, RIVER AND WOODS RESTAURANT

MAKES 12 servings

SUGGESTED DOSAGE: approximately 5 milligrams THC per egg half; approximately 10 milligrams THC per serving/whole egg.

CHEF DANIEL ASHER: Deviled eggs were one of the first things I made with my mother. Because of this, they offer a fond connection to my earliest food memories. If you bring them to a party or event, they are very popular and in high demand. Perhaps it's the fact that they are familiar and comforting. This infused version is a lovely way to enjoy a light, high-protein snack with the medicinal benefits of cannabis.

6 large organic cage-free brown eggs, room temperature

½ tablespoon white miso paste, or to taste

1 teaspoon stone-ground mustard

1 teaspoon sriracha, preferably McCauley Family Farm's Picaflor

1 teaspoon toasted sesame oil

6 (10 mg each THC) individual packets of Ripple Pure 10 Dissolvable THC

3 tablespoons organic mayonnaise, or to taste

GARNISHES

1 teaspoon black sesame seeds

⅛ cup scallion rings, thinly sliced on the bias

Smoked paprika

1. Place a large bowl of ice water near your cooking area.
2. To make the hard-boiled eggs: Place the eggs in a saucepan large enough to have them in a single layer. Cover the eggs with at least 1 inch of cold water and bring to a boil over medium-high heat. Turn off the heat, cover, and let stand until hard-boiled, about 10 to 11 minutes. Using a slotted spoon, remove the eggs and place them in the prepared water bath for 2 minutes. Remove from the water bath, then gently tap an egg on the counter to crack the shell. Peel under cold running water. Repeat with the remaining eggs. Transfer to a medium bowl. Cover with plastic wrap and place in the refrigerator until cold, about 15 minutes.
3. Slice the eggs in half lengthwise, then gently remove the yolks and transfer them to a bowl of a food processor. Place the egg whites on a decorative platter. Add the miso paste, mustard, sriracha, and sesame oil to the yolks and process until smooth and creamy. Add the Ripple packets and mayonnaise and process until fully incorporated. Adjust seasonings with additional mayonnaise and miso paste, if desired.
4. Using a pastry bag with a star tip, fill the bag with the egg yolk mixture, and pipe about 1½ teaspoons into the center of each egg white. If you don't own a pastry bag, you can also use a small spoon to fill the eggs.
5. Garnish with a sprinkle of black sesame seeds, a scattering of scallions, and a light dusting of smoked paprika. Serve at once.

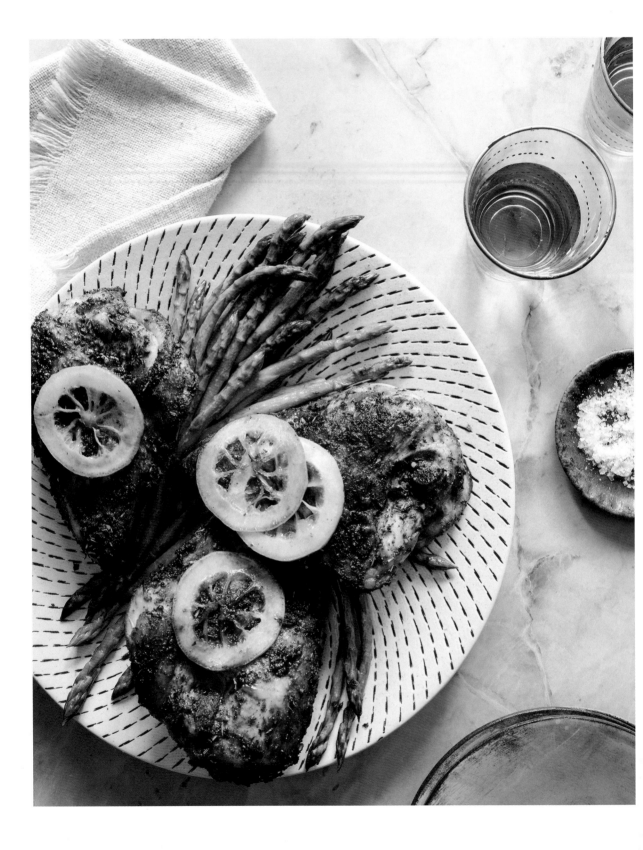

DAZED & INFUSED CITRUS HERB CHICKEN

CHEF DANIEL ASHER, RIVER AND WOODS RESTAURANT

MAKES 4 servings

SUGGESTED DOSAGE: approximately 5 milligrams THC per serving.

CHEF DANIEL ASHER: The bright flavors of the cannabis-infused citrus oil and glaze provides the perfect counterpoint to the tender chicken breasts. Serve this dish to your family and friends with the spirit of community, love, and mindful cooking.

DRY RUB

2 tablespoons Herbes de Provence

2 tablespoons Old Bay seasoning

2 tablespoons Cajun seasoning, such as Penzeys Spices

1 teaspoon fine sea salt

CANNABIS-INFUSED CITRUS OIL

¼ cup extra-virgin olive oil

1 capful infused olive oil, preferably Colorado Cannabis Company's Hybrid Olive Oil (10 milligrams THC)

3 tablespoons fresh lemon juice

CHICKEN

4 large (about 4 pounds) organic free-range split chicken breasts, bone-in, skin-on

¼ stick unsalted butter, melted

CANNABIS-INFUSED GLAZE

¼ cup local honey, melted

1¼ tablespoons lemon juice

1 capful of infused olive oil, preferably Colorado Cannabis Company's Hybrid Olive Oil (10 milligrams THC)

GARNISHES

2 teaspoons olive oil

1 medium lemon, thinly sliced

1. Preheat the oven to 400°F. Line a baking sheet with foil and set aside.

2. To make the dry rub: In a small bowl, stir together the Herbes de Provence, Old Bay seasoning, Cajun seasoning, and salt until well combined.

3. To make the cannabis-infused citrus oil: In a small bowl, whisk together the oils and lemon juice until well combined. Set aside.

4. Pat the chicken dry with paper towels. Place the chicken breasts skin-side up on the prepared baking sheet. Using a basting brush, spread the cannabis-infused citrus oil evenly over all sides of the chicken.

5. Evenly rub each chicken breast half with 1 tablespoon of the dry rub, over all sides, until well coated. Tip: Apply the rub to the bottom (bone sides) of each chicken first, ending with the skin-side to help prevent losing some of the rub on top.

6. Bake, skin-side up, until the internal temperature reaches 160°F, about 40 minutes.

7. Decrease the oven temperature to 350°F. Remove the chicken from the oven and drizzle the butter evenly over the top. Return the chicken to the oven and continue to bake until the internal temperature reaches 165°F and juices run clear, about 10 minutes, or depending on the size of the chicken breasts.

8. While the chicken is reaching an internal temperature of 165°F, make the cannabis-infused glaze. In a small

Recipe continues on next page

bowl, whisk together the honey, lemon juice, and oil. Set aside.

9. While the chicken is hot, apply the cannabis-infused glaze. Using a small pastry brush, gently dab the glaze evenly over the top of each breast half. Let the chicken rest for 5 minutes.

10. While the chicken is resting, quickly cook the lemon slices. Heat the oil in a medium skillet over medium heat. Add the lemon slices and cook for 1 minute. Using tongs, turn once and cook for another 1 minute.

11. To serve: Top each breast half with a slice of lemon. Serve with roasted organic vegetables and a grain of choice or the Thrifty Stuffing (page 339).

VARIATION

A whole chicken (about 3½ pounds), giblets and neck discarded, cut in half with the backbone removed and trimmed, is another option for this dish.

THRIFTY STUFFING

by CHEF DANIEL ASHER, RIVER AND WOODS RESTAURANT

MAKES 10 servings

CHEF DANIEL ASHER: The idea behind this unique stuffing is to make use of all those food items in your kitchen that seem to no longer have a purpose. Go through your pantry, refrigerator, and freezer grabbing all the random bits and pieces that are left over and looking like they have seen better days. It might be a few dried, wrinkled cranberries, or crystallized ginger left from the homemade granola that you made last month. Trail mix that the kids never finished, and a bunch of sad looking vegetables will do the trick. Use the trimmings from veggie peels to make vegetable stock. Even the leftover bits from the salt and vinegar and tortilla chips have a role. Remember, this is the time to make those leftovers shine instead of tossing them out!

BREAD CUBES

Note: You will need to oven dry the bread cubes at least 1 hour before you intend to make the stuffing.

1 (1-pound) day-old loaf of artisan bread, cut into ½-inch cubes, about 10 cups

STUFFING

2 tablespoons extra-virgin olive oil, or as needed

1 cup assorted mushrooms, cleaned, trimmed, and thinly sliced, preferably Mile High Fungi

½ cup diced organic red onion

½ cup diced organic celery, preferably Cure Organic Farm

½ cup diced organic carrots

1¼ cups diced zucchini, preferably Cure Organic Farm

2 medium cloves heirloom garlic, minced, preferably Toohey & Sons Organic

½ cup semisweet hard cider, preferably Big B's Delicious Orchards

½ cup assorted dried unsweetened fruits, such as cranberries or cherries

¼ cup assorted nuts, such as pistachios, Marcona almonds, or walnuts, coarsely chopped

1½ teaspoons fresh minced basil leaves

1½ teaspoons fresh minced sage leaves

1½ teaspoons fresh minced rosemary leaves

1½ teaspoons fresh minced thyme leaves

1½ teaspoons fresh minced oregano leaves

¾ teaspoon fine-grain sea salt, or to taste

½ teaspoon freshly ground black pepper, or to taste

2 large eggs, at room temperature, beaten

2 cups low-sodium organic vegetable stock, warm or as needed

Recipe continues on next page

1. To make the bread cubes: Preheat the oven to 275°F. Place the bread cubes on an ungreased baking sheet and oven dry, tossing occasionally, until well toasted and hard, about 45 minutes. Note: The cooking time will depend on the type and density of the bread. Remove from the oven and let cool.

2. Increase the oven temperature to 350°F. Note: If making 1 day ahead or baking with the Dazed & Infused Citrus Herb Chicken, skip this step.

3. While the bread cubes are toasting, sauté the vegetables. Heat the oil in a large skillet over medium heat. Add the mushrooms, onions, celery, and carrots and sauté until the onions are soft and translucent and some of the liquid from the mushrooms have evaporated, about 8 minutes. Add the zucchini, and sauté for 5 minutes. Add the garlic and sauté for 1 minute.

4. Remove the pan from the heat and carefully add the hard cider. Increase the heat to medium-high. Return the pan to the heat and bring the liquid to a simmer. Deglaze the pan, stirring frequently, scraping up the bits from the bottom, and continue to simmer until the liquid is reduced by half, about 5 minutes.

5. Lightly butter a 9×13-inch baking dish. Set aside.

6. Place the bread cubes in an extra-large bowl. Add the vegetable mixture, dried fruits, nuts, herbs, salt, and pepper, and gently mix all the ingredients together; do not overmix. Adjust seasonings with salt and pepper. Pour the eggs over the bread mixture and gently toss to coat.

7. Pour the stuffing into the prepared baking dish. Pour the stock just over the surface of the stuffing. If the mixture seems too dry, add more stock until the desired consistency is achieved. Let sit for 10 minutes before baking so that the bread can absorb some of the stock. Note: If you are making the stuffing 1 day ahead, cover with foil, then transfer to the refrigerator and bake off the next day.

8. Cover with foil and bake for 15 minutes, then remove the foil and bake uncovered until golden brown, about 15 minutes. Remove from the oven and let stand for 5 minutes before serving. Serve with Dazed & Infused Citrus Herb Chicken (page 337), if desired.

CHEF DANIEL ASHER'S NOTE

I also like to use STEM Ciders off-dry (as in not-so-dry) apple cider in this dish.

MAKE-AHEAD STUFFING NOTE

To save on time, you can make this stuffing 1 day ahead. Just remember to bake it in the oven 30 minutes before the Dazed & Infused Citrus Herb Chicken (page 337) is done.

RYAN SIMORANGKIR & TYLER PEEK

Co-owners, Sama Sama Kitchen

Tucked in the heart of Santa Barbara's downtown theater district, visitors will find Sama Sama, a Southeast Asian family-style restaurant. The eatery's Indonesian name has a dual meaning which can be defined as either "You're Welcome" or "Together." This very popular dining spot attracts residents and tourists alike, drawn to its flavorful, mouthwatering dishes.

Co-owner Ryan Simorangkir moved from Santa Barbara to Indonesia before he was a year old. It was there that he became childhood friends with his future business partner, Tyler Peek. The two developed a friendship which continued throughout their years in high school. They both returned to the United States after graduation to attend Pasadena's Le Cordon Bleu School. During this period in their lives, both men worked in commercial kitchens to gain much needed experience. Simorangkir did catering for Wolfgang Puck at the Grammy and Academy Awards, giving him expertise in cooking for large numbers of people, which was of great help when Sama Sama became a reality.

To further their culinary knowledge, both friends worked together at the W Hotel's restaurant in Puerto Rico and then ran the kitchen at Warung Kayu in Bali. As a child, Simorangkir was never crazy about Indonesian cuisine, always yearning for "kid food" like mac and cheese. Now, as an adult, his appetite for "street food" blossomed. Because his funds were limited while he was working in Bali, he found himself eating a steady diet of this type of cooking and, much to his surprise, discovered that he loved it! Both chefs decided that they needed to learn how to prepare this kind of fare, so Simorangkir reached out to his aunts for family recipes to guide them, which they generously shared.

Even though the two men loved Bali, they eventually felt that it was time to move back to the United States, where they could create their own concept of the delicious Indonesian street food that had become such an important part of their culinary lifestyle. For them, Santa Barbara seemed the ideal spot to put down roots, as its geographical location offered an abundance of readily available fresh fruits and vegetables. Both chefs felt it was extremely important that they combine the flavors of Indonesia with freshly sourced local ingredients. Living in a relatively small community like Santa Barbara made it easy to develop working relationships with the area's farmers, many of whom they saw each week at various farmers' markets. These connections would prove to be invaluable when they opened their own restaurant.

The two business partners transformed what had once been a sushi restaurant into a casual gathering place with a bright modern looking interior. Simorangkir's cousin who owns the Shelter Social Club, a local lodging business, selected the establishment's unique name. The owners thought that the title Sama Sama had a lilting, catchy sound that would be easy to remember. The restaurant's inviting back patio offers guests an arrangement of long communal tables which make a perfect gathering place for friends and family. This backyard area is colorfully accented by fresh herb and vegetable gardens illuminated by strings of sparkling lights. The cozy outdoor patio has been designated dog friendly, allowing pets to be part of the welcoming scene.

Sama Sama's crowd pleasing menu mixes Indonesian flavors with local ingredients, sourcing what is fresh and in season from farms in the Santa Barbara area and the surrounding Santa Ynez Valley. Some of the menu selections are based on Chef Simorangkir's family's recipes. Small-plate, family-style cuisine offers a variety of different dishes with gluten free, vegetarian friendly, and vegan options. The restaurant serves simple rustic food loaded with flavor and served with flair. Folks may partake of hot chicken bao, or crispy brussels sprouts, along with the always popular signature wings and pan-seared octopus. A pork butt porridge is sure to pique a visitor's curiosity. For those who want something lighter, there is crispy duck, green papaya, or market gado-gado salad which can be topped off with a mouthwatering dessert of banana donut fritters, or decadent black sesame tres leches with spiced rum milk. A relaxing Indonesian jasmine iced tea, with a touch of cream, is the ideal way to end a memorable evening. There are also exotic cocktails for those who desire something a bit stronger.

A friend of the owners of Sama Sama started a CBD wellness company called ONDA and invited Chefs Simorangkir and Peek to host a CBD dinner. This was the first occasion that the chefs had cooked with CBD which they thought lent a great, but subtle flavor to their savory creations. As many traditional dishes from Indonesia, especially Sumatra, use the cannabis plant as a cooking herb, the CBD paired perfectly with the restaurant's painstakingly prepared cuisine.

INDONESIAN CHICKEN SOUP
with Noodles and Cannabis (Soto Ayam)

by SAMA SAMA KITCHEN

MAKES 6 to 8 servings

Soto ayam is a deeply flavored Indonesian version of chicken soup. The broth has a beautiful aromatic flavor with multiple garnishes. The cannabis adds a satisfying flavor to this much-loved classic dish.

CHICKEN

2 tablespoons canola or peanut oil

6 boneless, skin-on chicken thighs, trimmed

1 tablespoon kosher salt

SOTO BROTH

2 stalks fresh lemongrass, trimmed and bruised with the handle of a heavy knife

5 lime leaves

2 Indonesian bay leaves (daun salam)

1 gallon water

1 tablespoon canola or peanut oil

2 cups organic unsweetened coconut milk (see cooking tip below)

1 teaspoon salt

SPICE PASTE

1 tablespoon coriander seeds

½ tablespoon cumin seeds

¼ teaspoon white peppercorns

½ cup coarsely chopped Asian or French shallots

6 medium garlic cloves, peeled and coarsely chopped

1 tablespoon cannabis flower, decarbed and ground (if using CBD oil, add 1 tablespoon just before serving)

1 tablespoon galangal root powder or 2 tablespoons fresh peeled and chopped

1. To make the Soto broth: Heat the canola oil in a large stockpot or Dutch oven (minimum 6-quart pot) over medium-high heat until hot but not smoking. Season the chicken with salt. Add the chicken thighs in batches if necessary, skin-side down, and sear, about 3 minutes. Using tongs, turn the pieces over and continue to sear, about 3 minutes. Repeat with the remaining chicken thighs.

2. Add the lemongrass stalks, lime leaves, bay leaves, and water and bring to a simmer over medium-high heat. Cover, and reduce the heat to maintain a simmer and cook until the chicken is tender, about 45 minutes.

3. While the chicken is simmering, make the spice paste. Heat a small skillet over medium heat. Add the coriander seeds, cumin seeds, and white peppercorns and toast, shaking the pan continuously, until fragrant, about 2 minutes. Set aside to cool for 5 minutes. Using a spice grinder, add the toasted coriander seeds, cumin seeds, and white peppercorns, and pulse until ground. Transfer the ground spice mixture to a blender. Add the shallots, garlic, cannabis, galangal, ginger, candlenuts, turmeric, fish sauce, and lime juice. Blend, stopping periodically to press down on the paste with a spoon, until well combined. Add the vegetable stock, and blend the mixture into a thick paste. **Note:** Alternatively, pound the spice paste with a pestle in a large mortar until smooth.

Ingredients list continues on next page

Recipe continues on next page

1 (2-inch) piece fresh ginger, peeled and
thinly sliced

1 ounce (¼ cup) whole candlenuts
(see Note on page 345)

½ teaspoon dried ground turmeric

3 tablespoons Asian fish sauce (nam pla
or nuoc mam) or to taste

3 tablespoons fresh lime juice, or to taste

⅓ cup vegetable broth, or as needed

SOFT-BOILED EGGS

Note: To save time, prepare the soft-
boiled eggs 1 day before you intend to use
them. Store the cooked and peeled eggs
in an airtight container in the refrigerator
(see step 4).

3 large organic eggs

CRISPY SHALLOTS

2 medium shallots, peeled and cut into
thin rings

1 tablespoon all-purpose flour, or as
needed

¼ cup canola or peanut oil, for frying

NOODLES

1 (14.11-ounce) package sweet potato
glass noodles, or vermicelli, or bihun
or bun

SUGGESTED GARNISHES

Lime wedges

Mung bean sprouts

4 scallions, thinly sliced into rounds

Celery or cilantro leaves

3 large soft-boiled eggs, halved

Crispy shallots

Sambal oelek chili paste, to taste

4. If you made the soft-boiled eggs 1 day ahead, skip this
step. While the chicken is simmering, make the soft-
boiled eggs. Place a small bowl of ice water near your
cooking area. Bring a saucepan large enough to have
the eggs in a single layer to a boil over medium-high
heat. Reduce the heat to a simmer. Using a slotted
spoon carefully add the eggs, one at a time, and
cook, maintaining a simmer, until soft-boiled, about
6½ minutes. Using a slotted spoon, remove the eggs and
place them in the prepared water bath for 2 minutes.
Remove from the water bath, then gently tap an egg on
the counter to crack the shells. Peel under cold running
water. Repeat with the remaining eggs. Transfer to a
small bowl. Cover with plastic wrap and place in the
refrigerator until ready to use as a garnish.

5. Using tongs, remove the chicken from the stock and
set aside to rest. Strain the stock, through a fine-mesh
strainer into a heat-resistant bowl and reserve, discarding
the lemongrass stalks, lime leaves, and bay leaves. Using
a large spoon, skim off any fat off the top.

6. Start boiling the water for the noodles.

7. While the chicken is resting, make the crispy shallot
garnish: Separate the shallots into rings and place in a
bowl. Lightly toss with flour. Heat the canola oil in a small
heavy-bottomed skillet over medium-high heat until hot,
but not smoking. Add the shallots in batches, and fry
until golden brown and crispy, about 1 minute. Using a
slotted spoon, remove the shallots and transfer them to a
paper-towel-lined plate and allow to cool. Repeat with the
remaining shallot rings.

8. While the crispy shallots are draining on a paper-towel-
lined plate, finish the Soto broth.

9. To finish the Soto broth: In the same stockpot used to
make the stock, heat the canola oil over medium-high
heat. Add the spice paste and cook, stirring often until
fragrant, about 1 minute. Pour in the coconut milk
and salt, stirring until the paste and the milk are well
combined. Stir in the reserved chicken broth and cook
until heated through, about 5 minutes. Adjust seasonings
with salt, if desired.

10. While the soup is heating through, prepare the noodles according to package directions. Drain and divide among soup bowls.

11. Remove the skin and fat from the thighs and discard. Shred the chicken and set aside. Slice the soft-boiled eggs in half lengthwise and set aside.

12. To serve: Divide the noodles evenly among the bowls, then top with shredded chicken. Ladle the broth over the top. Add a lime wedge and egg half to each bowl. Scatter mung bean sprouts, scallions, celery leaves, and crispy shallots over the top, to taste. Lightly drizzle sambal oelek chili paste over the top of each soup bowl, until desired heat is achieved.

NOTES

Candlenuts, Asian fish sauce, sweet potato glass noodles, mung bean sprouts, and sambal oelek are available in the Asian section of some supermarkets and at Asian markets. You may substitute raw, unsalted macadamia nuts for candlenuts.

1 tablespoon chopped fresh galangal = 1½ teaspoons galangal root powder.

TIP

Most canned coconut milk will separate into two layers: a solid white cream at the top and a watery liquid at the bottom. To recombine the two, either shake the can vigorously before opening it or carefully stir the milk once it has been opened.

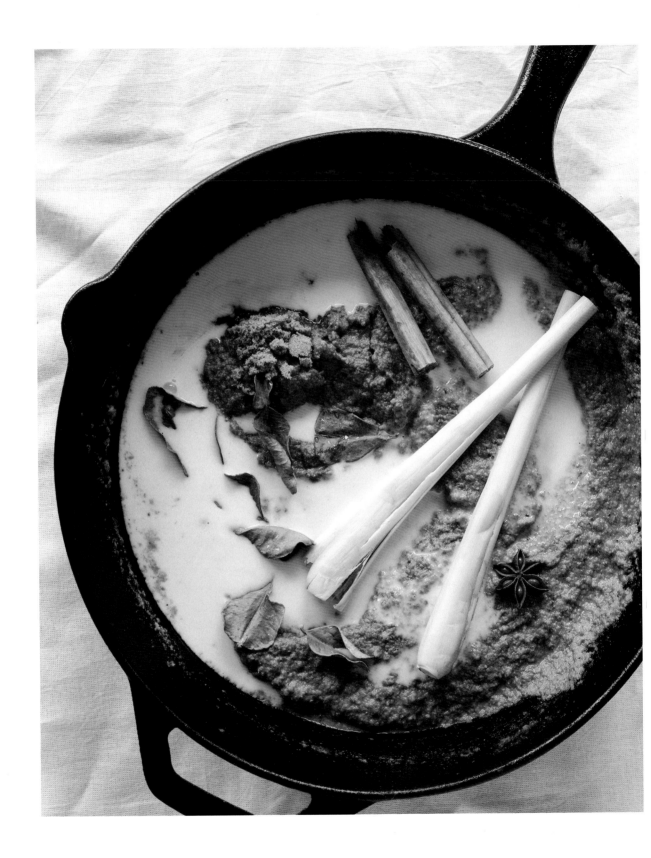

INDONESIAN STEW BEEF (RENDANG)

by SAMA SAMA KITCHEN

MAKES 4 servings

Rendang is a Malaysian meat dish that is "slow-simmered" in an Indonesian spice paste and curry. What gives this version an enriched aromatic flavor is the use of cannabis flower in the spice paste. The velvety sauce adds a welcome richness to the stew.

SPICE PASTE

5 whole cloves

1 whole nutmeg

6 red Fresnos peppers, stemmed, seeded and coarsely chopped (about ⅔ cup)

6 Asian or French shallots, coarsely chopped (about 1¼ cups)

1 ounce (¼ cup) whole candlenuts

4 medium cloves garlic, peeled and coarsely chopped (about ⅛ cup)

1 (2-inch) piece fresh ginger, peeled and coarsely chopped

1 tablespoon cannabis flower, decarbed and ground

1 tablespoon peeled and coarsely chopped fresh galangal root

1½ teaspoons ground turmeric

¼ cup vegetable oil, or as needed

BEEF

2 pounds boneless beef chuck roast, trimmed and cut into 1½-inch pieces

1 teaspoon salt

3 tablespoons vegetable oil or peanut oil

CURRY

2 stalks fresh lemongrass, trimmed and bruised with the handle of a heavy knife

2 cinnamon sticks

1. To make the spice paste: Heat a small skillet over medium heat. Add the cloves and whole nutmeg and toast, shaking the pan lightly and continuously, until fragrant, about 1 minute. Set aside to cool for 5 minutes. Slightly crush the nutmeg in a mortar and pestle or with the flat side of a large knife. Using a spice grinder, add the toasted cloves and nutmeg and pulse until ground. Transfer the ground spices to a blender. Add the peppers, shallots, candlenuts, garlic, ginger, cannabis, galangal, and turmeric and blend, scraping down the sides of the blender jar as needed, until well combined. Add the vegetable oil and blend the mixture into a paste. Set aside.

2. To prepare the beef: pat the meat dry with paper towels and season with salt.

3. Heat the oil in a 12-inch skillet or wok, over medium-high heat until hot but not smoking. Working in batches, brown the meat on all sides, about 6 minutes per batch. Remove the meat from the pot and set aside, reserving the drippings and oil in the skillet.

4. To make the curry: In the same skillet used to brown the meat, add the spice paste and cook, stirring continuously, over medium-high heat until fragrant, about 1 minute.

5. Lower the heat to medium-low and add the lemongrass stalks, cinnamon sticks, star anise, lime leaves, and sugar and cook, stirring continuously until the paste becomes dark brown in color and the oil just begins to separate, about 8 minutes. Remove the skillet from the heat and stir in the coconut cream, scraping up the bits from the bottom of the skillet, until well combined.

Ingredients list continues on page 349

Recipe continues on page 349

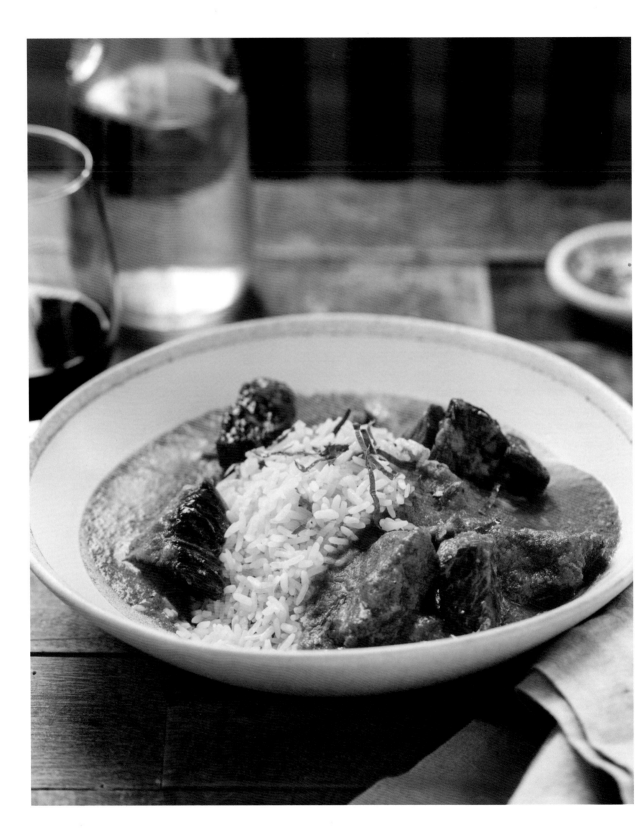

1 star anise

5 small fresh or frozen lime leaves, plus 5 thinly sliced for garnish

1 tablespoon grated palm sugar or brown sugar, or to taste

2¼ cups unsweetened coconut cream, or as needed

Jasmine or coconut rice, cooked according to package

6. Return the meat to the skillet along with any accumulated juices and bring to a boil. Reduce the heat to a low simmer and cook, stirring frequently to prevent the coconut cream from scorching, until the meat is fork-tender and most of the cream has been evaporated, about 2 hours. Discard the lemongrass stalks, cinnamon sticks, star anise, and lime leaves. Adjust seasonings with salt and pepper to taste. Note: Rendang is considered more of a dry curry because the dish is cooked down until most of the liquids have evaporated and the meat has become tender. Traditional curry dishes have more of a liquid base.

7. Thirty minutes before the rendang is done, start the rice. Cook the rice according to the package directions.

8. To serve: Place some of the rice in the center of each plate and top with rendang. Garnish with thinly sliced lime leaves. Serve at once.

NOTES

1 tablespoon chopped fresh galangal = 1½ teaspoons galangal root powder

You can adjust the heat by using more or less seeds from the chilies.

You may substitute raw, unsalted macadamia nuts for candlenuts.

Depending on the length of the stalks, you may need to trim the lemongrass a bit to get the stalks to fit in the skillet.

HOW TO STORE CANNABIS FLOWERS

It is important to purchase flowers that are fresh and not sitting too long on the shelf at the dispensary. The best way to store your cannabis flowers is in an airtight glass container. Always label and date the contents. Store in a cool, dry, dark place. Do not store in the refrigerator or freezer. If your cannabis is fresh, the flowers should last up to four months. When cannabis flowers begin to get a bit old, they will start to turn a golden yellow color, similar to old grass clippings.

JILL TRINCHERO

Founder, SDK Snacks

When Jill Trinchero was in her mid-twenties, she moved to Portland, Oregon, planning to stay for only five years to establish a career before moving on. Twenty-five years later, she is still there. Jill is the fourth generation of women in her family to live in Portland. Although raised in Northern California, during her childhood years she would, upon occasion, visit her mother's family who lived near Portland. Even then, she loved everything about the area and all it had to offer.

After marriage and motherhood, Jill found, as a stay-at-home mom, that eating healthy was one of her top priorities. Diagnosed with gluten intolerance over a decade ago, everything she cooks is gluten-free, made with quality local ingredients whenever possible. She has also been a vegetarian for twenty-eight years but is not opposed to cooking a roast for a special occasion. It is her belief that people really appreciate home-cooked foods, and, for Jill, cooking for others is an art form.

Jill enjoyed using recreational cannabis but could not find a tasty gluten-free, lightly dosed edible to suit her needs. This situation prompted her to begin experimenting with a variety of recipes seeking to develop a "socially dosed" single-serving edible. This quest resulted in the creation of a flavorful cookie that became very popular with her circle of friends.

All of Jill's research and hard work led to the development of SDK Snacks, a healthy cannabis edibles company that was created in 2015. She gathered market feedback from a segment of medical patients, which prepared her for being one of the first licensed processors in the state. On January 1, 2017, the business was officially opened as a designated recreational edibles company.

Jill Trinchero, the founder and CEO of SDK Snacks, is a pioneer in Oregon's cannabis scene, owning one of the state's first licensed edible companies. During the branding phase, the team concurred that the company's name should not be a reference to cannabis. The agreed-upon name, She Don't Know, or SDK, is based on Jill's philosophy, "The first step to enlightenment is admitting that you don't know." The flagship product was a THC-dosed, gluten-free chocolate chip cookie that was sold at dispensaries statewide. As of September 2018, there is a 50 milligrams dose of THC in each of the cookies that SDK makes.

SDK products now include a THC Chocolate Chip Cookie, THC Snickerdoodle, CBD-only Chocolate Chip Cookie and 1:1 THC: CBD Peanut Butter Cookie. Bernie's Kind Biscuits are now sold outside of the regulated market and can be shipped anywhere in the USA. Bernie's Kind Biscuits are a healthy medicated CBD-only dog treat named after Jill's beloved dog Bernie. The company's research has found that cannabis can be very helpful for many pet ailments.

The quality cannabis that infuses their product line had to come from a reputable source that would not compromise SDK's reputation or line of merchandise. Keeping this in mind, Jill has partnered with family-owned Moto Perpetuo Farm, which grows cannabis organically. The business also uses Bob's Red Mill gluten-free flours and Darigold's butter. Jill readily admits that she can taste quality and has found like-minded people to partner with. Not understanding why folks lower their standards when it comes to cannabis, it is her goal to educate and offer a superior product at a price that works for everyone.

Products are made in a gluten-free facility. No preservatives, corn syrup, sugar, or dyes are used. The snacks are small enough that they can be eaten in one bite. Every cookie is hand-weighed, five chips are added one by one to each of the chocolate chip cookies, then each edible is individually packaged. Every step is done by hand. Each cookie is infused with 50 milligrams of THC, making sure that the cookies and crackers are perfectly dosed. The SDK brand is designed to be unappealing to children. Jill feels very strongly about keeping cannabis products out of the hands of young people.

SDK Snacks is a woman-owned-and-operated company. Jill Trinchero provides mentorship and consultation for other rising female entrepreneurs. She serves on panels at industry events, championing the benefits of cannabis. This hardworking businesswoman is passionate about community service, art education advocacy, health-conscious cooking, and raising her two daughters. She actively participates in communities of women that are uplifting the power of cannabis to bring gender and economic equality to women everywhere.

SLOW-COOKER-STYLE CANNABIS-INFUSED OLIVE OIL

RECIPE FOR HIGH-TOLERANCE CONSUMERS; NOT FOR EDIBLES BEGINNERS OR CONSUMERS WITH LOW TOLERANCE

by JILL TRINCHERO, SDK SNACKS

MAKES approximately 2 cups

JILL TRINCHERO: I've made infused oils hundreds of times. There are many ways to do this successfully, but this is my favorite method. I skip the step of decarboxylating by doing a longer infusion time at a low temperature. This makes for a safe (low temp/no splatter) and effective way to infuse any oil.

It's hard to know the potency of the oil, unless you have it tested in an accredited cannabis testing lab. If you are new to cannabis edibles, I recommend trying a very small amount, ¼ teaspoon, wait an hour, and repeat. Continue doing this, before cooking with the oil, to see how you are affected.

You can adjust the potency of any dish to accommodate guests who are unsure or have a lower tolerance level. Do this by using a ratio of infused oil with non-infused oil, or leave the infused oil for the table for experienced users to drizzle on their own dish once it is served.

SUGGESTED DOSAGE: Approximately 800 milligrams per recipe or 25 milligrams THC per tablespoon.

Jill Trinchero's note: I love Kush strains and suggest using OG Kush or Mango Kush for this recipe.

4 grams cannabis flower

2 cups olive oil

1. Coarsely grind the cannabis flower with a handheld grinder or chop into pea-size pieces with a knife. Note: The plant matter should be fluffy and still resemble a flower. It is important not to use a coffee grinder or to grind into a fine powder.
2. Place the cannabis and olive oil in a slow cooker and set it on the lowest setting and cook for 8 to 24 hours, stirring only once or twice. Turn off the heat and let cool in the slow cooker until cool enough to handle.
3. Place a cheesecloth-lined fine-mesh strainer over a clean heat-resistant bowl. Carefully pour the oil mixture through the strainer and let sit over the bowl until it stops dripping. Gather up the corners of the cheesecloth and gently squeeze out any excess oil into the bowl with the infused oil; compost or discard the plant matter.
4. Pour the oil through a funnel into a clean bottle and cap or cork with a pourer spout. Label the bottle with the date and contents. Store in a cool dark place.

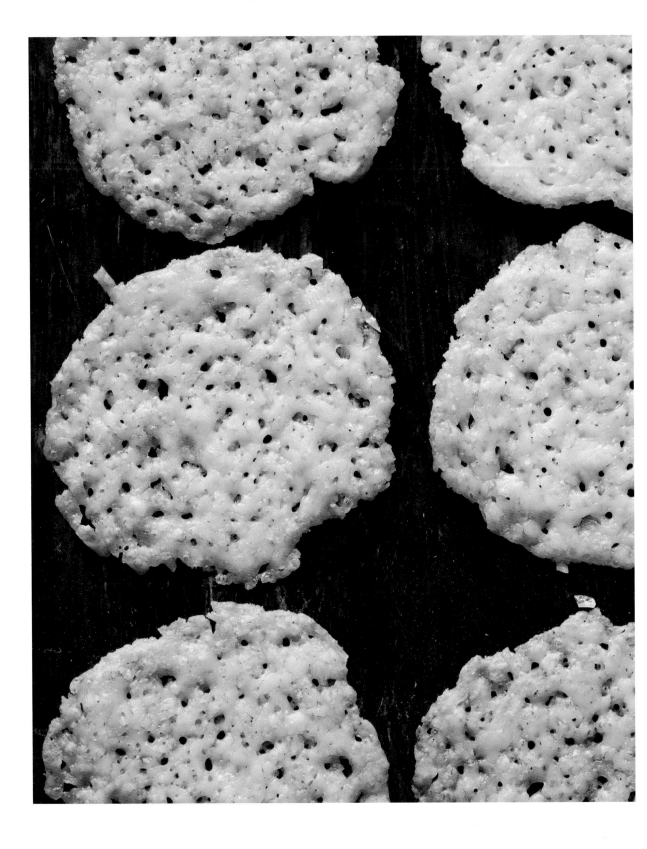

CANNABIS-INFUSED EGGLESS CAESAR SALAD

with Parmesan Crisps

(HIGH-DOSE RECIPE)

JILL TRINCHERO, SDK SNACKS

MAKES 6 servings

> **JILL TRINCHERO:** Because I love Caesar salad with lots of dressing, I make this recipe lightly infused. To be considerate of those folks who might not like as much dressing as I do, extra is served on the side. If you are serving someone that is vegetarian, omit the anchovy paste. The Parmesan crisps keep your creation gluten-free.
>
> **SUGGESTED DOSAGE:** Approximately 100 milligrams THC per recipe or 15–17 milligrams per serving.

PARMESAN CRISPS

Makes 6 crisps

½ cup grated Parmesan cheese

SALAD DRESSING

Makes 1⅓ cups

Note: To save on time, prepare the cannabis-infused oil 1 day before you intend to use it for the Caesar salad dressing.

3 medium cloves garlic

3 tablespoons lemon juice

1 tablespoon water

1 tablespoon anchovy paste

⅔ cup grated Parmesan cheese, plus extra for serving

¼ teaspoon kosher salt

¼ teaspoon freshly ground black pepper

¾ cup extra-virgin olive oil

¼ cup slow-cooker-style cannabis-infused olive oil (page 353)

LETTUCE

4 heads romaine lettuce, trimmed, washed, dried, and leaves separated

1. Preheat the oven to 400°F. Line a half-sheet-sized baking sheet with parchment paper. Set aside.
2. To make the Parmesan Crisps: Place the Parmesan cheese in the middle of the prepared baking sheet then separate it into 6 even piles spacing each about 3 inches apart. Using the edge of a knife, lightly pat each pile down to about 1½ to 2 inches in diameter. The pile should be flat but not pressed.
3. Bake in the oven until bubbling, crisp, and golden brown, approximately 5 minutes. Note: During baking, it is important to keep a close eye on the Parmesan Crisps to avoid burning. Allow to cool completely on the baking sheet, about 15 minutes.
4. While the Parmesan Crisps are cooling, start the salad dressing. Blend the garlic, lemon juice, and water in a blender until the garlic is minced. Add the anchovy paste and pulse for 1 minute. Add the Parmesan cheese, salt, and pepper, and blend until well combined. While the machine is running, gradually add the oils until emulsified and the desired thickness is achieved. Adjust seasonings with salt and pepper to taste.
5. To prepare the romaine lettuce leaves: Tear the leaves across the vein into pieces, about 1½ to 2 inches wide.

Recipe continues on next page

Note: There will be approximately 11 cups of torn lettuce leaves. Place in a large salad bowl. Set aside.

6. To serve: Add ¾ cup of the salad dressing to the lettuce pieces a little at a time, tossing to coat and adding more dressing as needed. Adjust seasoning with salt and pepper to taste. Using a thin spatula, carefully top the salad with the Parmesan Crisps.

7. Pour the extra dressing into a small container with a pour spout. Serve immediately, passing the remaining dressing at the table, if desired.

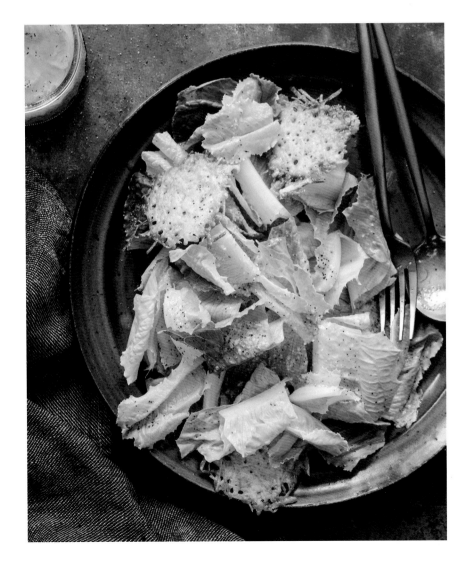

CANNABIS-INFUSED PESTO

(HIGH-DOSE RECIPE)

by JILL TRINCHERO, SDK SNACKS

MAKES just under 2 cups

> **JILL TRINCHERO:** I've always loved pesto! Loving nuts as well, I have found almonds to be my favorite. It has been my experience that any type of nut you favor can be substituted for, or combined with, the traditional pine nut.
>
> **SUGGESTED DOSAGE:** 1 cup of pesto is approximately 200 milligrams THC per recipe or 12.5 milligrams per tablespoon.

Note: To save on time, prepare the cannabis-infused oil 1 day before you intend to use it for the pesto.

2 cups fresh basil leaves, packed

⅛ cup coarsely chopped Marcona almonds

2 medium cloves garlic

¼ cup plus 2 tablespoons cannabis-infused olive oil (page 353)

2 tablespoons pine nuts

¼ cup freshly grated Parmesan cheese

½ teaspoon kosher salt

¼ teaspoon freshly ground black pepper

1. Place the basil, almonds, and garlic in the bowl of a food processor and process until the desired texture is achieved. While the motor is running, add the oil in a slow and steady stream. Spoon the pesto into a bowl. Stir in the pine nuts, Parmesan cheese, salt, and pepper until well combined. Use this pesto for the Baked Halibut recipe (page 358).

BAKED HALIBUT
with Cannabis-Infused Pesto
(HIGH-DOSE RECIPE)

by JILL TRINCHERO, SDK SNACKS

MAKES 6 servings

JILL TRINCHERO: This is a quick and easy dinner party main dish that is sure to impress your guests. I make it gluten-free, but you may use your favorite white, wheat, or sourdough bread. Salmon, or any white fish, can be substituted—the key is not to overcook. Even though you may feel that this recipe needs more oven time, it will continue to cook while you plate and serve. Be sure to have everything ready to go when you put the ingredients into the oven. Serve quickly! After it cools, it will overcook if reheated.

SUGGESTED DOSAGE: Approximately 150 milligrams THC per recipe or 25 milligrams per serving.

CANNABIS-INFUSED PESTO COATING

¾ cup cannabis-infused pesto, or to taste (page 357)

¾ cup bread crumbs

8 tablespoons unsalted butter, melted and divided

1 tablespoon Parmesan cheese

½ teaspoon kosher salt

¼ teaspoon freshly ground black pepper

HALIBUT FILLETS

6 (5-ounce) halibut fillets, about 1-inch thick

Kosher salt and freshly ground black pepper

GARNISH

Lemon wedges

1. Preheat the oven to 450°F. Line a baking sheet with parchment paper or foil. Set aside.
2. To make the cannabis-infused pesto coating: Combine the pesto, bread crumbs, 6 tablespoons of butter, cheese, salt, and pepper until well combined.
3. To make the halibut fillets: Arrange the fish in a single layer on the prepared baking sheet. Evenly brush the fish with the remaining 2 tablespoons of butter. Season with salt and pepper. Divide the pesto evenly on each fillet, making sure it sticks by gently pressing on the tops of the fish.
4. Roast the fish until opaque in the center, about 10 minutes, depending on the thickness of the fish. Do not overcook.
5. Transfer fillets to individual plates and garnish with lemon wedges. Serve immediately.

JILL TRINCHERO'S NOTE

25 milligrams per serving is quite a lot for an edible beginner or even an experienced consumer with a lower tolerance. Know your audience and adjust the amount of infused oil as necessary. You can use a ratio of inf[...] to non-infused oil to cut the potency [...] amazing results. Over consumption [...] edibles can be miserable.

CARLTON BONE

Owner, Upward Cannabis Kitchen

arlton Bone had always dreamed of moving out west, finally doing so when they went off to college in Portland, Oregon, which was a long way from their home in Florida. In 2016, they started their own business, Upward Cannabis Kitchen, located outside of Portland in a city called Clackamas. Already licensed to process cannabis concentrates into edible and topical products for adult use, Carlton shared space in a commissary-style kitchen with a variety of other great firms. This arrangement gave them a chance to connect with small farms and regional processors in the Portland area while also building their supply chain. They quickly decided to utilize concentrates and work with reputable firms who sourced from a variety of farms from across the state of Oregon.

The entrepreneur has always had a passion for crafting high-quality cannabis products. When not developing their own formulations, they help their mother, a cannabis physician and OB-GYN, develop treatment protocols and general integrative care practices in the Florida Medical Marijuana program. This has taught them a lot about the gendered effects of cannabis, particularly THC, and allowed them to integrate their personal identity as transgender into a lot of the work they are doing and the products they develop.

A branding and marketing firm from Portland proposed the Upward Cannabis name, which was the perfect fit for the new venture. The object was to destigmatize and celebrate all that cannabis has to offer. The Upward Cannabis Kitchen manufactures Junup (a cannabis kombucha), Piqmiup (an infused tea), and Beeup (an infused honey). These beverages and honey are formulated to deliver a wellness experience to consumers, offering them a source of relaxation and an opportunity to unwind, both physically and mentally. The hope is to create products that can only be obtained at specific dispensaries across the state.

The company's honey is sourced from a local honey farm in the Willamette Valley. The honey is raw processed, great to work with in a ferment, and nearly as aromatic and flavorful as the teas. Upward Cannabis Kitchen's kombucha is fermented from a honey substrate from this farm. Carlton explains that honey and cannabis have similar antimicrobial and antibacterial properties. Chemically these are the same as those we find in THC. Interestingly, culinary herbs and aromatics also have properties that are much like, or identical to, some that are found in the cannabis plant.

Carlton Bone is a big believer in community and the fact that we are all truly connected. Health and wellness have been the social justice issues that have most impacted their life. With easier access to cannabis because of changes in the law, Carlton hopes to share their experience and help their community to better understand the plant's value. Between their work on the Oregon Cannabis Association Legislative Committee, membership in the Minority Cannabis Business Association, and their work with the nonprofit People's Harm Reduction Alliance, they are helping the most vulnerable and targeted citizens. A portion of their company's proceeds support worthy causes that help these disadvantaged populations.

The owner of Upward Cannabis Kitchen has learned that the cannabis plant has a wealth of medical properties. THC is one of the molecules that have been studied and used to improve overall well-being. They believe that THC, along with cannabinoids, terpenes, and flavonoids has great potential for revolutionizing health care. It is their belief that we must continue to develop products for all types of consumers in order to find ways that cannabis can fit into people's lives. This business owner feels that beverages such as those they produce are a reliable and easy introduction into the world of THC and other cannabinoid edibles.

In light of the health concerns associated with mass-manufactured cannabis products, Upward Cannabis Kitchen's owner believes that the time has come to celebrate artisanal cannabis traditions. To this end, Carlton has begun working with farms and cultivators in Florida to develop new strategies for harvesting the potential of the cannabis plant and developing novel hemp products, culminating in the launch of the Upward Hemp Kitchen, which will provide hemp teas to consumers outside recreational and medical cannabis markets.

CANNABIS-INFUSED TEA

CARLTON BONE, UPWARD CANNABIS KITCHEN

MAKES 1 cup

This recipe uses ½ gram of cured cannabis bud, but the amount really depends on the potency of your cannabis. You can always add more or less depending on your tolerance.

2 teaspoons ground cannabis trim, stems, or buds

8 ounces cold filtered water

1 tea bag of any assamica black tea

Cannabis-infused honey, optional (page 363)

Cannabis-infused creamer, optional (page 364)

1. Place the cannabis into a tea infuser. Set aside.
2. Bring 8 ounces of cold filtered water to a boil. While the water is coming to a boil, warm the teacup by adding hot water halfway up the cup, and carefully swirl a few times. Once the teacup is warm, discard the water.
3. Place the tea infuser and tea bag into the teacup. Pour the boiling water over the tea and steep for 3 minutes. Carefully remove the tea infuser and tea bag, then compost or discard the plant matter. Serve at once with cannabis-infused honey or cannabis-infused creamer, if desired.

CANNABIS-INFUSED TISANE

by CARLTON BONE, UPWARD CANNABIS KITCHEN

MAKES 4 servings

> **CARLTON BONE:** Herbs and spices are homes to a variety of terpenes, the aromatic components of the plant, which allows for tremendous flexibility and control of flavoring the effects of tisane. The infusing of sweeteners and condiments with cannabinoids allows for fine-tuning dosing and enhancing bioavailability. This recipe explores ways to craft cannabis tisanes.

8 grams tea, such as green, oolong, or black

24 ounces water

Cannabis-infused creamer (page 364)

Cannabis-infused sweetener, such as honey or sugar (pages 363 and 365)

1. Place the tea in a stainless-steel bouquet garni ball. Bring the water to temperature, and steep tea for 2 to 3 minutes. Note: Water for green teas should be 170–185°F; Oolong should be brewed at 180–190°F; black teas and tisanes should be brewed at 208–212°F.

2. To serve: Warm teacups by adding hot water halfway up the cup, and carefully swirl a few times. Once the teacups are warm, discard the water. Add the tea, creamer, and/or infused sweetener of choice to desired dosage and taste.

NOTE

The cannabis-infused creamer and sweeteners will need to be made ahead of time.

WHAT IS CANNABIS DISTILLATE?

Also known as "the pure" in short: Refers to the cannabis extraction/purification process that removes and separates the cannabinoid, such as THC or CBD, into an odorless, tasteless, and viscous oil that is 99 percent pure concentrate.

CANNABIS-INFUSED HONEY

by CARLTON BONE, UPWARD CANNABIS KITCHEN

MAKES 16 ounces

This cannabis-infused honey is not only delicious, but also easy to make. Honey is a nutritious, natural sweetener that is full of antioxidants. In addition to complementing tea, infused honey is delicious when drizzled over blue cheese and figs, or mixed into yogurt or oatmeal.

SUGGESTED DOSAGE: There will be approximately 950 milligrams THC per batch and approximately 9.90 milligrams THC per teaspoon.

The Cannabis-infused Creamer counterbalances the tannins in the tea recipes found on pages 361 and 362. The creamer adds a richer, sweeter taste and a smooth, silky texture, offsetting the bitter notes and neutralizing the tannins.

2 cups local, raw honey

1 gram cannabinoid, such as THC or CBD distillate

Herbs, aromatics, or spices of choice, optional

1. Place the honey into the top pan of a double boiler. Set aside.

2. Pour about 1 inch of water into the bottom pan and bring to a simmer, making sure the top bowl does not touch the simmering water.

3. Bring the honey to 180°F. Remove from heat and stir in the cannabinoid concentrate until fully incorporated.

4. Pour into a heat-resistant jar with a lid and let cool, uncovered, to room temperature. Add herbs, aromatics, or spices if desired. Tightly seal the lid and label the jar with the date and contents. Store in a cool dark place for up to 1 month.

CANNABIS-INFUSED CREAMER

by CARLTON BONE, UPWARD CANNABIS KITCHEN   **MAKES** 2½ cups

The Cannabis-infused creamer counterbalances the tannins in strong teas. The creamer adds a richer, sweeter taste and a smooth, silky texture, offsetting the bitter notes and neutralizing the tannins.

SUGGESTED DOSAGE: There will be approximately 950 milligrams THC per batch and approximately 7.92 milligrams THC per teaspoon.

16 ounces heavy cream or nut milk

100 grams (¾ cup packed) powdered sugar

1 gram cannabinoid, such as THC or CBD distillate

1 teaspoon of pure vanilla extract

⅛ teaspoon freshly grated nutmeg

1. Place the cream into the top pan of a double boiler. Set aside.
2. Pour about 1 inch of water into the bottom pan and bring to a simmer, making sure the top pan does not touch the simmering water.
3. Bring the cream to a simmer, about 10 minutes. Whisk in the sugar, cannabinoid, vanilla, and nutmeg, until well combined.
4. Transfer the creamer into a clean heat-resistant jar with lid and let cool, uncovered, to room temperature, about 2 hours. Tightly seal the lid and label the jar with date and contents. Store in the refrigerator for up to 7 days.

CANNABIS-INFUSED TAPIOCA MALTODEXTRIN SUGAR

by CARLTON BONE, UPWARD CANNABIS KITCHEN

MAKES 2¼ cups

SUGGESTED DOSAGE: There will be approximately 950 milligrams THC per batch and approximately 8.8 milligrams THC per teaspoon.

1 tablespoon (10 grams) culinary-grade apricot kernel oil

1½ teaspoons (2 grams) sunflower lecithin

1 gram cannabinoid, such as THC or CBD distillate

1½ cups (40 grams) tapioca maltodextrin, lightly packed

1⅓ cups (300 grams) sugar

1. In a small saucepan, combine the apricot kernel oil, sunflower lecithin, and cannabinoid concentrate, stirring until well combined. Cook over low heat until it reaches a temperature of 160°F, about 3 minutes.
2. Place the tapioca maltodextrin in the bowl of a food processor. While the motor is running on the medium speed setting, add the apricot kernel oil mixture in a slow and steady stream.
3. Reduce the food processor setting to low speed then add the sugar, blending until the mixture is well combined.
4. Transfer the cannabis-infused sugar to a clean jar and tightly seal with a lid. Label the jar with date and contents. Store in a cool dark place.

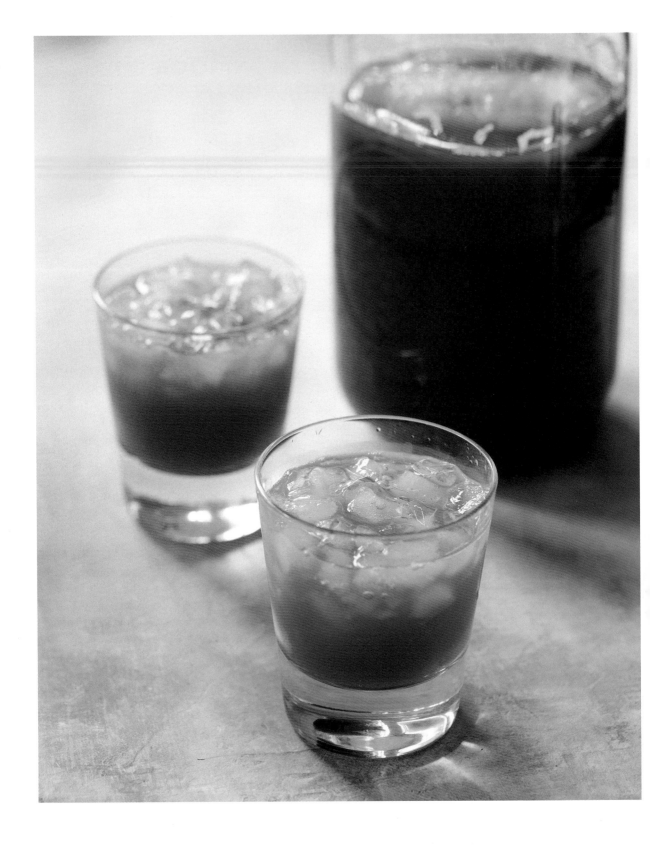

UPWARD CANNABIS KITCHEN'S KOMBUCHA

by CARLTON BONE, UPWARD CANNABIS KITCHEN

MAKES 14½ cups

SUGGESTED DOSAGE: Approximately 11 milligrams THC per bottle.

CARLTON BONE: There are a plethora of ways to ingest cannabis. From delicious baked treats to refined tinctures, manufacturers are pushing to create a myriad of creative options for consumers looking to nourish their endocannabinoid system. One area that has rapidly grown in popularity is cannabinoid beverages. This class of products spans the gamut from mixable concentrates to ready-to-drink formulas, and innovation shows no signs of abetting.

The Upward Cannabis Kitchen was founded in Portland, Oregon, in 2016 with the hope of "giving rise to culinary wonders." Central to this mission were carefully crafted beverage recipes the founders spent years perfecting. The most popular was a cannabis-infused kombucha, the recipe for which can be found below. However, before jumping into crafting beverages, it's worth understanding all the wonderful potential benefits of this product!

Kombucha is a fermented, slightly alcoholic, lightly effervescent, sweetened black or green tea drink commonly intended as a functional beverage. The pre- and probiotic elements of the beverage, combined with the antioxidant capacities of *Camellia sinensis* (tea) create a powerful platform for enhancing the bioavailability of cannabinoids. The Upward process takes this a step further by utilizing locally sourced wildflower honey to ferment our beverage instead of the usual refined sugar. This different style of ferment is called Jun, and has its roots in ancient Tibet, similar to the cannabis plant.

8 grams tea

1 gallon spring or distilled water

¼ cup distilled white vinegar

155 milligrams cannabis concentrate (THC or CBD, assumes 99% distillate)

420 grams (about 1⅓ cups) honey, warmed

Jun SCOBY (SCOBY = symbiotic colony of bacteria and yeast)

1. Place the tea in a clean cheesecloth bag. Set aside.

2. To make the tea: In a large stainless-steel pot, bring the water to a boil over medium-high heat. Remove the pot from the heat, then add the tea and let steep for 10 minutes. Remove the cheesecloth bag with the tea and let cool completely until it reaches room temperature, about 2 hours. Transfer all but 2 cups of the tea to a clean heat-resistant glass gallon jar, reserving the 2 cups.

3. To infuse the honey: Place the vinegar in a small saucepan and bring to a boil over medium-high heat. Carefully

Recipe continues on next page

transfer 150 milligrams (about ¼ teaspoon) vinegar (while still hot) to a heat-resistant bowl, discarding the remaining vinegar. Stir in the cannabis distillate until completely dissolved. Add the honey and stir until smooth and well combined.

4. Transfer the honey to the same fermenting jar with the tea and gently stir with a stainless-steel spoon until the honey is completely dissolved.

5. When the tea is around 26°C (78°F), add the SCOBY and its starter liquid into the jar with the tea, then top off with the reserved 2 cups of tea. Note: Do not put your SCOBY and starter liquid in hot tea, because this could kill the SCOBY.

6. Cover the jar with a lint-free cloth, such as a coffee filter, and secure with a rubber band or canning jar ring. Ferment at room temperature, out of direct sunlight. Note: Ideal temperature is 68–80°F.

7. Ferment for 5 to 8 days, checking on the kombucha and the SCOBY periodically. After 5 days, begin tasting the kombucha daily by pouring a little out of the jar and into a cup. When the desired balance of sweetness and tartness has been reached, the kombucha is ready to be bottled.

8. To decant the tea: Line a small fine stainless-steel strainer with a coffee filter. Use the strainer and a funnel over each clean bottle. Using a stainless-steel ladle, ladle the kombucha from the gallon jar through the strainer into each bottle, leaving about ½ inch to 1 inch of headroom in each bottle. Note: When you are near the bottom, gently lift the baby SCOBY and place it in a clean mason jar with the mother along with 1 cup of the kombucha brew to cover them for the next batch.

9. Allow conditioning for 24 to 48 hours to improve carbonation before refrigerating. (See sidebar on Kombucha Stages for definition of conditioning found on page 371, Stage 4).

NOTES

SCOBY cultures sometimes sink to the bottom or sit sideways. This does not indicate a problem with the SCOBY or kombucha brew. A moldy or dead SCOBY will be white, black, or colorful, fuzzy, and dry. If mold develops, it is very important to discard the whole batch of the kombucha brew, including the SCOBY.

The baby SCOBY (developing SCOBY) initially looks like a layer of slime, a bit gunky, growing on the top of the kombucha brew; this is completely normal.

Honey can sometimes leave sediment of a brownish color in the jar if this gets on the SCOBY and can make it appear to be discolored, even if it is not.

Upward Cannabis Kitchen

TEA

Avoid teas with any oils or flavoring agents, as they can cause your ferment to sour or mold in a number of ways.

Teas that are naturally flavored, however, such as some varieties of jasmine green tea, are an option for bringing more flavor into your final product. Much of this can be controlled during the final bottling.

JUN SCOBY culture (SCOBY=symbiotic colony of bacteria and yeast)

Can be acquired from a number of outlets like Kombucha Kamp and some larger retail establishments, or it can be grown from a store-bought bottle of Jun.

In addition to the culture, a small amount of liquid (about 1 cup) is needed from the prior ferment to help adjust pH and jump-start yeast cultures.

HONEY

Wild honeys are recommended, while artificially flavored honey should be avoided.

TOOLS AND SUPPLIES NEEDED

- Gallon jar
- pH strips or meter
- Muslin, cheesecloth, or hemp cloth
- Six 18-ounce classic swing-top glass bottles with flip-top stoppers. Otherwise, any combination of bottles that can be sealed.
- A heating mat or wrap. Optional, depending on the time of year and your fermentation setup.

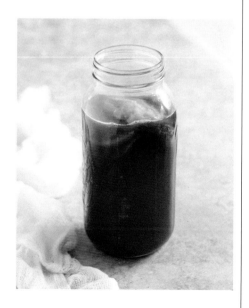

Upward Cannabis Kitchen

Stage One: Preparing Your Materials

1. Sanitize your workstation, tools, and fermenting equipment. Kombucha is highly sensitive to pH and bacteria, and mistakes here may not show themselves until your ferment is almost finished. In addition, do not use any metals, aside from stainless steel, when handling your kombucha and culture, as they will destroy your SCOBY. Alternative materials like glass, porcelain, and food-grade plastics are acceptable so long as they are clean.

2. If you are growing your culture, you will want to begin this process a few days before starting your fermentation, as it will take a little bit of time. To do this, add a scant tablespoon of honey to roughly ⅓ of the contents of a bottle of store-bought Jun. Looking for raw and unpasteurized products will help your chances of success. Reseal and place in a cool, dry area. Monitor until you start to see the development of the SCOBY culture, which should look like an opaque or white disk floating at the top of the drink.

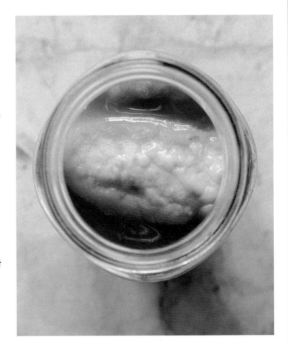

3. To maximize your success when fermenting it is important that you have an environment that is temperature and light controlled. The ideal temperature for the tea when fermenting is 23–29°C (73–84°F) and should not fall below 15°C (59°F), as this will cause the culture to go dormant. Light is not necessary. As the culture may be damaged by exposure to bright sunlight, place it somewhere partially covered, such as the corner of your kitchen counter.

Stage Two: Preparing Your Ingredients

1. The first and most integral stage of this process is developing your infused substrate, or honey. This is the vehicle for the cannabinoids to eventually get into the finished product, and so an improper infusion will be amplified in the end product.

Stage Three: Fermenting Your Jun

1. The longest and most important part of this process happens largely out of sight and mind, as the Jun SCOBY works its magic to transform the sweetened tea into a vibrant and delicious fermented beverage.

2. The fermentation should last anywhere from 5–8 days, depending on the temperature and health of your SCOBY. The higher the ambient temperature, the faster the fermentation is; while newer SCOBYs can take longer to ferment.

3. During the process of fermentation, the honey is broken down by the yeast and converted into carbon dioxide gas (CO_2), various organic acids, and other compounds. The vessel is left semi-porous to create an anaerobic environment for our microbiome, and it is the combination of these processes that gives the Jun its characteristic flavor.

4. The infusion is at first sweet, but this sweetness disappears as the honey is broken down. At the same time, an acidic flavor will develop as a result of the activities of the bacterium. One visual indicator of successful fermentation is the growth of a new SCOBY over the course of the fermentation. The most important indicator however will be your pH, which should finish between 2.7 and 3.4, as this will ensure only healthy cultures in your brew.

5. Given the nature of this ferment, it is important to note that your beverage can spoil in a number of potential ways. If you notice an uncharacteristically pungent odor or green, blue, or black growths or feel uncomfortable with the quality of your ferment, you can search for tips and guides online, for guidance on how to problem solve an array of issues. The wonderful resources at Kombucha Kamp are a great place to start.

Stage Four: Bottling Your Jun

1. The importance of bottling your brew is principally to improve carbonation, but it also serves as an opportunity to add flavor. This process is known as conditioning, and takes place due to the fact that the activity of the bacterium

is stopped when the bottling excludes the air, while the yeast continues to work away.

2. While pH range is most important in creating a safe beverage, there is a lot of flexibility when choosing when to bottle. For instance, if a slightly sweet drink is preferred, the fermentation can be stopped early. For a drier or slightly more acidic flavor, it can be continued longer.

3. If you want to make another batch, set aside 1 cup of unstrained liquid to use as your "starter liquid" for next time. You can also store your SCOBY(s) in this liquid to preserve its health between batches.

4. When bottling, make sure to leave at least ½ inch to 1 inch of room between the surface of the liquid and bottle cap. This space, known as headroom, will influence the rate of carbonation. Less room will generally have less carbonation potential due, but too much can lead to continued fermentation during the conditioning phase, affecting the beverage's taste.

5. If flavor is desired, between one teaspoon and a tablespoon of the fruit juice of choice can be added to each bottle along with the Jun. Juices, as well as small pieces of fruit, are great additions to the bottling step as their sugars can help yeasts work, creating a more effervescent and flavorful beverage.

6. Jun tea will keep in bottles for months when kept in a cool place. Be careful to monitor for continued fermentation if bottles get above 15°C in order to avoid a foamy mess!

Stage Five: Serving Tip

1. Remove from refrigerator and let come to slightly under room temperature before carefully opening, in order to prevent rapid pressure loss and excessive foaming. Jun is best served over ice, as this will maintain its ideal temperature range for longer as well as provide an aqueous base that increases overall effervescence.

2. Sediment is normal and is due to the growth of yeasts. While some consumers like to strain yeasts from the mixture when drinking, they do have some desirable positive effects when ingested.

SOUTH

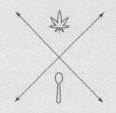

JAZMINE MOORE

Chef/Owner, Green Panther Chef

Chef Jazmine Moore grew up in a unique household. Her mother was both a restaurateur who cooked a wide variety of food, and a firm believer in homeopathic remedies. Chef Jazz, as she is known, grew up knowing that foods had their own medicinal properties and that eating well was the foundation of good health. Her beliefs were put to the test in 2006 when she was diagnosed with Crohn's disease during her last year at Baltimore International Culinary College. Finding that the medicine she was prescribed caused her to feel worse prompted the chef to research the subject.

Eventually returning to her homeopathic roots, the chef started experimenting with cannabis and CBD until she found the strain and method that worked best for her. This took great perseverance and extensive trial and error, but her efforts paid off. Within a year she was able to stop her prescription medicines and began to look and feel like her healthy self again. By 2008, she was in full remission.

Green Panther Chef is the result of Chef Jazz's efforts to find a solution to her Crohn's disease, along with the desire to help folks who are experiencing similar health problems. Starting out as a catering company, the business soon expanded and began offering private cooking lessons in people's homes. During these sessions, the chef demonstrates how to make meals infused with cannabis. The company now offers cooking demonstrations online, private and group classes, workshops, and full-service catering. The chef's ongoing blog posts share cannabis cooking tips and recipes for CBD-infused sauces, along with other useful informational tidbits. She agrees that knowledge is critical. Chef Jazz aims to destigmatize cannabis and encourages the average cannabis consumer to experiment.

The company's home base is a commercial kitchen located in Takoma Park, Maryland. Green Panther Chef has now expanded to include a full line of culinary CBD products, wellness consulting, and educational cooking classes. The focus now includes micro-dosing as well as health and wellness. Micro-dosing cannabis is the act of consuming small doses of cannabinoids which are so low that they are unlikely to cause psychoactive effects in the mind. This is becoming more popular because of its discretion and lasting effects and benefits, especially for those who are dealing with chronic pain and high levels of stress. Chef Jazz emphasizes that low and slow is the way to go.

With more than a decade of experience, the veteran cannabis chef and culinary artist continues to host dinners and teach others the proper way to cook with cannabis. Her favorite method of cannabis consumption is ingesting via food. Chef Jazz has a great deal of love and admiration for her company's namesake, the panther. She feels that they are understated animals, with endless elegance, that in a unique way is representative of her brand.

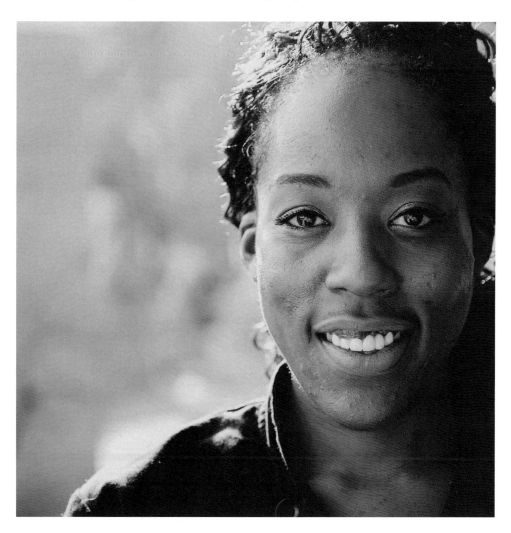

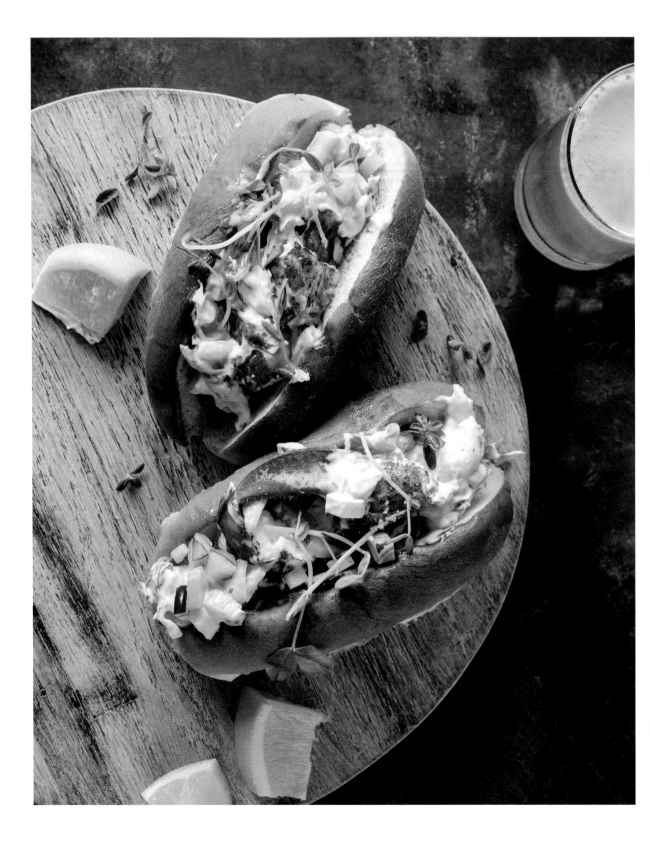

CLASSIC LOBSTER ROLLS

by JAZMINE MOORE, GREEN PANTHER CHEF

SERVES 4 as a main dish

These lobster rolls shine with sweet chunks of fresh lobster meat tossed in a mixture of celery, red onions, thyme, and mayonnaise. Split-top hot dog buns slathered with cannabis-infused butter adds a delicious twist to this summertime classic.

SUGGESTED DOSAGE: Approximately 52 milligrams of THC per recipe; serving; Approximately 13 milligrams THC per serving; 21% THC.

3 (1¼ pounds each) fresh live Maine lobsters (about 2 cups of meat)

½ cup finely diced celery

½ cup finely diced red onion

½ cup mayonnaise, homemade or store-bought

½ tablespoon fresh minced thyme

½ tablespoon fresh lemon juice

Salt and freshly ground black pepper

2 tablespoons cannabis-infused unsalted butter, melted, homemade or store-bought

4 New England–style split-top hot dog buns

Microgreens

Lemon wedges

1. Place a large bowl of ice water near your cooking area. Place a rimmed baking sheet near the ice-water bath.

2. To steam the lobsters: Fill a large stockpot with 2 inches of salted water. Bring to a boil. Using tongs, carefully lower the lobsters, one at a time, headfirst into the boiling water. Cover the pot and return the water to a boil, about 4 minutes. Steam until the outer shells of the lobsters turn bright red and an internal temperature of the lobster meat reaches 135°F, about 9 minutes.

3. Using tongs, carefully plunge the lobsters into the ice-water bath for about 2 minutes, replenishing the ice in the bowl of water as necessary. Transfer the chilled lobsters to the baking sheet. Repeat with the remaining lobsters.

4. Remove the meat from the lobsters and cut into ½-inch chunks. Pat the lobster meat dry with paper towels, then transfer to a medium bowl. Cover with plastic wrap and place in the refrigerator until the meat is very cold, about 2 hours.

5. In a separate large bowl, stir together the celery, red onions, mayonnaise, thyme, and lemon juice until well combined. Fold in the lobster meat. Adjust seasonings with salt and pepper.

6. To grill the buns: Preheat a skillet over medium-low heat. Brush the outside of each bun with the cannabis-infused butter and grill until golden brown, about 2 minutes on each side.

Recipe continues on next page

7. To assemble: Evenly divide the lobster meat mixture among the buns and top with microgreens, to taste. Serve with a lemon wedge, a bowl of chowder or chips and pickles on the side.

VARIATION

Serve the lobster meat mixture on 8 toasted mini potato rolls, such as Martin's, for the perfect-party appetizer.

NOTE

If you can't find microgreens, an alternative garnish is lining each bun with 1 to 2 lettuce leaves before adding the lobster salad.

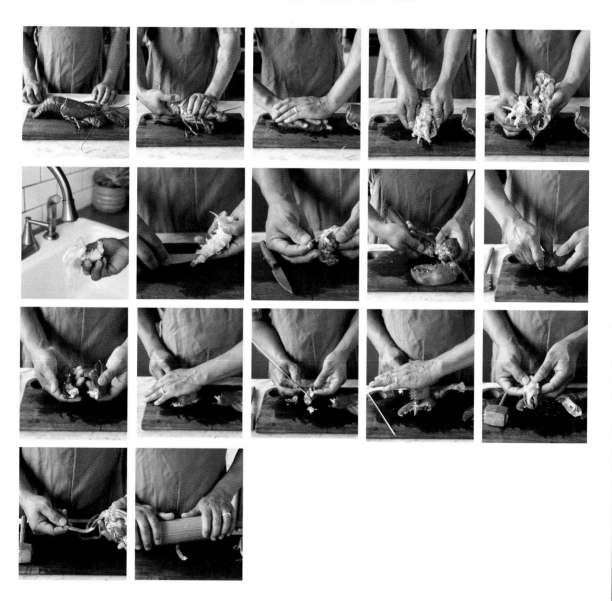

GRILLED SEA BASS OVER TABBOULEH
with Herb "Pesto"

by JAZMINE MOORE, GREEN PANTHER CHEF

MAKES 4 servings

> If you can't find sustainably raised sea bass, opt for snapper, striped bass, cod or grouper fillets with skin on, which have a similar flavor and texture.
>
> **SUGGESTED DOSAGE:** Approximately 52 milligrams of THC per recipe; approximately 13 milligrams THC per serving; 21% THC.

PEARL BARLEY

2 cups water

1 cup pearl barley

½ teaspoon salt

TABBOULEH WITH HERB "PESTO"

Makes 1 quart and ½ cup

1 cup (about 1 bunch) fresh parsley, thick stems removed

1 cup (about 1 bunch) fresh mint, thick stems removed

½ tablespoon fresh thyme leaves

4 tablespoons extra-virgin olive oil, divided

2½ tablespoons fresh lemon juice, divided, or to taste

1 tablespoon THC-infused extra-virgin olive oil, divided

Salt and freshly ground black pepper

1 large green bell pepper, seeded and diced

1 large red bell pepper, seeded and diced

1 small red onion, diced

1 medium clove garlic, peeled and minced

1. To make the pearl barley: In a medium saucepan, bring 2 cups of water, barley, and ½ teaspoon of salt to a boil. Cover and reduce the heat to a simmer. Cook, stirring occasionally, until most of the water is absorbed and the barley is tender, about 35 minutes. Transfer to a mesh strainer and rinse under cold running water, then allow to drain completely. Place in a medium decorative bowl and fluff with a fork. Set aside.

2. To make the tabbouleh with herb "pesto:" While the barley is cooking, in a bowl of a food processor with the standard "S" blade add the parsley, mint, thyme, 2 tablespoons of extra-virgin olive oil, and 1 tablespoon of the lemon juice and process until well combined. Add ½ tablespoon of the THC-infused olive oil and process for 30 seconds. Adjust seasonings with salt and pepper to taste. Set aside.

3. Add the remaining 1½ tablespoons of lemon juice, the remaining ½ tablespoon of THC-infused oil, and the remaining 2 tablespoons of extra-virgin olive oil to the bowl with the barley. Fold in the chopped herbs, bell peppers, red onions, garlic, and walnuts until well combined. Adjust seasoning with additional lemon juice, olive oil, salt and pepper to taste, if desired.

4. Allow the tabbouleh to sit at room temperature for about 15 minutes, before serving.

5. To make the sea bass: Heat 2 tablespoons of the olive oil in a large grill pan over medium-high heat. Brush the fish with the remaining 2 tablespoons of olive oil. Sprinkle both sides of each of the fillets with lemon zest and season

15 whole walnuts, toasted and coarsely chopped

SEA BASS

4 tablespoons extra-virgin olive oil, divided

4 (6-ounce) sea bass fillets, skin on, preferably sustainably harvested

Zest from 1 large lemon

4 lemon twists or slices, for garnish

with salt and pepper. When the grill pan is hot but not smoking add the fish skin-side down, and grill until the skin is crispy, about 3 to 4 minutes. Using a spatula, gently turn the fillets over and cook until opaque in the center and browned, about 5 minutes.

6. To serve: Place the tabbouleh on a large serving platter and top with the sea bass fillets. Garnish each fillet with a lemon twist or slice. Serve at once.

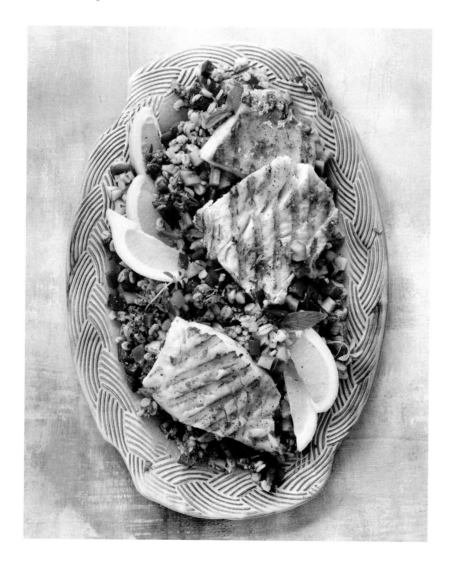

MINI PEACH BOURBON POUND CAKE PANINIS

by JAZMINE MOORE, GREEN PANTHER CHEF   **MAKES** one (9×5-inch) cake; 5 paninis

Peaches simmered in bourbon until fork-tender make for a delicious filling, elevating this pressed sandwich into an oh-so-good dessert!

SUGGESTED DOSAGE: Approximately 52 milligrams of THC per recipe; Approximately 13 milligrams of THC per serving; 21% THC.

POUND CAKE

1¾ sticks unsalted butter, softened at room temperature, plus extra for greasing loaf pan

¼ stick unsalted cannabis-infused butter (page 384), softened at room temperature

1½ cups cane sugar

¼ pound cream cheese, cut into pieces, softened

3 organic eggs, room temperature

¾ teaspoon pure vanilla extract

1½ cups all-purpose flour

⅛ teaspoon fine sea salt

PEACH BOURBON FILLING

2 tablespoons unsalted butter

2 medium fresh ripe peaches, pitted and cut into ⅓-inch-thick slices

¼ cup bourbon

½ teaspoon ground cinnamon, or to taste

¼ tablespoon fresh thyme leaves, minced

Organic extra-virgin olive oil cooking spray, for panini press

GARNISHES

Crème fraîche

2 tablespoons thinly sliced fresh mint leaves

1. Position an oven rack in the lower third of the oven. Preheat the oven to 320°F. Grease a 9×5-inch loaf pan. Cut a length of parchment paper long enough to line the bottom of the loaf pan and place in the pan. Lightly grease the parchment paper. Set aside.

2. To make the pound cake: In a bowl of a stand mixer fitted with a paddle attachment, cream the 1¾ sticks of butter, ¼ stick cannabis-infused butter, and sugar together on medium-low speed until light, fluffy, and creamy, scraping down the sides of the bowl as needed. While the stand mixer is running, carefully add the cream cheese, 1 piece at a time, and mix until well combined, scraping down the sides of the bowl as needed. Add the eggs one at a time, mixing each one well before adding the next egg. Add the vanilla and mix for another 30 seconds, scraping down the sides of the bowl as needed.

3. In a large bowl, sift together the flour and salt. Working in batches, add the flour mixture to the butter mixture and mix on low speed until smooth. Do not overwork the batter.

4. Add the batter to the prepared loaf pan and smooth the top with a spatula. Place the pan in the center of the lower third rack of the oven and bake until a toothpick inserted into the center of the cake comes out clean, about 1 hour and 40 minutes. Let the cake cool in the pan for 15 minutes before turning out onto a wire rack. Allow the cake to cool completely.

5. Once the cake has cooled completely, make the peach bourbon filling. Melt the butter in a medium saucepan

over medium heat. Add the peaches and bourbon then bring to a simmer over medium-high heat, stirring often. Stir in the cinnamon and thyme and continue to simmer, reducing the heat if necessary, gently stirring frequently, until the peaches are fork-tender, about 10 minutes, or depending on the thickness and ripeness of the slices.

6. Preheat a panini press according to the manufacturer's directions. Lightly spray the panini press with cooking spray.

7. To assemble: Cut the cake into twelve ½-inch slices, removing the end slices from the loaf, reserving for another use. Overlap the peach slices across one side of a cake slice. Drizzle some of the leftover bourbon sauce evenly over the peaches. Note: The amount of leftover bourbon sauce will depend on how juicy and ripe the peaches are. Top with a second slice of cake.

8. Place on the panini press and grill according to the manufacturer's directions or until golden brown, about 4 minutes. Transfer to a plate and top with a dollop of crème fraîche and sprinkles of mint. Repeat with the remaining cake slices and filling. Serve at once.

NOTE

If you don't own a panini press, a waffle iron is a good substitute.

Jazmine Moore, Green Panther Chef

MAKES approximately 1 stick of cannabutter

Chef Jazmine Moore: I get this question from patients and recreational users alike: "How can I make and properly dose my edibles?" The answer is simple: Dosing is not accurate and is an approximate number with a margin of a few milligrams. Edibles are more than the traditional brownies, gummies, and other sweets that saturate the market. I'm here to make you comfortable with unfamiliarity of cannabis and show you how to unlock the medicinal benefits of the cannabis plant. This process is a labor of love but has yielded the most consistent product and makes it easy to dose.

Let's get started:

This is a concentrated cannabutter that can be "cut" with non-infused oil to achieve desired effects. My suggested strains are Charlotte's Web (hemp-derived/high-CBD and low-THC content) or GSC (elevated THC levels averaging between 25 and 28 percent) because of the cannabinoid and terpene profiles. The amount of THC changes per harvest, so you can't say all of one strain has this set amount of THC. That is why you should work with a budtender to get accurate numbers. The strain I used for this calculation has 21 percent THC.

What you will need:

French press (large enough to accommodate soaking the cannabis)
Cheesecloth
Fine-mesh strainer
Spoon
Baking dish
Foil
Parchment paper
Baking sheet
Saucepan
Mason jar with a tight-fitting lid or heat-resistant storage container

7 grams of cannabis
Filtered water, or as needed

1⅓ sticks unsalted organic grass-fed butter, preferably Trickling Springs Creamery butter, melted

1. To clean the cannabis: Coarsely break apart the cannabis into even pea-size pieces. Place the bud pieces and stems into a French press. Slowly pour enough filtered water over the cannabis to soak. Note: If some of the cannabis clumps at the top, use a spoon to gently stir the water. Place the plunger on top, making sure not to press down yet. Change the water twice a day for 36 hours, or until the water runs clear, pressing down slowly on the plunger for each water change. Note: The cannabis will not break down in the water and will yield a lighter tasting product.

2. Strain the cannabis through a cheesecloth-lined fine-mesh strainer, pressing on the cannabis with the back of a spoon. Gather the corners of the cheese-cloth and gently squeeze out any excess water.

3. Spread the cannabis out in a single layer in a baking dish and loosely cover with foil. Set aside on the counter overnight to allow the cannabis to dry completely.

4. Decarboxylate the cannabis. See page (page 387) on how to decarboxylate the cannabis.

5. After the cannabis has been decarboxylated, weigh it to calculate the potency of your cannabutter.

6. To make the cannabutter: Place the decarboxylated cannabis and melted butter into a clean French press. Press down on the plunger, stopping just above

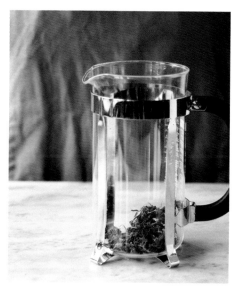
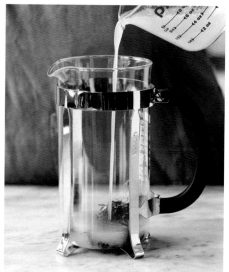

the butter line. Set the French press in a saucepan. Pour enough hot water in the saucepan to come halfway up the sides of the French press. Simmer for 3 hours, adding additional water as needed. Note: Do not allow it to boil.

7. Press down on the plunger evenly and slowly, making sure to lower it all the way down. Carefully pour the cannabutter into a clean mason jar and seal the lid, discarding the leftover debris.

8. Refrigerate the cannabutter until it solidifies, about 24 hours. Once solidified, pat dry with paper towels to absorb any residual moisture. Using the back of a knife, remove any green film from the butter and discard. Tightly seal the lid and label the jar with the date and contents. The cannabutter can be stored in the refrigerator for up to 2 months or frozen for up to 5 months.

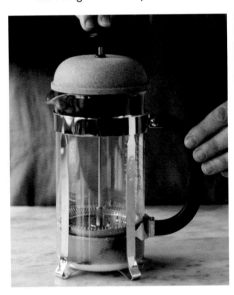 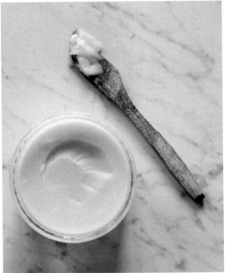

Decarboxylation is a heating technique in which THCA (Tetrahydrocannabinolic acid), the raw, nonpsychoactive acid form of THC, is transformed into the psychoactive delta-9 tetrahydrocannabinol (commonly referred to as "THC"). THC is the chemical compound found in cannabis that makes you high. So before making edibles, decarboxylating, or "decarbing" is a must. This process can be done in several ways. Below is one suggested method.

Preheat the oven to 245°F. Line a baking sheet with parchment paper. Spread the cannabis out in a single layer on the prepared baking sheet. Bake until the cannabis is completely dry and its color has changed from green to light brown, but not burned, approximately 25 to 30 minutes. Allow to cool completely on the baking sheet before using, about 15 minutes.

Note: It is important to check on the cannabis periodically to make sure it is not burning.

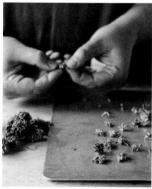 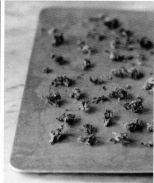 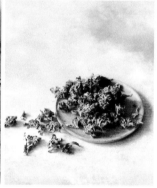

JESSICA COLE

Founder, White Rabbit High Tea

Jessica Cole, founder of White Rabbit High Tea, has always had a desire to bring people together. As a young girl, she was the one who loved organizing parties, documenting these special moments with the camera that she constantly carried with her. In those early days, many weekends were spent with her grandmother, who taught Jessica all about makeup and glamour, showing her how to do things with style and grace. While growing up in Ashland, Oregon, one of her favorite stories was the classic tale of Alice in Wonderland. Years later, the memory of this strange fantasy motivated Jessica to weave snippets from that story into the workings of her new cannabis party planning venture, which she named after the fabled White Rabbit.

When Jessica was in her early twenties, a broken ankle and subsequent surgeries resulted in her rejection of the opiate prescriptions that the doctors had given her for pain. Instead, she got a medicinal marijuana license at age twenty-one and grew cannabis for herself. She has always found cannabis to be a source of creativity, calmness, and pain relief.

After moving to Los Angeles, California, Jessica decided to put her talent for party organizing and planning to good use. She intended to merge the city's evolving cannabis scene with its mainstream culture in a refined yet whimsical way. It was her idea to bring cannabis out of the closet, on a silver platter, and enjoy it with a cup of her favorite beverage, tea. Presto! White Rabbit High Tea hopped into its place in society. The company specializes in the highest High Tea and Garden Parties in the Los Angeles area. These occasions have become known as high-class cannabis-infused events.

At its inception, in 2016, the company's events were held at a little boutique hotel in West Hollywood. From that point on, the owner of White Rabbit High Tea has searched for additional interesting and inspiring locations to keep events fresh and fun. Her goal is to bring a love of teatime and cannabis together, sharing the experience with folks who want to go down the rabbit hole.

Guests are asked to come dressed in formal attire or their Sunday best. Costumes are encouraged as they help to set the tone for the occasion. Upon arrival, there is a costume box available that guests may hunt through if they feel the need to add a little extra pizazz to their outfits. Some participants have been known to come dressed as characters from "Alice in Wonderland," wearing top hats and white rabbit costumes, which adds a touch of childhood nostalgia to the festivities.

Visitors are seated around a long table where they meet new friends and make joyful memories. The goal is to create an amazing experience for everyone, which is sometimes less about cannabis and more about tea. The table is carefully set with an emphasis on detail and visuals. To create a lasting impression, Jessica uses a floral designer for each event, most notably Tanya Argüelles from Superette Studio. Keeping with the party's theme, one unique arrangement had cannabis flowers cleverly tucked among its classic floral art. Often, when space allows, guests will pull out a croquet set between sips of tea and play a relaxing game, enthusiastically paying homage to the spirit of the Lewis Carroll fantasy.

Guests who attend these special events come from all walks of life: artists, journalists, businesspeople, and celebrities—the list varies with each occasion. All are treated to a traditional high tea experience with bite-size sandwiches, scones, and desserts such as petits fours, tarts, and custards. Servers, called "Tea Tarts," walk around with vintage pots full of tea and pour for guests throughout the afternoon. The cannabis is laid out along the table where guests can choose from the products that the event's sponsors have to offer. Jessica is extremely proud of these brand partners, who are pleased to have this opportunity to showcase their merchandise. Pretty much any cannabis item you can think of is on display including edibles, vape pens, joints, and tinctures. Each sponsor is given an opportunity to share information about their product. As the afternoon draws to a close, goodie bags full of items such as cannabis skin rub, tinctures, and pre-rolls are distributed to the guests as a tangible reminder of a lovely fairy tale–like afternoon.

Jessica Cole believes that we all need to take time from our busy schedules to incorporate play back into our lives. Doing so enables us to unwind and regroup. Dressing up for High Tea as a play character from our imagination takes us to another place, allowing a brief respite from the everyday routine. White Rabbit High Tea offers its guests the opportunity to indulge in this fantasy for one delightfully magical afternoon.

CANNA CREAM

by JESSICA COLE, WHITE RABBIT HIGH TEA

MAKES approximately 2 cups

Canna cream is a versatile ingredient and can be used in a variety of sweet and savory dishes. With just a splash, canna cream can add creaminess to scrambled eggs, or give your stand-by pasta sauces a hint of richness, mashed potatoes a lavish texture, and more.

SUGGESTED DOSAGE: 18 milligrams per cup.

CANNA CREAM

⅛ ounce cannabis, trimmed, coarsely ground, decarboxylated

2 cups (1 pint) organic heavy whipping cream

WHIPPED CANNABIS- INFUSED CREAM

2 cups canna cream (See recipe above)

2 tablespoons confectioners' sugar, or as needed

1 teaspoon pure vanilla extract, or as needed

1. To make the cream infusion: Place the cannabis and cream into the top pan of a double boiler. Pour about 1 inch of water into the bottom pan and bring to a simmer over medium heat, making sure the top pan does not touch the simmering water. Place the top pan with the cannabis-cream mixture on top, and cover partially with a lid. Gently simmer, stirring occasionally, for 45 minutes. Remove from the heat and let cool completely. Note: Do not let the cream come to a boil.

2. Once cooled, transfer to a clean container with a pour spout, cover, and label with contents. Place in the refrigerator and allow to steep overnight.

3. Strain the infused cream through a cheesecloth-lined fine-mesh strainer into a clean container with a pour spout. Note: A large measuring cup works well.

4. Gather the corners of the cheesecloth and gently squeeze out any excess cream into the container, discarding or composting the plant matter. Use the cream right away or label with the date and contents and store in the refrigerator for up to 3 days. Use the canna cream to make whipped cannabis-infused cream, if desired.

5. To make the whipped cannabis-infused cream: Before you plan to make the whipped cream, place a metal mixing bowl and metal whisk attachments from a handheld mixer into the freezer for about 15 minutes.

6. Remove the metal mixing bowl and whisks from the freezer. Place the canna cream, 2 tablespoons confectioners' sugar, or to taste and vanilla into the chilled bowl then whisk on medium-high speed, scraping down the sides of the bowl as needed, until stiff peaks form.

DATE SCONES

by JESSICA COLE OF WHITE RABBIT HIGH TEA

MAKES 18 to 20 scones, depending on the size of cutter used

JESSICA COLE: Being in sunny southern California, we love using the local produce. Dates have always conjured up visions of sunshine, palm trees, and wide-open spaces ready to roam. This West Coast take on a British classic will transport any tea party to sunny southern California. In this recipe, one can use cannabis butter or cannabis-infused milk in the actual baking of the recipe for an even more modern twist, or use a cannabis butter or canna cream (see page 390) or an infused clotted clotted cream to top it off when serving.

3 cups self-rising flour, plus extra for dusting

1 tablespoon sugar, plus extra for sprinkling tops of scones

1 teaspoon organic ground ginger

1 teaspoon ground cardamom

1 teaspoon salt

4 tablespoons unsalted butter, cold and cut into small pieces

4 tablespoons cannabis-infused butter, cold and cut into small pieces

7 individual pitted dates (about 2 ounces) chopped into pea-sized pieces

1 cup whole milk, or as needed, plus 1 tablespoon for brushing tops of scones

Orange marmalade and raspberry jam, to serve

Clotted cream, to serve

1. Preheat the oven to 400°F. Line a baking sheet with parchment paper. Set aside.

2. In a large bowl, sift together the flour, sugar, ginger, cardamom, and salt.

3. Using a pastry cutter or fork, cut the butters into the flour until mixture resembles small peas or bread crumbs. Add the dates and using your fingers, mix them into flour mixture. Note: The dates are prone to stick together and using your fingers to separate the pieces is helpful when mixing them into the flour mixture.

4. Make a well in the center of the flour mixture, then add the milk. Using a wooden spoon, mix the flour and milk together until a soft dough forms, adding more milk, if needed.

5. Knead the dough inside the mixing bowl, making sure to pull all the dry ingredients into itself until it comes together. Alternately, turn the dough out onto a lightly floured work surface and knead gently until it comes together. Note: It is important not to overwork the dough because the scones will become tough.

6. Lightly dust a clean work surface with flour.

7. Pat the dough out into a circle, about ¾ inches thick. Using a 2-inch round biscuit cutter, cut out the rounds, then

Recipe continues on page 393

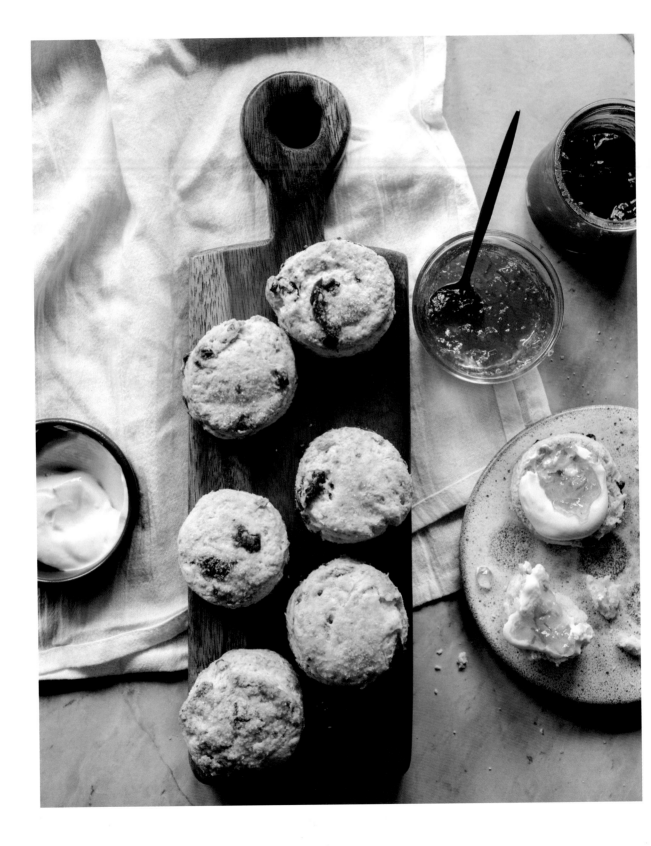

gently knead the scraps of dough and cut out into rounds. Note: If you do not have a 2-inch round biscuit cutter, the rim of a drinking glass, or the rim of a jar or a jar lid, or something that would be close to 2 inches works well.

8. Place the scones on the prepared baking sheet, about 1 inch apart. Brush the tops of the scones with the remaining 1 tablespoon of milk. Sprinkle the tops evenly with sugar, or to taste.

9. Bake until golden brown, about 18 to 20 minutes. Transfer to a wire rack and allow the scones to cool completely, about 20 minutes.

10. Serve with orange marmalade, raspberry jam, and clotted cream.

JESSICA COLE'S SUGGESTED STRAINS

I prefer the strawberry strains such as Strawberry Fields, Strawberry Ice, Strawberry Cough, Sour Patch Kiss, Bruce Banner, FPOG, Brian Berry Cough, Strawberry Banana, Strawberry Diesel, or anything else that has a fruity palate.

NOTE

If you don't have self-rising flour on hand, make your own by sifting together 3 cups all-purpose flour with 1½ tablespoons of baking powder, and ¾ teaspoon of salt. Make sure to reduce the salt amount listed in the ingredient section to ½ teaspoon instead of 1 teaspoon.

DIRECTORY

B

Blue Sparrow Coffee
3070 Blake Street
Unit 180
Denver, CO 80205
www.bluesparrowcoffee.com

Brent Harrewyn
121 LaFountain Street
Winooski, VT 05401
www.brentharrewyn.com

Clare Barboza Photography
www.clarebarboza.com

C

Jessica Catalano
www.jessicacatalano.com

Cloud Creamery
Framingham, MA
www.cloudcreamery.co

D

deadhorse hill
281 Main Street
Worcester, MA 01608
www.deadhorsehill.com

De Angelis USA Corp (SFOGLINI)
25 Vermilyea Lane
West Coxsackie, NY 12192
www.sfoglini.com

Desert Green Hemp
71290 Holmes Road

Sisters, OR 97759
www.desertgreenhemp.com

Destino Distribution & Canna Ocho
1829 SW 8th Street
Miami, FL 33135-3417
www.destinodistri.com

E

East Fork Cultivars
10325 Takilma Road
Cave Junction, OR 97523
www.eastfokcultivars.com

Eaton Hemp, LLC
543 East 5th Street
New York, NY 10009
www.eatonhemp.com

Elmore Mountain Therapeutic
4373 Elmore Mountain Road
Elmore, VT 05661
www.emtcbd.com

Entente Chicago
700 N Sedgwick
Chicago, IL 60654
www.ententechicago.com

Euphoric Food
193 Grove Street
Apt. 2
Haverhill, MA 01832
www.eateuphoria.com

F

Carly Fisher
www.carlyfisher.com

5 Birds Farm
3300 Hartland Hill Road
Woodstock, VT 05091
www.5birdsfarm.com

Franny's Farmacy
22 Franny Farm Road
Leicester, NC 28748
www.frannysfarmacy.com

Flour Child Collective
www.flourchild.org

G

Garden Society
840 N Cloverdale Blvd.
Cloverdale, CA 95425
www.thegardensociety.com

Green Goddess Café
618 South Main Street
Stowe, VT 05672
www.greengoddessvt.com

The Green Lady Dispensary
11 Amelia Drive
Nantucket, MA 02554
www.thegreenladydispensary.com

Green Panther Chef
1032 15th Street NW
Washington, DC 20005
www.greenpantherchef.com

H

House of Spain
P.O. Box 86642
Portland, OR 97286
www.houseofspainwellness.com

Hudson Hemp/Treaty
67 Pinewood Road
Hudson, NY 12534
www.hudsonhemp.com

www.ourtreaty.com

J

Jenny's BAKED At Home
953 Greene Avenue
Brooklyn, NY 11221
www.jennybakedathome.com

L

Local 111 Restaurant C.U.B. Food Inc.
111 Main Street
Philmont, NY 12565
www.local111.com

Love's Oven
225 Mariposa Street
Denver, CO 80223
www.choosethelove.com

Luce Farm Wellness
170 Luce Road
Stockbridge, VT 05773
www.lucefarmwellness.com

LUVN Kitchn
www.luvnkitchn.com

M

Maria Hines
8548 17th Avenue NW
Seattle, WA 98117

Mason Jar Event Group
582 Locust Place
Boulder, CO 80304
www.masonjareventgroup.com

Tracey Medeiros
www.traceymedeiros.com

O

Opulent Chef
633 Larkin Street
#201
San Francisco, CA 94109
www.opulentchef.com

OrcaSong Farm
280 Dolphin Bay Road
Eastsound, WA 98245
www.orcasong.com

P
The Pantry Company Inc.
13912 Old Harbor Lane
Marina del Rey, CA 90292
www.pantryfoodco.com

Plant People
49 Elizabeth Street
Floor 3
New York, NY 10013
www.plantpeople.co

Poppy Bee Surfaces
www.poppybeesurfaces.com

Prank Bar
1100 South Hope Street
Los Angeles, CA 90015
www.prankbar.com

Provender Kitchen + Bar
112 Main Street
Ellsworth, ME 04605
www.eatprovender.com

R
The Regional
130 South Mason Street
Fort Collins, CO 80524
www.theregionalfood.com

River and Woods
2328 Pearl Street
Boulder, CO 80302
www.riverandwoodsboulder.com

Rose Glow Tea Room
305 19th Street NE
Washington, DC 20002
www.roseglowtearoom.com

Gretchen Rude
Food Stylist

S
Sama Sama Kitchen
1208 State Street
Santa Barbara, CA 93101
www.samasamakitchen.com

She Don't Know, LLC (SDK)
P.O. Box 2106
Portland, OR 97208
www.sdksnacks.com

T
Tasty High Chef
www.tastyhighchef.com

U
Upward Cannabis Kitchen
16641 SE 82nd Drive
Ste 102
Clackamas, OR 97015

V
VegeNation
10075 S Eastern Avenue
Henderson, NV 89052
www.vegenationlv.com

W
Jordan Wagman
125 Maplewood Avenue
Toronto, ON M6 1J7
www.jordanwagman.com

White Rabbit High Tea
2427 Burson Road
Topanga, CA 90290
www.whiterabbithightea.com

Z
ZenBarn
179 Guptil Road
Waterbury Center, VT 05677
www.zenbarnvt.com

CONVERSION CHARTS

METRIC AND IMPERIAL CONVERSIONS

(These conversions are rounded for convenience)

Ingredient	Cups/Tablespoons/Teaspoons	Ounces	Grams/Milliliters
Butter	1 cup/ 16 tablespoons/ 2 sticks	8 ounces	230 grams
Cheese, shredded	1 cup	4 ounces	110 grams
Cream cheese	1 tablespoon	0.5 ounce	14.5 grams
Cornstarch	1 tablespoon	0.3 ounce	8 grams
Flour, all-purpose	1 cup/1 tablespoon	4.5 ounces/0.3 ounce	125 grams/8 grams
Flour, whole wheat	1 cup	4 ounces	120 grams
Fruit, dried	1 cup	4 ounces	120 grams
Fruits or veggies, chopped	1 cup	5 to 7 ounces	145 to 200 grams
Fruits or veggies, puréed	1 cup	8.5 ounces	245 grams
Honey, maple syrup, or corn syrup	1 tablespoon	0.75 ounce	20 grams
Liquids: cream, milk, water, or juice	1 cup	8 fluid ounces	240 milliliters
Oats	1 cup	5.5 ounces	150 grams
Salt	1 teaspoon	0.2 ounce	6 grams
Spices: cinnamon, cloves, ginger, or nutmeg (ground)	1 teaspoon	0.2 ounce	5 milliliters
Sugar, brown, firmly packed	1 cup	7 ounces	200 grams
Sugar, white	1 cup/1 tablespoon	7 ounces/0.5 ounce	200 grams/12.5 grams
Vanilla extract	1 teaspoon	0.2 ounce	4 grams

OVEN TEMPERATURES

Fahrenheit	Celsius	Gas Mark
225°	110°	¼
250°	120°	½
275°	140°	1
300°	150°	2
325°	160°	3
350°	180°	4
375°	190°	5
400°	200°	6
425°	220°	7
450°	230°	8

INDEX